T0226521

Tropical Diseases

Guest Editors

ALIMUDDIN ZUMLA, MD, MSc, PhD
JENNIFER KEISER, MSc, PhD

INFECTIOUS DISEASE CLINICS OF NORTH AMERICA

www.id.theclinics.com

Consulting Editor
ROBERT C. MOELLERING Jr, MD

June 2012 • Volume 26 • Number 2

SAUNDERS an imprint of ELSEVIER, Inc.

W.B. SAUNDERS COMPANY

A Division of Elsevier Inc.

1600 John F. Kennedy Blvd., Suite 1800, Philadelphia, PA 19103-2899.

http://www.theclinics.com

INFECTIOUS DISEASE CLINICS OF NORTH AMERICA Volume 26, Number 2
June 2012 ISSN 0891–5520, ISBN-13: 978-1-4557-3880-9

Editor: Stephanie Donley
Developmental Editor: Teia Stone

Infectious Disease Clinics of North America (ISSN 0891–5520) is published in March, June, September, and December by Elsevier Inc., 360 Park Avenue South, New York, NY 10010-1710. Periodicals postage paid at New York, NY and additional mailing offices. Subscription prices are $271.00 per year for US individuals, $463.00 per year for US institutions, $134.00 per year for US students, $321.00 per year for Canadian individuals, $573.00 per year for Canadian institutions, $383.00 per year for international individuals, $573.00 per year for international institutions, and $185.00 per year for Canadian and international students. To receive student rate, orders must be accompanied by name of affiliated institution, date of term, and the *signature* of program/residency coordinator on institution letterhead. Orders will be billed at individual rate until proof of status is received. Foreign air speed delivery is included in all *Clinics* subscription prices. All prices are subject to change without notice. **POSTMASTER**: Send address changes to *Infectious Disease Clinics of North America*, Elsevier Health Sciences Division, Subcription Customer Service, 3251 Riverport Lane, Maryland Heights, MO 63043. **Customer Service: 1-800-654-2452 (US). From outside of the US and Canada, call 1-314-447-8871. Fax: 1-314-447-8029. E-mail: JournalsCustomerService-usa@elsevier.com (print support) or JournalsOnlineSupport-usa@elsevier.com (online support).**

Infectious Disease Clinics of North America is also published in Spanish by Editorial Inter-MÅdica, Junin 917, 1ᵉʳ A 1113, Buenos Aires, Argentina.

Reprints. For copies of 100 or more, of articles in this publication, please contact the Commercial Reprints Department, Elsevier Inc., 360 Park Avenue South, New York, New York 10010-1710. Tel. (212) 633-3812, Fax: (212) 462-1935, E-mail: reprints@elsevier.com.

Infectious Disease Clinics of North America is covered in *MEDLINE/PubMed (Index Medicus), Current Contents/Clinical Medicine, Science Citation Alert, SCISEARCH,* and *Research Alert.*

Printed and bound by CPI Group (UK) Ltd, Croydon, CR0 4YY
Transferred to Digital Print 2012

Contributors

CONSULTING EDITOR

ROBERT C. MOELLERING Jr, MD
Shields Warren-Mallinckrodt Professor of Medical Research, Harvard Medical School; Department of Medicine, Beth Israel Deaconess Medical Center, Boston, Massachusetts

GUEST EDITORS

ALIMUDDIN ZUMLA, MD, MSc, PhD(Lond), FRCP(Lond), FRCP(Edin), FRCPath
Professor of Infectious Diseases and International Health, Division of Infection and Immunity, University College London Medical School; Consultant Infectious Diseases Physician, University College London Hospitals NHS Foundation Trust, London, United Kingdom.

JENNIFER KEISER, PhD
University of Basel; Professor, Department of Medical Parasitology and Infection Biology, Swiss Tropical and Public Health Institute, Basel, Switzerland

AUTHORS

RON H. BEHRENS, MB ChB, MD, FRCP
Senior Lecturer, Department of Clinical Research, London School of Hygiene & Tropical Medicine, London, United Kingdom

IDIR BITAM, PhD
Service d'Ecologie et des Systèmes Vectoriels, Institut Pasteur d'Algérie, Algiers, Algeria

JOHANNES BLUM, MD
Director, Outpatient Clinic, Department Medical Services and Diagnostics, Swiss Tropical and Public Health Institute, Basel, Switzerland

RETO BRUN, PhD
Professor of Biology, Department Medical Parasitology and Infection Biology, Swiss Tropical and Public Health Institute, Basel, Switzerland

ENRICO BRUNETTI, MD
Staff Physician, Division of Infectious and Tropical Diseases, San Matteo Hospital Foundation, Co-Director, WHO Collaborating Centre for Clinical Management of Cystic Echinococcosis, Assistant Professor of Infectious Diseases, University of Pavia, Pavia, Italy

JOFFRE MARCONDES DE REZENDE, MD
Emeritus Professor, Faculty of Medicine, Federal University of Goiás, Goiânia, Goiás, Brazil

ERMIAS DIRO, MD
Department of Clinical Sciences, Institute of Tropical Medicine, Antwerp, Belgium; Department of Internal Medicine, University of Gondar, Gondar, Ethiopia

URS DUTHALER, PhD
University of Basel; Postdoctoral Fellow, Department of Medical Parasitology and Infection Biology, Swiss Tropical and Public Health Institute, Basel, Switzerland

THOMAS FÜRST, MA
University of Basel; Research Fellow, Department of Epidemiology and Public Health, Swiss Tropical and Public Health Institute, Basel, Switzerland

HIRO GOTO, MD, PhD
Associate Professor, Department of Preventive Medicine, Faculdade de Medicina; Laboratory of Soroepidemiology and Immunobiology, Instituto de Medicina Tropical de São Paulo, Universidade de São Paulo, São Paulo, Brazil

EDUARDO GOTUZZO, MD
Instituto de Medicina Tropical Alexander von Humboldt, Universidad Peruana Cayetano Heridia, Lima, Peru

BRUNO GRYSEELS, MD, PhD
Professor and Director, Institute of Tropical Medicine, Antwerpen, Belgium

RUMINA HASAN, MBBS, PhD, FRCPath
Professor, Department of Pathology and Microbiology, Aga Khan University, Karachi, Pakistan

CHRISTOPH HATZ, MD
University of Basel; Professor, Department of Medical Services and Diagnostic, Swiss Tropical and Public Health Institute, Basel; Professor, Institute of Social and Preventive Medicine, University of Zurich, Zurich, Switzerland

LI YANG HSU, MBBS, MRCP, MPH
Department of Medicine, National University Health System, Singapore, Singapore

JENNIFER KEISER, PhD
University of Basel; Professor, Department of Medical Parasitology and Infection Biology, Swiss Tropical and Public Health Institute, Basel, Switzerland

TAHAR KERNIF, VetD
URMITE, UMR CNRS-IRD 6236, WHO Collaborative Centre for Rickettsial Diseases and Other Arthropod-borne Bacterial Diseases, Aix Marseille University, Marseille, France; Service d'Ecologie et des Systèmes Vectoriels, Institut Pasteur d'Algérie, Algiers, Algeria

STEFANIE KNOPP, PhD
University of Basel; Postdoctoral Fellow, Department of Epidemiology and Public Health, Swiss Tropical and Public Health Institute, Basel, Switzerland

JOSÉ ANGELO LAULETTA LINDOSO, MD, PhD
Laboratory of Soroepidemiology and Immunobiology, Instituto de Medicina Tropical de São Paulo, Universidade de São Paulo; Laboratório de Investigação Médica, Hospital das Clínicas da Faculdade de Medicina da Universidade de São Paulo; Instituto de Infectologia Emílio Ribas, Secretaria do Estado da Saúde do Estado de São Paulo, São Paulo, Brazil

JOSÉ EDUARDO LEVI, PhD
Virology Laboratory, Institute of Tropical Medicine, University of São Paulo, São Paulo, Brazil

CLARISSE MARTINS MACHADO, MD
Virology Laboratory, Institute of Tropical Medicine, University of São Paulo; Hematopoietic Stem Cell Transplantation Program, Amaral Carvalho Foundation, Jaú, São Paulo, Brazil

EYAL MELTZER, MD, DTM&H
Department of Medicine C and Center for Geographic Medicine, Sheba Medical Center, Tel Hashomer; Sackler School of Medicine, Tel Aviv University, Tel Aviv, Israel

BEHZAD NADJM, MB ChB, MD, DTM&H
Clinical Lecturer, Department of Clinical Research, London School of Hygiene & Tropical Medicine, London, United Kingdom

ESTHER SHU-TING NG, MBBS, MRCP
Department of Medicine, National University Health System, Singapore, Singapore

PHILIPPE PAROLA, MD, PhD
URMITE, UMR CNRS-IRD 6236, WHO Collaborative Centre for Rickettsial Diseases and Other Arthropod-borne Bacterial Diseases, Aix Marseille University, Marseille, France

BOBBI S. PRITT, MD, MSc, (D)TMH
Assistant Professor of Laboratory Medicine and Pathology, Clinical Parasitology and Virology, Division of Clinical Microbiology, Department of Laboratory Medicine and Pathology, Mayo Clinic, Rochester, Minnesota

DIDIER RAOULT, MD, PhD
URMITE, UMR CNRS-IRD 6236, WHO Collaborative Centre for Rickettsial Diseases and Other Arthropod-borne Bacterial Diseases, Aix Marseille University, Marseille, France

ANIS RASSI Jr, MD, PhD
Chief, Division of Cardiology, Anis Rassi Hospital, Goiânia, Goiás, Brazil

ANIS RASSI, MD
Emeritus Professor, Faculty of Medicine, Federal University of Goiás, Goiânia, Goiás, Brazil

JON E. ROSENBLATT, MD
Professor of Medicine and Microbiology, Division of Clinical Microbiology, Department of Laboratory Medicine and Pathology, Mayo Clinic, Rochester, Minnesota

BRYAN H. SCHMITT, DO
Instructor in Laboratory Medicine and Pathology, Division of Clinical Microbiology, Department of Laboratory Medicine and Pathology, Mayo Clinic, Rochester, Minnesota

SADIA SHAKOOR, MBBS, FCPS
Department of Pathology and Microbiology, Aga Khan University, Karachi, Pakistan

CRISTINA SOCOLOVSCHI, MD, PhD
URMITE, UMR CNRS-IRD 6236, WHO Collaborative Centre for Rickettsial Diseases and Other Arthropod-borne Bacterial Diseases, Aix Marseille University, Marseille, France

BANCHOP SRIPA, PhD
Professor, Tropical Disease Research Laboratory, Department of Pathology, Khon Kaen University, Khon Kaen, Thailand

PETER STEINMANN, PhD
University of Basel; Postdoctoral Fellow, Department of Epidemiology and Public Health, Swiss Tropical and Public Health Institute, Basel, Switzerland

ANDREW USTIANOWSKI, PhD(Lond), FRCP(Lond), DTM&H
Director, Regional Infectious Diseases Unit, North Manchester General Hospital, Manchester, United Kingdom

JÜRG UTZINGER, PhD
University of Basel; Professor, Department of Epidemiology and Public Health, Swiss Tropical and Public Health Institute, Basel, Switzerland

JOHAN VAN GRIENSVEN, MD, PhD, MSc
Department of Clinical Sciences, Institute of Tropical Medicine, Antwerp, Belgium

DAVID A. WARRELL, DM, DSc, FRCP, FRCPE, FMedSci
Emeritus Professor of Tropical Medicine, Nuffield Department of Clinical Medicine, John Radcliffe Hospital, University of Oxford, Headington, Oxford, United Kingdom

A. CLINTON WHITE Jr, MD, FACP, FIDSA
Paul R Stalnaker Distinguished Professor and Director, Infectious Diseases Division, Department of Internal Medicine, University of Texas Medical Branch, Galveston, Texas

LIMIN WIJAYA, MBBS, MRCP, DTM&H
Department of Infectious Diseases, Singapore General Hospital, Singapore, Singapore

STEPHEN G. WRIGHT, FRCP
Consulting Physician, King Edward VII Hospital Sister Agnes, The Hospital for Tropical Diseases; Honorary Senior Lecturer, Department of Infectious & Tropical Diseases, London School of Hygiene & Tropical Medicine, London, United Kingdom

ANITA K.M. ZAIDI, MD, SM, FAAP
Professor, Department of Paediatrics and Child Health, Aga Khan University, Karachi, Pakistan

ALIMUDDIN ZUMLA, MD, MSc, PhD(Lond), FRCP(Lond), FRCP(Edin), FRCPath
Professor of Infectious Diseases and International Health, Division of Infection and Immunity, University College London Medical School; Consultant Infectious Diseases Physician, University College London Hospitals NHS Foundation Trust, London, United Kingdom

Contents

> The term tropical diseases encompasses all diseases that occur principally in the tropics. This term covers all communicable and noncommunicable diseases, genetic disorders, and disease caused by nutritional deficiencies or environmental conditions (such as heat, humidity, and altitude) that are encountered in areas that lie between, and alongside, the Tropic of Cancer and Tropic of Capricorn belts. In tropical countries, apart from noncommunicable diseases, a severe burden of disease is caused by an array of different microorganisms, parasites, land and sea animals, and arthropods.

> This article discusses the epidemiology, prevention, clinical features, first aid and medical treatment of venomous bites by snakes, lizards, and spiders; stings by fish, jellyfish, echinoderms, and insects; and poisoning by fish and molluscs, in all parts of the world. Of these envenoming and poisonings, snake bite causes the greatest burden of human suffering, killing 46,000 people each year in India alone and more than 100,000 worldwide and resulting in physical handicap in many survivors. Specific antidotes (antivenoms/antivenins) are available to treat envenoming by many of these taxa but supply and distribution is inadequate in many tropical developing countries.

> Blood transfusion and transplantation may represent efficient mechanisms of spreading infectious agents to naive populations. In the developed countries, as a consequence of globalization, several factors such as international commerce, tourism, and immigration have acted as important features for the emergence or reemergence of infectious diseases previously referred to as tropical. This article reviews the relevant bacterial, protozoan and viral infections that are more frequently associated with blood transfusion and/or solid organ or marrow transplantation and may affect susceptible populations worldwide.

> Malaria remains the most important parasitic infection in humans. There have been significant advances in the treatment of both nonsevere and

severe malaria with the advent of artemisinin combination therapies and parenteral artesunate, but the optimum supportive management of severe malaria is unclear. A broadly acceptable therapy for the prevention of relapses in *Plasmodium* vivax infection has not been discovered. Globally, the priority remains to prevent infection in the vulnerable, to move toward elimination where feasible, and to ensure that effective treatment is available to all. In developed settings, prevention of infection and its early recognition are crucial.

Human African trypanosomiasis (sleeping sickness) is caused by the unicellular parasite *Trypanosoma brucei* and transmitted by tsetse flies. It occurs exclusively in sub-Saharan Africa, usually in rural areas affected by civil conflicts and neglected health systems. Reported cases are fewer than 10,000/year, which classifies it as one of the most neglected tropical diseases. Because sleeping sickness is fatal if not treated, it has to be included in the differential diagnosis of every febrile traveler returning from a game park in East Africa. Elimination of the disease is considered feasible provided better tools for diagnosis and treatment can be made available.

Chagas disease, also known as American trypanosomiasis, is a chronic infection caused by *Trypanosoma cruzi*, a protozoan parasite. It is transmitted to human beings mainly through the feces of infected triatomine bugs. The disease affects an estimated 8 to 10 million people in the Americas, putting them at risk of developing life-threatening cardiac and gastrointestinal complications. This article provides a brief update on the epidemiology, clinical manifestations, diagnosis, and treatment of Chagas disease.

Tegumentary leishmaniases are caused by approximately 15 species of protozoa of the genus *Leishmania*. They prevail in tropical and subtropical areas of the Old and New World but human mobility also makes them a medical problem in nonendemic areas. Clinical manifestations may comprise cutaneous and mucocutaneous forms that may be localized, disseminated, or diffuse in distribution and may differ in Old and New World leishmaniases. Diagnosis and treatment vary according to the clinical manifestations, geographic area, and *Leishmania* species involved. This article highlights the diversity and complexity of tegumentary leishmaniases, which are worsened by human immunodeficiency virus/*Leishmania* coinfection.

Visceral leishmaniasis (VL) is a vector-borne parasitic disease targeting tissue macrophages. It is among the most neglected infectious diseases.

Classical manifestations of VL include chronic fever, hepatosplenomegaly, and pancytopenia. Most cases can be detected through serologic and molecular testing. Although therapy has historically relied on antimonials, newer therapeutic options include conventional or liposomal amphotericin B, paromomycin and miltefosine. Coinfection with human immunodeficiency virus (HIV) is increasingly reported and comes with additional diagnostic and therapeutic challenges. This article provides an up-to-date clinical review of VL focusing on clinical presentation, diagnosis, management, and issues related to HIV coinfection.

The review provides current views on human protozoan parasites of the gut. The recognition of the importance of cryptosporidium, cyclospora and microsporidia over the last three decades emphasises the possibility that more pathogenic intestinal protozoa are presently unrecognized. Each of these is a zoonotic infection and the potential for a zoonotic element to the transmission of giardiasis has been recognized. A common theme in increased understanding of the biology and pathological mechanisms involved in causing disease is the application of molecular techniques to the various stages of the parasite life cycle. Molecular methods are increasingly contributing to laboratory diagnosis of these conditions with increased yields of positive results though in the tropics it is likely that fecal microscopy will remain the standard for some time to come. The nitroimidazole compounds are the mainstay of treatment for giardia and amebiasis with no major advance in therapeutics since their role was appreciated. Nitazoxanide was shown to be effective for cryptosporidiosis in the 1990s.

Infection with soil-transmitted helminths occurs via ingestion of nematode eggs with contaminated food and water, via hands, or inhalation of dust, or by penetration of larvae through the skin. Trichinella infections are caused by the ingestion of larvae contained in undercooked meat. In highly endemic areas, preventive chemotherapy (ie, regular administration of anthelmintic drugs to at-risk populations) is the key strategy against soil-transmitted helminthiasis. Integrated control approaches, including improved hygiene, sanitation, and water, are required for lasting effects. Because of growing tourism, travel, and migration, clinicians and specialized travel clinics must remain aware of the diagnosis, prevention, and treatment of soil-transmitted helminth and Trichinella infections.

More than 150 million people, mainly in developing countries, are affected by filarial nematode infections that cause debilitating and disfiguring diseases. Although transmission is restricted to the tropics and subtropics, imported infections sometimes occur in Europe and North America among immigrants and refugees from endemic countries, and rarely among long-term travelers. This article reviews the epidemiology of the most important human filarial nematodes, their current distribution, life cycles, clinical features, and disease burden. Diagnosis, treatment, and tools for prevention and control are discussed. Protective measures for travelers are summarized, and vulnerable groups and case numbers in North America identified.

Schistosomiasis is a tropical parasitic disease, caused by blood-dwelling worms of the genus *Schistosoma*. The main human species are *S mansoni* (occurring in Africa and South America) and *S japonicum* (South and East Asia) causing intestinal and hepatosplenic schistosomiasis, and *S haematobium* (Africa) causing urinary schistosomiasis. Severe symptoms develop in predilected people with heavy and long-standing infections. Acute schistosomiasis, a flulike syndrome, is a regular finding in travel clinics. Although prevalences can be high, most infected people show limited, intermittent, or aspecific symptoms. The diagnosis of schistosomiasis relies on microscopic examination of stools or urine, serologic tests, and imaging. Praziquantel is the drug of choice, active against all species in a single or a few oral doses. Current control strategies consist mainly of preventive therapy in communities or groups at risk.

Food-borne trematodiases are an emerging public health problem in Southeast Asia and Latin America and of growing importance for travel clinics in Europe and North America. The disease is caused by chronic infections with liver, lung, and intestinal flukes. This article focuses on the most important liver and lung flukes that parasitize man, namely *Clonorchis sinensis*, *Fasciola gigantica*, *Fasciola hepatica*, *Opisthorchis felineus*, *Opisthorchis viverrini*, and *Paragonimus* spp. The article describes the epidemiology of major liver and lung fluke infections, including current distribution, burden, life cycle, clinical signs and symptoms, diagnostic approaches, and current tools for prevention, treatment, and control.

Although humans can be definitive hosts for cestodes (tapeworms), major pathologic conditions occur during cestode larval stages when humans serve as the intermediate host for these parasites. The most relevant forms of human disease caused by cestode larvae are echinococcosis, caused by *Echinococcus granulosus* (cystic echinococcosis) and *Echinococcus multilocularis* (alveolar echinococcosis), and cysticercosis, caused by *Taenia solium*. These infections occur worldwide, but their relevance is particularly high in developing countries, where poor hygiene conditions facilitate the transmission of the parasites. The therapeutic approach is often complex, requiring surgery and/or chemotherapy or, in the case of cystic echinococcosis, percutaneous treatments.

The bacterial gastrointestinal infections cholera, salmonellosis, shigellosis, campylobacteriosis, and diarrheagenic *Escherichia coli* are prevalent in tropical regions. These diseases impose an immense cost and contribute significantly to childhood morbidity and mortality. Management is hampered by limited access to diagnostic facilities and by antimicrobial drug resistance. Rapid point-of-care assays aim to reduce treatment delay and encourage rational use of antimicrobial agents. Control through safe drinking water, good sanitation, and vaccination against typhoid and cholera in high-risk populations is recommended. Vaccines against other *Shigella* and diarrheagenic *E coli* infections are under development.

The purpose of this article is to overview vector-borne rickettsioses in North Africa, focusing on epidemiologic aspects, clinical features, diagnosis procedures, and treatment. The protective measures, the exposure to risk, and the dynamics of endemic emerging and re-emerging diseases in the region are detailed to minimize the risk when traveling in this area. In addition, the article describes the scientific contribution on the rickettsial field of North-African researchers from the beginning of the 20th century until today.

The viral hemorrhagic fever (VHF) syndrome is a potentially life-threatening infection typified by a combination of a capillary leak syndrome and bleeding diathesis. Most but not all agents causing VHF are arboviruses, with transmission to humans resulting from an arthropod bite. Agents of VHF affect humans on all continents. Population growth, urbanization, human activities, and even climate change all contribute to a continual flux in the epidemiology of many arboviruses. This review provides an overview of the epidemiology of arboviral infections and VHF, the main clinical syndromes, and their diagnosis and treatment.

Fungal infections are more common and diverse in the tropics but are also increasingly seen in returning travelers and migrants as international travel becomes easier. They are conventionally classified into superficial, cutaneous, subcutaneous, and systemic mycoses. This article provides an overview of superficial, cutaneous, and subcutaneous mycoses that are more prevalent and/or geographically restricted to the tropics and briefly discusses fungal infections in returning travelers. Systematic data on such infections as travel-associated diseases are currently lacking, and enhanced surveillance for fungal infections may lead to early diagnosis and an understanding of the epidemiology of the fungal infections among travelers.

INFECTIOUS DISEASE CLINICS OF NORTH AMERICA

Preface

Tropical Diseases

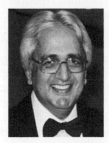 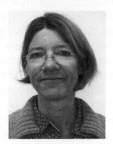

Alimuddin Zumla, MD, MSc, PhD(Lond),   Jennifer Keiser, PhD
FRCP(Lond), FRCP(Edin), FRCPath
Guest Editors

The term "Tropical Diseases" encompasses all communicable and noncommunicable diseases, and disorders and disease due to nutritional deficiencies or environmental conditions (such as heat, humidity, and altitude) that are encountered in geographical areas that lie between, and alongside, the Tropic of Cancer and Tropic of Capricorn belts. In tropical countries, apart from noncommunicable diseases, a severe burden of disease is caused by an array of different types of micro-organisms, parasites, land and sea animals, and arthropods. Approximately 15 million people die each year due to tropical infectious and parasitic diseases, the vast majority living in developing countries. Increased international air travel, migration, tourism, and employment visits to and from tropical regions have contributed to an increased incidence of such diseases being seen in the United States, United Kingdom, and Europe.

Climate change and global warming are causing tropical diseases and vectors of disease to spread to higher altitudes and latitudes. The last decade of the 20th century has seen a resurgence in tropical diseases being encountered in the countries outside the tropics such as the United States. These diseases include Chagas disease and vector-borne viral encephalitides, trypanosomiasis, giardiasis, and viral hemorrhagic fevers. Bites from several animal species including snakes, scorpions, and jellyfish cause much morbidity and mortality from envenomation and secondary infections. Skin diseases in returning traveller from the tropics are frequent. The rising success rates of solid organ and hematopoietic stem cell transplantations, with associated immunosuppression, have started to face the impact of neglected tropical diseases transmitted via infected donor tissue. More posttransplantation respiratory viral, bacterial, protozoal, and fungal infections are being recognized.

This wide array of diseases is compounded and made worse by the common issues of poverty, poor living conditions, malnutrition, HIV/AIDS, and poor health systems, which afflict a large proportion of the population of developing countries across the tropics. Although, over the past decade, lifestyle issues and changes in diet have led

Infect Dis Clin N Am 26 (2012) xv–xvii
doi:10.1016/j.idc.2012.03.012
0891-5520/12/$ – see front matter © 2012 Elsevier Inc. All rights reserved.

to an increase in the number of noncommunicable diseases such as hypertension, diabetes, chronic obstructive airways disease, myocardial infarction, and cerebrovascular accidents in resource-poor tropical countries, tropical infectious diseases remain one of the major causes of preventable morbidity and mortality. Schistosomiasis is the second most important parasitic disease after malaria, with 207 million people infected and 700 million at risk in over 70 countries. In addition to these, leishmaniasis, onchocerciasis, filariasis, Chagas' disease, African trypanosomiasis, rickettsioses, enteric fever, helminthiases, viral hemorrhagic fevers, and diarrheal diseases affect billions of people each year, have extremely high public health impact, and cause significant morbidity and mortality in adults and children. These diseases share population targets, ecological niches, and wide geographical distribution. Respiratory tract infections are common globally and are caused by a variety of bacterial, viral, and fungal pathogens, some of which have restricted geographical distributions.

The number and range of tropical and infectious diseases prevalent worldwide is extremely large and broad. It is imperative that physicians globally are aware of the wide spectrum of tropical, infectious, and parasitic diseases their patients may have been exposed to. This issue of *Infectious Diseases Clinics of North America* is aimed at giving an up-to-date and comprehensive overview of tropical, infectious, and parasitic diseases through 19 articles written by authoritative experts from all around the world. For practical clinical purposes, specific listings and classifications are useful for streamlining the microbiological and clinical assessment of the patient's illness. Alimuddin Zumla and Andy Ustianowski in the introductory article present several practical classifications of infectious and tropical diseases, which will serve as "aid memoirs" or "checklists" for guiding clinicians, microbiologists, pathologists, and laboratory staff. Migrant populations living in the west are part and parcel of blood and organ transplant donor and recipient programs and a wide range of infectious and tropical diseases that are transmitted via these routes are described by Machado and Levy. Every year millions of people present to hospitals and health care centers with venomous bites, stings, and poisoning encountered from a variety of land and sea animals. David Warrell in his article vividly illustrates a range of clinical conditions as a result of bites and poisoning from snakes, lizards, jellyfish, scorpions, and ingestion of seafood.

Diseases due to protozoa affect over a billion people each year and these are covered in the articles on protozoal infections of the gut by Stephen Wright; malaria by Drs Behzad Nadjm and Ron Behrens; African trypanosomiases by Reto Brun and Johannees Blum; American trypanosomiases by Anis Rossi Sr, Anis Rossi Jr, Joffre Marcondes, and De Rezende; cutaneous and mucocutaneous leishmaniases by Hiro Goto, Jose Angelo, and Lauletto Lidonso; and visceral leishmaniases by Johan van Griensven and Ermias Diro. More than one-third of the world's population are infected with a range of helminths and these are comprehensively described in articles that cover nematode infections, filariases, soil-transmitted helminths, and Trichinella (Stefanie Knopp and colleagues); trematode infestations: blood flukes (schistosomiases) by Bruno Gryseels and lung and liver flukes (Thomas Fürst, Urs Duthaler, Banchop Sripa, Jürg Utzinger, and Jennifer Keiser); cestode infestations, hydatid disease, and cysticercosis by Enrico Brunetti and Clinton White. The diagnosis and management of rickettsial, viral, and fungal infections remain an important challenge in medical inpatient and outpatient practice in Europe, United States, and developing countries. These diseases are covered in the articles on rickettsial infections by Philippe Parola, arboviral and viral hemorrhagic fevers by Eyal Metzer; and fungal infections by Lil Yang Hsu, Limin Wijaya, Esther Shu-Ting-Ng, and Eduardo Gotuzzo. Since many tropical diseases have high mortality rates, it has become important that accurate and rapid clinical diagnosis is made. Rapid and accurate diagnosis of tropical diseases remains an important challenge in medical inpatient and outpatient practice in Europe, United States, and developing countries. The identification and diagnosis of a range of tropical diseases are covered extensively in the comprehensive and highly illustrated article on Laboratory Diagnosis by Jon Rosenblatt, Bryan Schmitt, and Bobbi Pritt.

This *Infectious Diseases Clinics of North America* volume on "Tropical Diseases" illustrates vividly that a range of tropical diseases present to the physician in a variety of clinical situations and settings. It is imperative that clinicians in the United States and Europe have a high degree of clinical awareness of the possibility of a "tropical disease" to diagnose and treat the disease quickly, thus reducing morbidity and mortality.

We are extremely grateful to all the contributors for their contributions to this excellent and comprehensive volume on Tropical Diseases. Our sincere thanks to Stephanie Donley, Clinics Editor, and Jeannette Forcina, Editorial Assistant, Elsevier Publishing, and their staff for their kind assistance and diligence throughout the development of this special issue. Dr Robert Moellering, Consulting Editor for *Infectious Disease Clinics of North America*, gave his enthusiastic and unflinching support to this project. Adam Zumla provided administrative support to Professor Zumla. We thank our families for their support and patience during the many long hours spent on this project.

Alimuddin Zumla, MD, MSc, PhD(Lond), FRCP(Lond), FRCP(Edin), FRCPath
Department of Infection
Division of Infection and Immunity
University College London Medical School
University College London Hospitals
NHS Foundation Trust
London WC1E 6AJ, United Kingdom

Jennifer Keiser, PhD
Swiss Tropical and Public Health Institute
Medical Parasitology and Infection Biology Department
Socinstr. 57
CH-4051 Basel, Switzerland

E-mail addresses:
a.zumla@ucl.ac.uk (A. Zumla)
jennifer.keiser@unibas.ch (J. Keiser)

Tropical Diseases
Definition, Geographic Distribution, Transmission, and Classification

Alimuddin Zumla, MD, MSc, PhD(Lond), FRCP(Lond), FRCP(Edin), FRCPath[a],*,
Andrew Ustianowski, PhD(Lond), FRCP(Lond), DTM&H[b]

KEYWORDS

- Classification • Tropical disease • Infectious diseases

KEY POINTS

- The term tropical diseases encompasses all communicable and non-communicable diseases that occur principally in the tropics.
- Approximately 15 million people die each year because of tropical infectious and parasitic diseases.
- Tropical diseases are not restricted to the tropics. Increasing migration, international air travel, tourism, and work visits to tropical regions have contributed to an increased incidence of such diseases being seen in the United States, United Kingdom, and Europe.
- Classification of tropical diseases is useful for microbiologists, pathologists, laboratory staff and practicing infectious diseases physicians.
- This article gives an overview of the definition, geographical distribution, transmission and practical classification of tropical infectious diseases.

The term tropical diseases encompasses all diseases that occur principally in the tropics. This term covers all communicable and noncommunicable diseases, genetic disorders, and disease caused by nutritional deficiencies or environmental conditions (such as heat, humidity, and altitude) that are encountered in areas that lie between, and alongside, the Tropic of Cancer and Tropic of Capricorn belts. In tropical countries, apart from noncommunicable diseases, a severe burden of disease is caused by an array of different microorganisms, parasites, land and sea animals, and arthropods.[1–3]

Approximately 15 million people die each year because of tropical infectious and parasitic diseases, most living in developing countries.[4] This wide array of diseases is compounded and made worse by the common issues of poverty, poor living conditions, malnutrition, human immunodeficiency virus (HIV)/acquired immune deficiency

[a] Department of Infection, Division of Infection and Immunity, University College London Medical School, University College London Hospitals NHS Foundation Trust, London WC1E 6AJ, UK; [b] Regional Infectious Diseases Unit, North Manchester General Hospital, Manchester, UK
* Corresponding author.
E-mail address: a.zumla@ucl.ac.uk

Infect Dis Clin N Am 26 (2012) 195–205
doi:10.1016/j.idc.2012.02.007
0891-5520/12/$ – see front matter © 2012 Elsevier Inc. All rights reserved.

syndrome (AIDS), and poor health systems (consequential on poverty, mismanagement, and corruption) that afflict a large proportion of developing countries across the tropics. Although, in the past decade, lifestyle issues and changes in diet have led to an increase in the number of noncommunicable disease such as hypertension, diabetes, chronic obstructive airways disease, myocardial infarction, and cerebrovascular accidents in resource-poor tropical countries, tropical infectious diseases remain one of the major causes of preventable morbidity and mortality.[5] Tuberculosis, HIV/AIDS, and malaria alone are currently responsible for an estimated 6 million deaths annually.[1–4] Schistosomiasis is the second most important parasitic disease after malaria, with 200 million people infected and 779 million at risk in more than 70 countries. In addition to these, leishmaniasis, onchocerciasis, filariasis, Chagas disease, African trypanosomiasis, rickettsioses, enteric fever, helminthiases, viral hemorrhagic fevers, and diarrheal diseases have extremely high public health impacts, and cause significant morbidity and mortality in adults and children. These diseases share population targets, ecological niches, and wide geographic distribution.[1–4] Respiratory tract infections (RTIs) are caused by a variety of bacterial, viral, and fungal pathogens. RTIs remain major causes of morbidity and mortality in adults and children worldwide, causing millions of deaths each year.[6,7] The identification and diagnosis of acute and chronic bacterial (including tuberculosis), viral, and fungal respiratory infections remain an important challenge in medical inpatient and outpatient practice in Europe, the United States, and developing countries. Respiratory infectious diseases such as severe acute respiratory syndrome (caused by coronavirus) and the avian influenza[8] are frequently causes of major concern. The Global Surveillance Network of the International Society of Travel Medicine (ISTM) and the Centers for Disease Control (CDC) established a worldwide communications and data collection network of travel/tropical medicine clinics in 1995, and their valuable Web site gives regularly updated information on geographic and temporal trends in disease-associated morbidity among travelers, immigrants, and refugees.[9]

TROPICAL DISEASES IN THE UNITED KINGDOM, EUROPE, AND THE UNITED STATES

Tropical diseases are not restricted to the tropics. Increasing migration, international air travel, tourism, and work visits to tropical regions have contributed to an increased incidence of such diseases being seen in the United States, United Kingdom, and Europe.[9,10] Climate change and global warming (with a resulting increase in average and nadir temperatures) may be causing tropical diseases and vectors to spread to higher altitudes in mountainous regions, and to higher latitudes that were previously spared, such as the southern United States and the Mediterranean area. The last decade of the twentieth century was marked by a resurgence in tropical diseases being encountered in countries outside the tropics, such as the United States, including Chagas disease, a chronic, systemic, parasitic infection caused by the protozoan *Trypanosoma cruzi*, and vector-borne viral encephalitides.[3,9] Other previously rare, but presently emerging, diseases from particular geographic areas include leptospirosis, trypanosomiasis, giardiasis, and viral hemorrhagic fever. Bites from several animal species, including snakes, scorpions, and jellyfish, cause much morbidity and mortality from envenomation and secondary infections. Skin diseases are common in travelers returning from the tropics.[3]

The increasing success rates of solid organ and hematopoietic stem cell transplantations, with advances in immunosuppression, make transplants an early therapeutic option for many diseases affecting a considerable number of people worldwide. Thus, transplant programs in Western countries, as well as those in developing countries, have started to face the impact of neglected tropical diseases transmitted via the donor tissue.[11] More posttransplantation respiratory viral, bacterial, protozoal, and fungal infections are being recognized. It is imperative that physicians globally are aware of the wide spectrum of tropical, infectious, and parasitic diseases to which their patients may have been exposed. It is prudent to enquire about travel history and geographic origins early in consultations, to aid early diagnosis and treatment and thereby prevent poor outcomes in many patients. An extensive enquiry into the travel history is prudent because certain tropical infectious diseases can first present years or even decades after the last tropical travel, including malaria (*Plasmodium ovale* and *Plasmodium vivax*), trypanosomiases (*T cruzi* and *Trypanosoma brucei gambiense*), strongyloidiasis (*Strongyloides stercoralis*), filariases, and schistosomiasis (any *Schistosoma* spp). It is imperative to consider the possibility of a tropical disease in cases that are difficult to diagnose, even potentially in those without a suggestive travel history. For example, malaria can occur in patients who have not traveled overseas, being acquired near city airports where mosquitoes imported on aircraft arriving from the tropics can survive and transmit the infection during the summer months.[12] A high degree of clinical awareness of the possibility of a tropical disease enables an early diagnosis to be made and enables effective treatment measures to be initiated, reducing morbidity and mortality.

CLASSIFICATION OF TROPICAL DISEASES

The number and range of tropical and infectious diseases prevalent globally is extremely large and broad ranging.[1–3] Thus, for practical purposes, specific listings and classifications are useful for streamlining the microbiological and clinical assessment of the patient's illness. Classification of tropical diseases can also serve as aidemémoires or checklists for guiding clinicians, microbiologists, pathologists, and laboratory staff. For the practicing infectious diseases physician, there are several ways in which tropical/infectious diseases are presented in century-old classic tropical diseases textbooks like *Manson's Tropical Diseases* or other major treatises that present the classification of tropical diseases with a combination of clinical and microbiological approaches. The classification of infectious and tropical diseases, and their treatment, control, and prevention, have historically involved the joint efforts of epidemiologists, microbiologists, and clinicians.

Table 1 gives a basic classification of common infectious pathogens for clinical use. Physicians also tend to classify infectious diseases according to the most important organ or organ system to be affected, or the important clinical manifestations of the specific disease (**Table 2**).[13,14] Microbiologists tend to prefer classifying infectious diseases according to the classic microbiological nomenclature codes of kingdom, phylum, class, order, family, genus, and species and have large standard textbooks that give detailed classification and nomenclature.[15] They relate information according to microscopic appearance after staining or culture characteristics, to advise the clinician on the most appropriate antibiotic therapy and management. However, with advances in molecular technology, microorganisms are frequently being reclassified and renamed. For example *Rickettsia tsutsugamushi*, the causal agent for scrub typhus, has been reclassified into the genus *Orientia*. DF-2 is now known as *Capnocytophaga canimorsus*.[16] Epidemiologists usually describe tropical disease in terms of person, place, time, and exposure, with a view to developing control and prevention strategies to limit the spread of the diseases in the community. They often classify infectious diseases according to their distribution, their means of transmission, and according to their reservoirs in nature. Such classifications use the routes of transmission or acquisition of the infectious disease (**Table 3**).

Table 1
Basic microbiological classification of common infectious pathogens for clinicians

Microbiological or Clinical Grouping	Parasitologic Grouping and Examples
Bacteria	**Protozoa**
Morphologic descriptions	Flagellates
Cocci, bacilli, vibrios	i. *Trypanosoma* spp *(T cruzi, T brucei rhodesiense, T brucei gambiense, T rangeli)*
Gram staining	
Gram-positive (high or low GC)	
Gram-negative	ii. *Giardia lamblia*
Oxygen requirements	iii. *Leishmania* spp
Aerobes and anaerobes	iv. *Trichomonas* spp
Chlamydia	Ameboids
Chlamydia pneumoniae	i. *Entamoeba histolytica*
Chlamydia trachomatis	ii. *Acanthamoeba* spp
Mycoplasma	iii. *Naegleria fowleri*
Mycoplasma pneumoniae	Ciliates
Mycoplasma arthritidis	i. *Balantidium coli*
Mycoplasma genitalium	Sporozoans
Spirochetes	i. *Plasmodium* spp *(Plasmodium falciparum, Plasmodium malariae, Plasmodium vivax, Plasmodium ovale)*
Treponema spp *(Treponema pallidum, Treponema pertenue, Treponema carateum)*	
Leptospira spp *(Leptospira icterohaemorrhagica, Leptospira canicola)*	ii. *Babesia microti*
	iii. *Toxoplasma gondii*
	iv. *Microsporidium* spp
Borrelia spp *(Borrelia recurrentis, Borrelia burgdorferi)*	v. *Cryptosporium* spp
Spirillum minus	**Helminths**
Rickettsia	Nematodes (roundworms, pin/threadworms, whipworms, hookworms)
Rickettsia spp	i. Gut nematodes (*Ascaris lumbricoides, Enterobius vermicularis, Trichuris trichiuria, Ancylostoma* spp, *Necator americanus*)
Spotted fever group	
Typhus group	
Scrub typhus group (now *Orientalis*)	
Viruses	ii. Tissue/muscle nematode (*Dracunculus medinensis, Trichinella spiralis, Gnathostoma spinigerum, Linguatella serrata, Armillifer armillatus*)
DNA viruses	
Group 1: double-stranded DNA (pox, herpes, papova, hepadna)	
Group II: single-stranded DNA (parvo)	iii. Central nervous system nematodes (*Angiostrongylus cantonensis*)
RNA viruses	Trematodes (flatworms/flukes)
Group III: double-stranded (reo)	i. Liver flukes (*Fasciola hepatica, Fasciolopsis buski, Clonorchis sinensis, Opisthorchis* spp)
Group IV: single-stranded (positive sense: orthomyxo, rhabdo, picorna, toga)	
Group V: single-stranded (negative sense: Ebola, Marburg)	ii. Blood flukes (*Schistosoma haematobium, Schistosoma mansoni, Schistosoma japonicum, Schistosoma intercalatum, Schistosoma mekongi*)
Fungi	
Ascomycetes (sac fungi)	iii. Lung flukes (*Paragonimus westermani*)
Basidiomycetes (club fungi)	Cestodes (tapeworms)
Zygomycetes (mucor fungi)	i. Intestinal tapeworms (*Taenia solium, Taenia saginata, Diphyllobothrium latum, Hymenolepis nana*)
Phycomycetes (algal fungi)	
Morphology	ii. Intestinal tapeworm larval infections in organs:
Unicellular (*Candida* spp, *Histoplasma* spp)	a. Cysticercosis (*Taenia solium* larvae)
Multicellular (*Aspergillus* spp, *Rhizopus* spp, *Fusarium* spp)	b. Echinococcosis (larvae of dog tapeworms *Echinococcus granulosus*, and *Echinococcus multilocularis*)
Dimorphic (*Penicillium marneffei*)	

Abbreviation: GC, guanine and cytosine.

Table 2
Some examples of tropical infectious diseases by main organ system involved

Main Organ System Involved	Common Pathogens
Gastrointestinal	Bacterial: all gastroenteritides, tuberculosis Protozoal: Chagas disease, amebiasis, *Giardia*, coccidia Helminthic: multiple
Hepatic	Bacterial: leptospirosis, polymicrobial, anaerobes Protozoal: amoebic hepatitis/abscess, malaria, trypanosomiasis Helminthic: schistosomiasis, liver trematodes, hydatidosis Viral: hepatitis A–E, yellow fever, herpes viruses
Respiratory	Bacterial: tuberculosis, pneumococcal pneumonia, legionnaires, mycoplasma pneumonia Fungal: aspergillosis, histoplasmosis, coccidioidomycosis, blastomycosis Helminthic: paragonimiasis, strongyloides hyperinfection, hydatid, tropical pulmonary eosinophilia Protozoal: *Plasmodium falciparum*
Cardiovascular	Bacterial: endocarditis, rheumatic fever, tuberculosis, syphilis Protozoal: Chagas disease Helminthic: schistosomiasis
Renal tract	Bacterial: poststreptococcal, tuberculosis Helminthic: schistosomiasis Protozoal: *Plasmodium falciparum*
Neurologic	Bacterial: *Neisseria meningitidis* and other bacterial meningitis, leprosy, botulism, diphtheria Protozoal: *Naegleria fowleri*, Acanthamoebae, trypanosomiasis, *Plasmodium falciparum* Helminthic: cysticercosis, hydatid, *Angiostrongylus cantonensis*, gnathostomiasis Viral: HIV, HTLV-1, Japanese encephalitis, enteroviruses, rabies
Dermatologic	Bacterial: tropical ulcers, syphilis, mycobacteria (eg, leprosy, tuberculosis, *Mycobacterium ulcerans*), anthrax Fungal: sporotrichosis, mycetoma, *Penicillium* Protozoal: leishmaniasis Helminthic: acute schistosomiasis, *Loa loa*, *Gnathostoma*, onchocerciasis, cutaneous larva migrans, larva currens Arthropods: bites and stings, scabies, myiasis, tungiasis
Musculoskeletal	Pyomyositis, trichinosis, cysticercosis, tuberculosis, hydatid

Many tropical infectious diseases are characterized by chronic inflammation as the battle between the host and pathogen becomes protracted. Pathologic reports often describe the presence of a granuloma in biopsy tissue and the tissue may be processed with special stains, molecular methods, or culture to try to identify further. A granuloma[17–19] is defined as a chronic, compact collection of inflammatory cells in which mononuclear cells predominate, usually formed as a result of an undegradable product, in the case of tropical infectious diseases; examples are given in **Table 4**. Some of the organisms contained within the granuloma remain viable, and these can reactivate to cause active disease when the patient becomes immunosuppressed from HIV or immunosuppressive therapy. Tuberculosis in HIV-infected individuals or in those on anti-TNF-α therapy, and Chagas disease in transplant recipients, are classic examples. Infectious diseases transmitted through medical procedures (eg, transfusion of blood

Table 3
Main routes of transmission of tropical and parasitic diseases

Route/Mode of Transmission	Disease (Examples)
Mother to child	
Congenital/vertical	
Transplacental transmission via blood	TORCHES group of infections (toxoplasmosis, rubella, cytomegalovirus, *Herpes simplex*, syphilis), HIV, hepatitis viruses, malaria, trypanosomiases, bacterial infections
Perinatal	
Vaginal/cervical contact during delivery	Bacterial, viral, fungal infections
Contact via breast milk	Sexually transmitted diseases
Airborne/inhalational	
Inhalation of air, aerosol, fomite contaminated by microbes	RTIs caused by bacteria, viruses, fungi, *Chlamydia* spp and *Mycoplasma* spp (eg, lobal pneumonia, influenza, pneumonic plague, tuberculosis)
Contact of skin/mucosa	
Direct (touching, kissing, sex)	Sexually transmitted diseases, mycosis, scabies, MRSA
Indirect (indirect contact with infected fomite, body fluid, secretions, stool, blood, plasma, or pus)	Boils, MRSA, sexually transmitted diseases, respiratory infections, *C difficile* and so forth
Ingestion	
Ingestion of any food or water contaminated with:	
Microorganisms	Infections caused by bacteria (eg, typhoid, cholera, dysentery), viruses (eg, hepatitis A, B, and C), mycobacteria (eg, *Mycobacterium xenopi*), protozoa (eg, *Entamoeba histolytica*, *Cryptosporidium* spp)
Toxins	Staphylococcal, botulism, *Bacillus cereus*, scrombrotoxin, mushroom (*Amanita phalloides*)
Parasite ova/cysts	Infections caused by nematodes, trematodes, cestodes, protozoa (*Entamoeba histolytica*, *Cryptosporidium* spp)
Insect/arthropod-borne injection through skin penetration	
Mosquitoes and disease transmission	
Anopheles spp	Malaria (all *Plasmodium* spp), bancroftian filariasis (*Wuchereria bancrofti*)
Culicine spp	Arbovirus encephalitis (eg, Japanese B encephalitis, St Louis encephalitis, West Nile virus)
Aedes spp	Yellow fever, filariasis (bancroftian)
Sandfly and disease transmission (*Phlebotomus* spp, *Lutzomyia* spp)	Leishmaniasis (all forms), sandfly fever (or Pappataci 3 day fever; Toscana, Sicilian, and Naples virus infections), bartenellosis (*Bartonella bacciliformis*)
Tsetse flies and disease transmission (*Glossina* spp)	Sleeping sickness (*Trypanosoma brucei rhodesiense*, *T brucei gambiense*)
Black flies (*Simulium* spp)	Onchocerciases (river blindness) (*Onchocerca volvulus*)

(continued on next page)

Table 3
(continued)

Route/Mode of Transmission	Disease (Examples)
Horse/deer flies (*Chrysops* spp)	Filariasis (*Loa loa*), tularemia (*Francisella tularensis*)
Lice	Pediculosis Trench fever, bacillary angiomatosis and endocarditis (*Bartonella quintana*), epidemic typhus (*Rickettsia prowazekii*), louse-borne relapsing fever (*Borrelia recurrentis*)
Fleas	Plague (*Yersinia pestis*), endemic/murine typhus (*Rickettsia typhi*), bartonellosis, and cat scratch disease (*Bartonella henselae*), dwarf tapeworm (*Hymenolepis nana*)
Arachnids	
Mites	Chiggers, scrub typhus (*Orientia tsutsugamushi*) Scabies
Ticks	Lyme disease (*Borrelia burgdorferi*), tick typhus (Rocky Mountain spotted fever), ehrlichiosis (*Anaplasma phagocytophilum*), relapsing fever (*Borrelia recurrentis*), tularemia (*Francisella tularensis*), arboviruses (eg, Crimean-Congo hemorrhagic fever, Omsk hemorrhagic fever, babesiosis (*Babesia microti*)
Insect feces rubbed into skin	
Reduvid bugs (*Rhodnius* spp, *Triatoma* spp, *Panstrongylus* spp)	Chagas disease: feces of reduvid bugs with *T cruzi* spp are rubbed into skin by scratching)
Direct penetration through skin	
Helminth larvae	Helminth larvae penetration into subcutaneous tissue: swimmers itch (*Schistosoma* spp), hookworm and roundworm larvae
Fly larvae	Fly (bots and warbles) larvae (cutaneous myiases)
Innoculation or injection	
Breach of skin or mucous membrane caused by needles, tattoos, ear piercing, acupuncture, cupping, traditional scarification via blades	Viruses, bacteria, or fungal infections
Animal and human bites	Viruses (rabies, HIV, hepatitis B, hepatitis C, *Herpes* spp), bacterial infections (anaerobic and aerobic) including tetanus, actinomycosis, rat bite fever (*Spirillum minus*), *Pasteurella multocida*, *Capnocytophaga canimorsus*
Multiple modes of transmission	
Insect bites and airborne	eg, Plague: *Y pestis* flea bite (bubonic plague), airborne (pneumonic plague)
Direct contact, airborne, and ingestion of contaminated meat	eg, Anthrax: *Bacillus anthracis* skin contact with animal hides (cutaneous anthrax), airborne (pulmonary anthrax), ingestion of contaminated meat (gastrointestinal anthrax)
Insect bites, blood transfusion, needles, and congenital	eg, Malaria: *Plasmodium* spp
Skin/mucosa contact, needles, blood transfusion	eg, HIV, hepatitis B

Table 4
Infectious causes of granulomas

Class of Organism	Examples	Clinical Disease and Site of Granulomas
Bacteria		
Mycobacteria spp	*Mycobacterium tuberculosis*	Tuberculosis (any organ)
	Mycobacterium leprae	Leprosy (skin and nerves)
	Mycobacterium kansasii	Pneumonia (lung)
	Mycobacterium marinum	Fish tank granuloma (skin)
	Mycobacterium bovis	BCGiosis (skin)
Brucella spp	*Brucella abortus, Brucella mellitensis, Brucella suis*	Brucellosis (any organ)
Yersinia spp	*Y pestis*	Plague (skin, lung)
Listeria spp	*Listeria monocytogenes*	Listerioses (brain)
Spirochetes	*Treponema pallidum*	Primary syphilis (skin)
	Treponema carateum	Yaws (skin/mucous membranes)
Fungi	*Histoplasma capsulatum*	Histoplasmosis (any organ)
	Coccidioides immitis	Cocciodomycoses (any organ)
	Aspergillus fumigatus	Pulmonary aspergillosis (lung)
	Cryptococcus neoformans	Cryptococcosis (any organ)
Protozoa	*Toxoplasma gondii*	Toxoplasmosis (eye or brain)
	Leishmania spp	Leishmaniases (skin, mucous membranes, spleen, liver)
Helminth ova/larvae		
Trematodes	*Schistosoma* spp	Granulomas (any organ)
	Fasciola spp, *Opisthorchis* spp	Granulomas (liver, bile duct)
Cestodes	*Clonorchis sinensis*	Granuloma around cysticerci (muscle, brain, subcutaneous tissue)
	Taenia solium	
Helminth larvae	*Ascaris lumbricoides, Ancylostoma* spp, *Necator americanus*	Granulomas (cutaneous and visceral) around dead larvae

or blood-related products[20] and via transplantation) can also be classified microbiologically according to the type of microorganism (**Box 1**).

GEOGRAPHIC DISTRIBUTION OF TROPICAL DISEASES

There are geographic differences in the distribution and intensity of tropical infectious diseases and knowledge of these in relation to travel history or country of origin may increase the likelihood of making an accurate and rapid diagnosis. The incidence and prevalence of each disease varies with time, and therefore published World Health Organization data and map resources can rapidly become outdated because of the lag between data collection and publication. The Global Health Observatory (GHO)[21] is a unique and useful service providing a gallery of global maps illustrating the prevalence of an extensive list of major health topics including tropical diseases, which are updated on a regular basis. These maps are classified by disease themes, including all major infectious and parasitic diseases. Each theme page provides information on the global situation, prevalence, and trends, using core indicators, database views, publications, and links to relevant Web pages. The GHO also issues analytical reports

> **Box 1**
> **Classification of infections related to transfusion (of blood, platelet, immunoglobulin, clotting factors, or plasma)**
>
> *Parasites*
>
> *Plasmodium* spp
>
> *Babesia microti* ssp
>
> *Trypanosma cruzi*
>
> *Trypanosoma brucei* ssp
>
> *Leishmania donovani*
>
> *Toxoplasma gondii*
>
> *Viruses*
>
> HIV-1, HIV-2
>
> Human T-lymphotropic virus (HTLV) type I, HTLV type II
>
> Hepatitis A, B, C, D, E
>
> Epstein B virus, cytomegalovirus
>
> Kaposi sarcoma herpesvirus (HHV-8)
>
> Parvovirus
>
> West Nile virus
>
> Severe acute respiratory syndrome
>
> *Bacteria*
>
> Gram-negative bacteria (eg, *Pseudomonas* spp, *Yersinia* spp, *Salmonella* spp)
>
> Gram-positive bacteria (eg, *Staphylococcus* spp, *Streptococcus* spp, *Brucella* spp)
>
> *Spirochetes*
>
> Spirochetes (eg, *Treponema pallidum*, *Leptospira* spp, *Borrelia burgdorferi*)
>
> Ehrlichia
>
> *Fungi*
>
> *Candida* spp
>
> *Other*
>
> New variant Creutzfeldt-Jakob disease prion

on the current situation and trends for priority health issues. A key output of the GHO is the annual publication *World Health Statistics*, which compiles statistics for key health indicators and also includes a brief report on progress toward health-related Millennium Development Goals. In addition, the GHO provides analytical reports on cross-cutting topics such as the report on women and health and burden of disease.

SOURCES OF LITERATURE ON TROPICAL DISEASES

Ongoing research and surveillance continues to yield new information. Advances in tropical medicine, as with all clinical specialties, tend to be distributed throughout the general medical and scientific literature, and sole reliance on such sources for specialist tropical medicine information does not usually suffice. There are several major textbooks focusing on clinical and laboratory aspects of tropical and parasitic diseases.[1-3] The information they contain is comprehensive, but some details may become outdated rapidly because of new developments, and readers are advised to look up more current sources of literature on each subject area.[22] It is important that any comprehensive search encompasses general and specialist sources, including journals, books, databases, and Web sites. Many traditional print resources, such as journals, indexes, and, increasingly, books, are now available online.

This issue of *Infectious Diseases Clinics of North America* on tropical diseases covers the epidemiologic, clinical, laboratory, and management aspects of most of the common tropical infectious and parasitic diseases that may present to the physician in the west. Diseases caused by venomous bites, stings, and poisoning are also described to emphasize that not all tropical diseases are caused by microorganisms.

REFERENCES

1. Cook GC, Zumla A, editors. Manson's tropical diseases. 22nd edition. London: Saunders; 2009. p. 1830.
2. Guerrant R, Wag DH, Weller PF, editors. Tropical infectious diseases. Principles, pathogens and practice. 3rd edition. London: Elsevier Saunders; 2011.
3. Hunters tropical medicine and emerging infectious diseases. 2000.
4. WHO Report 2008. The Global Burden of Disease 2004 update: 1. Cost of illness. 2. World health - statistics. 3. Mortality - trends. I. World Health Organization. Geneva: World Health Organization; 2008 (NLM classification: W 74).
5. Mabey D, Gill G, Whitty C, et al, editors. Principles of medicine in Africa. 4th edition. Cambridge (UK): Cambridge University Press; 2012.
6. Zumla A, Yew WW, Hui D, editors. Infectious Diseases Clinics of North America. Emerging respiratory infections of the 21st century, vol. 24. New York: Elsevier Saunders; 2010. Issue 3.
7. Zumla A. Emerging respiratory infections of the 20th century. Curr Opin Pulm Med 2010;16:165–7.
8. Zhong NS, Zeng GQ. Pandemic planning in China: applying lessons from severe acute respiratory syndrome. Respirology 2008;13(Suppl 1):S33–5.
9. The Global Surveillance Network of the ISTM and CDC. A worldwide communications and data collection network of travel/tropical medicine clinics. Available at: http://www.istm.org/geosentinel/main.html. Accessed September 26, 2011.
10. Odolini S, Parola P, Gkrania-Klotsas E, et al. Travel-related imported infections in Europe, EuroTravNet 2009. Clin Microbiol Infect 2011. DOI: 10.1111/j.1469-0691.2011.03596.x.
11. Muñoz P, Valerio M, Puga D, et al. Parasitic infections in solid organ transplant recipients. Infect Dis Clin North Am 2010;24(2):461–95.
12. Gratz NG, Steffen R, Cocksedge W. Why aircraft disinsection? Bull World Health Organ 2000;78(8):995–1004.
13. Gill GV, Beeching NJ. Lecture notes in tropical medicine. ISBN: 9781405180481. Blackwell Publishing; 2009. p. 402.
14. Eddleston M, Davidson R, Brent A, et al. Oxford handbook of tropical medicine. ISBN: 9780199204090. 3rd edition. Oxford University Press; 2008. p. 843.
15. Boone DR, Garrity GM, Castenholz RW, editors. Bergey's manual of systematic bacteriology. 2nd edition. London (UK): Springer; 2001.
16. McCarthy M, Zumla A. DF-2 infection (may follow dog bites and hazardous to the immunosuppressed). BMJ 1988;297:1355–6.
17. Zumla A, James DG. Granulomatous infections - aetiology and classification. Clin Infect Dis 1996;23:1–13.

18. James DG, Zumla A, editors. Granulomatous disorders 616. Cambridge (United Kingdom): Cambridge University Press; 1999.
19. Zumla A, James DG. Granulomatous infections - an overview. In: James DG, Zumla A, editors. Granulomatous disorders. Cambridge (UK): Cambridge University Press; 1999. p. 103–21.
20. Bates I, Owusu-Ofori S. Blood transfusion. Chapter 14. In: Manson's tropical diseases. 21st edition, 2009. p. 229–35.
21. Global Health Observatory World Map. WHO website. Available at: http://www.who.int/gho/map_gallery/en/. Accessed December 5, 2011.
22. Schoonbaert D, Eyers AE, Eyers J. Sources of literature on tropical medicine. Manson's Tropical Diseases. International Edition. In: Cook G, Zumla A, editors. 22nd edition. London (UK): Elsevier; 2009. p. 1829.

Venomous Bites, Stings, and Poisoning

David A. Warrell, DM, DSc, FRCP, FRCPE, FMedSci

KEYWORDS

- Snake bite • Lizard bite • Fish sting • Jellyfish sting • Seafood poisoning
- Scorpion sting • Spider bite • Antivenom

KEY POINTS

- Venomous snake bites are an environmental hazard to agricultural workers, preventable by wearing protective footwear, using lights at night and by sleeping under a mosquito net.
- Snake bite first aid involves immobilization and rapid evacuation to the hospital for treatment with specific antivenoms that are indicated for systemic or severe local envenoming.
- The agonising pain of marine stings is relieved by hot (45°C) water but marine poisons are not destroyed by cooking.
- Fatal bee, vespid and ant sting anaphylaxis can be provoked by a single sting, while mass attacks by these Hymenoptera can kill by direct envenoming.
- Scorpion stings cause severe local pain and potentially fatal "autonomic storm" especially in children while spider bites can cause either necrotic (loxoscelism) or neurotoxic envenoming.

VENOMOUS SNAKES

Dangerously venomous snakes of medical importance inhabit most parts of the world, and are members of 4 families: Elapidae (cobras, kraits, mambas, coral snakes, Australasian snakes, sea snakes); Viperidae (old-world vipers and adders, American rattlesnakes, moccasins, lance-headed vipers, Asian pit vipers); Atractaspidinae (burrowing asps); and Colubridae (arboreal back-fanged snakes).

Epidemiology

Although snake bite is a frequent medical emergency in many parts of the rural tropics, its incidence is underestimated because most victims are treated by traditional practitioners and are therefore unrecorded. Focal community studies in Africa and Asia

No funding.
The author has nothing to disclose.
Nuffield Department of Clinical Medicine, John Radcliffe Hospital, University of Oxford, Headley Way, Headington, Oxford OX3 9DU, UK
E-mail address: david.warrell@ndm.ox.ac.uk

Infect Dis Clin N Am 26 (2012) 207–223
doi:10.1016/j.idc.2012.03.006
0891-5520/12/$ – see front matter © 2012 Published by Elsevier Inc.

id.theclinics.com

indicated 4 to 162 snake bite deaths per 100,000 population per year. Recently, well-designed, nationally representative surveys in India and Bangladesh produced direct estimates of 46,000 and 6000 deaths each year, respectively.[1,2] In Western countries, envenoming by exotic snakes kept as pets (often illegally), is an increasing challenge for poisons centers.[3] Most bites occur in rural areas of tropical developing countries, inflicted on the lower limbs of agricultural workers and children. Asian kraits (*Bungarus* sp) and African spitting cobras bite people who are asleep on the floors of their houses. Seasonal peaks of incidence coincide with rain and agricultural activity.

Prevention

Snakes should be avoided. In snake-infested areas, boots, socks, and long trousers/pants should be worn for walks in undergrowth or deep sand. A light should be used at night. The dangers of sleeping on the ground are mitigated by sleeping under a mosquito net.[4] Fishermen should avoid touching sea snakes caught in nets or on lines.

Venom

Snake venoms are complex, each containing more than a hundred different proteins and peptides. Venom enzymes include digestive hydrolases, hyaluronidase spreading factor, and procoagulants. Neurotoxins cause paralysis by blocking transmission at neuromuscular junctions presynaptically or postsynaptically.

Clinical Features

Effects of anxiety and prehospital treatment may obscure direct effects of envenoming. Immediate local pain and bleeding from the fang punctures are followed by tenderness, swelling, and bruising that extend up the limb and tender enlargement of regional lymph nodes. Nausea, vomiting, and syncope are early indications of systemic envenoming.

Elapids

Bites by most elapids produce minimal local effects, but African spitting cobras and Asian cobras cause painful local swelling, blistering, and superficial necrosis (**Fig. 1**). However, elapid venoms are better known for their paralytic effects, first detectable as bilateral ptosis and external ophthalmoplegia appearing from 15 minutes to 10 hours after the bite (**Fig. 2**). Pupils, face, palate, jaws, tongue, vocal cords, neck muscles, and muscles of deglutition and respiration are affected progressively over the next few hours. In addition, envenoming by terrestrial Australasian elapids causes hemostatic disturbances and sometimes generalized rhabdomyolysis and acute kidney injury (AKI). Sea snake envenoming results in generalized myalgia, trismus, myoglobinuria, and generalized flaccid paralysis.

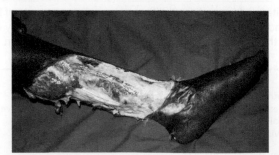

Fig. 1. Extensive superficial necrosis of skin following a bite by a black-necked spitting cobra (*Naja nigricollis*) in Nigeria. (Copyright © Prof D.A. Warrell.)

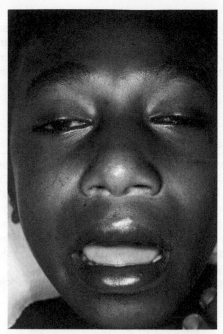

Fig. 2. Ptosis, external ophthalmoplegia, facial paralysis, and inability to open the mouth in a boy bitten by a Papuan taipan (*Oxyuranus scutellatus*) in Papua New Guinea. (The parents gave full permission for this image to be published.) (Copyright © Prof D.A. Warrell.)

Some elapids spit their venom into the eyes of perceived aggressors, provoking intense pain, blepharospasm, palpebral edema, and leukorrhea (**Fig. 3**). Corneal erosions, hypopyon, anterior uveitis, secondary infections, and blindness may ensue.

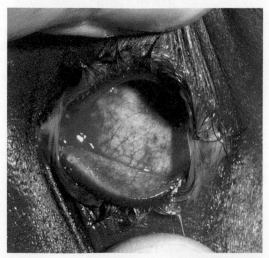

Fig. 3. Inflammation, blepharospasm, and leukorrhea caused by venom spat into the eye by a back-necked spitting cobra (*Naja nigricollis*) in Nigeria. (Copyright © Prof D.A. Warrell.)

Vipers and pit vipers

Local envenoming may be severe, affecting the whole limb, adjacent trunk and, in children, the whole body. Bruising and blistering appears within hours, tissue necrosis within days (**Fig. 4**). Hypotension, shock, and hemostatic abnormalities are common. Spontaneous bleeding occurs from gums (**Fig. 5**), nose, gastrointestinal tract, and lungs, and into the skin, conjunctivae, and brain. Some viper venoms cause neuromyotoxicity. AKI is an important complication.

Laboratory Investigations

Peripheral neutrophil leukocytosis is common. Consumption coagulopathy is detected quickly with the 20-minute whole blood clotting test (20WBCT). A few milliliters of venous blood is placed in a new, clean, dry, glass vessel, left undisturbed for 20 minutes, then tipped once to see if it has clotted. Incoagulable blood suggests a plasma fibrinogen concentration of less than 0.5 g/L.[5] Laboratory assessment of blood coagulation and fibrinolysis, and a platelet count are also useful. Raised serum creatine kinase, myoglobin, and potassium levels indicate rhabdomyolysis. Dark red, brown, or black urine may contain erythrocytes, hemoglobin, or myoglobin. Electrocardiographic (ECG) abnormalities include ST-T changes, atrioventricular block, and arrhythmias.

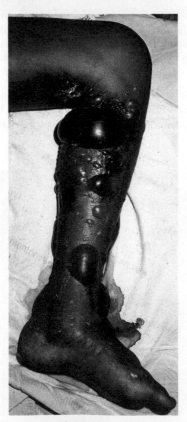

Fig. 4. Swelling, bruising, blistering, and necrosis of the leg of a boy bitten by a Malayan pit viper (*Calloselasma rhodostoma*) in Thailand. (Copyright © Prof D.A. Warrell.)

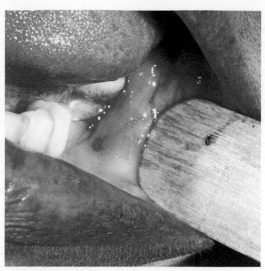

Fig. 5. Bleeding from the gingival sulci in a patient bitten by a common lancehead (*Bothrops atrox*) in Peru. (Copyright © Prof D.A. Warrell.)

Management of Snake Bite

First aid

Patients should be moved to the hospital as quickly, passively, and immobile as possible. Traditional first-aid methods (local incisions, suction, vacuum extractors, tourniquets, cryotherapy, electric shock, instillation of chemicals and herbs) are dangerous and ineffective.

Compression of superficial veins and lymphatics in the whole bitten limb at a pressure of about 55 mm Hg can be achieved using long elasticated bandages and a splint (pressure-immobilization method). This method prolonged the lives of experimental animals and did not increase local necrosis after rattlesnake venom injection.[6] Local pressure can be applied by the pressure-pad method, which is simpler and has proved to be effective in a field trial.[7] Applying nitroglycerin ointment to the bitten limb may slow lymphatic spread of venom.[8]

Antivenom treatment

Antivenom (antivenin), the only specific antidote for envenoming, has proved effective in reducing mortality, correcting coagulopathies caused by Viperidae and Australian Elapidae, and reversing postsynaptic neurotoxicity. Antivenom is whole or enzyme-digested immunoglobulin G (IgG) of horses or sheep that have been hyperimmunized with selected venoms. Antivenoms are widely unavailable in sub-Saharan Africa, New Guinea, and other developing countries.

Indications for antivenom

Antivenom is indicated if there are hemostatic abnormalities, neurotoxicity, hypotension, shock, new ECG abnormalities, generalized rhabdomyolysis, hemolysis, rapidly spreading local swelling, or extensive blistering/bruising especially involving the digits.

Antivenom administration

Intradermal/conjunctival hypersensitivity tests do not predict antivenom reactions. Pretreatment with subcutaneous adrenaline (epinephrine) reduces the risk of severe early reactions (adult dose 0.25 mL of 0.1% solution).[9] Polyspecific (polyvalent) antivenoms appropriate for the geographic region and clinical features are recommended because of the difficulty in identifying the species responsible for bites. The antivenom should be administered as soon as these indications are fulfilled. Benefit can be expected as long as signs of systemic envenoming persist, but local necrosis is not preventable unless antivenom is given within a few hours of the bite. Antivenom should be diluted in approximately 5 mL of isotonic fluid per kilogram body weight and infused intravenously over 30 to 60 minutes. Ideally, the initial dose should be based on results of clinical trials, but in most countries it is judged empirically. Children must be given the same dose as adults.

Repeated dosing is indicated if blood coagulability (20WBCT) is not restored within about 6 hours or if cardiovascular effects or paralysis progress after 1 to 2 hours. Recurrent systemic envenoming may occur hours or days after an initially good response to antivenom, especially if a rapidly cleared Fab fragment antivenom is used (eg, CroFab for North American pit viper bites).

Antivenom reactions

Early (anaphylactic) reactions develop 10 to 180 minutes after starting antivenom. Risk increases with dose and speed of administration. The mechanism is complement activation by immune complexes or IgG aggregates, rather than acquired immunoglobulin E (IgE)-mediated type I hypersensitivity.

At the first sign of a reaction, early reactions should be treated with adrenaline (epinephrine): adults 0.5 to 1.0 mL (children 0.01 mL/kg) of 0.1% (1 in 1000, 1 mg/mL) by intramuscular injection.

Late (serum sickness type) reactions develop between 5 and 24 (mean 7) days after antivenom. Risk and speed development increases with the dose of antivenom. Clinical features include fever, itching, urticaria, arthralgia, lymphadenopathy, periarticular swellings, mononeuritis multiplex, and albuminuria.

Treatment of late reactions consists of oral histamine-H1 blocker such as chlorphenamine (adults 2 mg every 6 hours, children 0.25 mg/kg per day in divided doses) or oral prednisolone (adults 5 mg every 6 hours, children 0.7 mg/kg per day in divided doses) for 5 to 7 days.

Supportive treatment

Bulbar and respiratory paralysis threatens aspiration, airway obstruction, respiratory failure, and death. A cuffed endotracheal tube or laryngeal mask airway should be inserted to maintain the airway as soon as there is pooling of secretions or respiratory distress.

Anticholinesterases are given if the patient responds to a test dose of (ideally) edrophonium and atropine.[10] Hypotension and shock are treated with plasma expanders or vasoconstrictors.

Oliguria and AKI may require dialysis or hemoperfusion. Local infection at the site of the bite may be caused by unusual bacteria from the snake's venom or fangs. Tetanus immunity is boosted. Prophylactic antibiotics are not indicated unless the wound has been tampered with. Blisters and bullae are left unpunctured. Excessive elevation of the bitten limb increases the risk of intracompartmental ischemia. Once signs of necrosis have appeared, surgical debridement, immediate split-skin grafting, and broad-spectrum antibiotic cover are indicated.

Compartment syndrome is uncommon, but many unnecessary fasciotomies are performed. Snake-bitten limbs may be painful, tensely swollen, cold, cyanosed, and apparently pulseless, signs suggesting compartment syndrome. However, intracompartmental pressures (**Fig. 6**) are rarely high enough (more than 45 mm Hg) to suggest

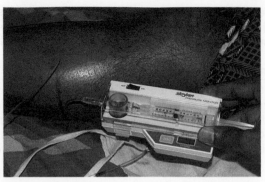

Fig. 6. Direct measurement of pressure in the anterior tibial compartment in a man bitten by a Russell's viper (*Daboia russelii*) in India. (Copyright © Prof D.A. Warrell.)

a risk of ischemic necrosis justifying fasciotomy. Fasciotomy is absolutely contraindicated until blood coagulability has been restored by adequate antivenom treatment followed by clotting factors.

Ophthalmia caused by spitting elapids is treated by irrigating the eyes with generous volumes of water, relieving pain with adrenaline/epinephrine (0.1% eye drops) or topical anesthetics such as tetracaine (with caution), and excluding corneal abrasion by fluorescein staining/slit-lamp examination or by treating it presumptively with topical antimicrobials (eg, tetracycline, chloramphenicol, or fluoroquinolone).[11]

VENOMOUS LIZARDS

Mexican beaded lizards (*Heloderma horridum*) of western to southern Mexico and Gila monsters (*Heloderma suspectum*) of the southwestern United States and adjacent areas of Mexico are the only lizards of medical importance.[12] Venom from submandibular glands is inoculated by grooved mandibular teeth. This venom contains a tissue-kallikrein–like enzyme that releases bradykinin and several peptides, including exendin-4, a glucagon-like peptide-1 homologue.

Clinical Features

These inoffensive animals bite only those who provoke them, and cling on tenaciously. Pain and swelling develop rapidly, radiating up the bitten arm to the shoulder and trunk. Dizziness, weakness, nausea, vomiting, profuse generalized sweating, breathlessness, hypotension, tachycardia, and angioedema may evolve, accompanied by neutrophil leukocytosis, thrombocytopenia, mild coagulopathy, and ECG changes.

Treatment

The lizard's bulldog grip is disengaged by levering the jaws apart with a screwdriver or by running cold water over the animal. Severe pain is relieved by local or systemic analgesia. Tetanus immunity is boosted and the wound observed for evidence of sepsis. No antivenom is available. Hypotension is treated with plasma expanders and vasoconstrictors. Angioedema responds to epinephrine, antihistamine, and hydrocortisone.

VENOMOUS FISH

Tropical oceans have the richest venomous fish fauna but dangerous sharks, chimeras, and weeverfish also occur in temperate northern waters.[13] Some rivers in

South America, West Africa, and Southeast Asia are inhabited by freshwater stingrays (*Potamotrygon* sp). Venom glands are embedded in grooves in the spines or beneath a membrane covering the long barbed precaudal spines of stingrays.

Incidence and Epidemiology

Each year, some 1500 stings by rays (*Dasyatis* sp) and 300 by scorpionfish (*Scorpaena* sp) occur in the United States, while hundreds of weeverfish (*Trachinus* sp) stings are recorded in the United Kingdom. Stonefish (*Synanceja* spp) stings are frequent in Southeast Asia. Most fish stings are inflicted on the ankles and soles of people wading near the shore or in the vicinity of coral reefs. Tropical aquarium enthusiasts may be stung by their pet lion fish (*Pterois* and *Dendrochirus* spp) **(Fig. 7)**.

Prevention

Adopt a shuffling gait when wading, avoid handling living or dead fish, and keep clear of fish in the water, especially in the vicinity of tropical reefs. Footwear protects against most species except stingrays.

Venom Composition

Stingray and weeverfish venoms contain thermolabile peptides, enzymes, and a variety of vasoactive compounds such as kinins, 5-hydroxytryptamine, histamine, and catecholamines.

Clinical Features

There is immediate agonizing pain and tender, hot, erythematous swelling that spreads up the stung limb. Wounds may be infected by marine *Vibrio* spp (eg, *Vibrio vulnificus*), freshwater *Aeromonas hydrophila*, and other unusual bacteria, particularly if the spine remains embedded. Stingray spines, up to 30 cm long, can cause severe lacerating injuries especially to the ankles, but if the victim inadvertently falls onto the ray, its spine may penetrate the thoracic or abdominal cavities with fatal results.

Systemic effects are uncommon after weeverfish stings, but people stung by rays or Scorpaenidae (scorpionfish and stonefish) may develop nausea, vomiting, diarrhea, sweating, hypersalivation, cardiac arrhythmias, hypotension, respiratory distress, neurologic signs, and generalized convulsions.

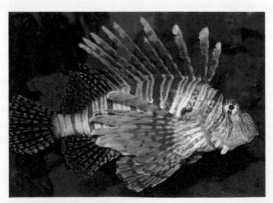

Fig. 7. Lion fish (*Pterois volitans*) a popular tropical aquarium fish from the Indo-Pacific ocean. (Copyright © Prof D.A. Warrell.)

Treatment

Pain is alleviated rapidly by immersing the stung limb in uncomfortably hot but not scalding water. Temperature is assessed using the unstung limb. Fragments of stinger spine and membrane should be removed as soon as possible. Stonefish (*Synanceja*) antivenom manufactured in Australia has paraspecific activity against the venoms of North American scorpionfish and some other Scorpaenidae. Ancillary treatments for severe hypotension are adrenaline (epinephrine) or atropine if there is bradycardia. Antibiotic treatment of secondary infections should include doxycycline or cotrimoxazole to cover marine *Vibrio* and *Aeromonas* spp.

POISONOUS FISH AND SHELLFISH

Acute gastrointestinal symptoms (food poisoning) after eating seafood are caused by allergy, bacterial or viral infections, or seafood poisoning.[14]

Gastrointestinal and Neurotoxic Syndromes

Nausea, vomiting, abdominal colic, and watery diarrhea usually precede neurotoxic symptoms: paresthesia of lips, mouth, and extremities, reversed temperature perception, myalgia, progressive flaccid paralysis, dizziness, ataxia, cardiovascular disturbances, bradycardia, and rashes. The commonest causes of this syndrome are as follows.

1. *Ciguatera fish poisonings*. Global incidence exceeds 50,000 per year, and in 50% of Pacific islands, up to 2% of the population are affected each year with 0.1% case fatality. Causative ion channel toxins (ciguatoxins, maitotoxin, scaritoxin) are acquired through the food chain from reef bacteria and benthic dinoflagellates such as *Gambierdiscus toxicus*. The toxins are concentrated in the liver, viscera, and gonads of tropical shore or reef fish (grouper, snapper, parrotfish, mackerel, moray eel, barracuda, jack), which are increasingly marketed in the West. Symptoms develop 1 to 6 hours after ingestion. Gastrointestinal symptoms resolve within a few hours, but paresthesia and myalgia may persist for weeks or months.
2. *Tetrodotoxin poisoning*. Scaleless sunfish, pufferfish, toadfish, and porcupine fish (**Fig. 8**) (order: Tetraodontiformes) may contain tetrodotoxin, which blocks Na^+ channels, producing neurotoxic and cardiotoxic effects. It is also found in some amphibians and marine invertebrates. Pufferfish (fugu) is popular in Japan where, despite stringent regulations, poisoning still occurs. Neurotoxic symptoms develop rapidly, causing death from respiratory paralysis as soon as 30 minutes after ingestion.

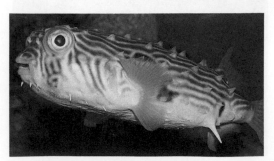

Fig. 8. Striped burrfish (*Chilomycterus schoepfi*), a tetrodotoxic porcupine fish (Diodontidae) from the western Atlantic. (Copyright © Prof D.A. Warrell.)

3. *Paralytic shellfish poisoning.* Bivalve mollusks acquire neurotoxins such as saxitoxin from dinoflagellates (*Alexandrium* spp), which may bloom in sufficient abundance to produce "red tides" causing die-offs of fish and marine birds and mammals. Symptoms develop within 30 minutes of ingestion, sometimes progressing to fatal respiratory paralysis.
4. *Neurotoxic shellfish poisoning.* Gastroenteritis followed by paresthesia is caused by ingestion of mollusks contaminated by brevitoxins from *Gymnodinium breve* microalgae, which bloom as a red tide.
5. *Amnesic shellfish poisoning* develops after ingestion of mussels containing domoic acid from diatoms (*Pseudonitzschia* spp). Gastroenteritis starts within 24 hours of exposure. Headache, coma, and short-term amnesia may ensue.

Histamine-Like Syndrome (Scombrotoxic Poisoning)

Dark-fleshed scombroid fish (tuna, mackerel, bonito, and skipjack) and also sardines and pilchards may be decomposed by bacteria (*Proteus morgani* and *Klebsiella pneumoniae*), releasing histamine. Toxic fish may produce a tingling or smarting sensation in the mouth when eaten. Symptoms develop rapidly: flushing, burning, sweating, urticaria, pruritus, headache, abdominal colic, nausea, vomiting, diarrhea, bronchial asthma, giddiness, and hypotension.

Treatment

No specific treatments or antidotes are available. Gastrointestinal contents should be eliminated by emetics and purges if this can be achieved safely and within 1 to 2 hours of ingestion. Activated charcoal adsorbs saxitoxin and other shellfish toxins. Paralytic poisoning is treated by endotracheal intubation, mechanical ventilation, and cardiac resuscitation. Scombrotoxic poisoning is treated with adrenaline/epinephrine, bronchodilators, and antihistamines.

Prevention

Cooking does not prevent marine seafood poisoning because the toxins are heat-stable. Scaleless fish should be regarded as potentially tetrodotoxic and very large fish, particularly Moray eels (**Fig. 9**) and parrotfish (Scaridae), are likely to be ciguatera-toxic. Scombroid poisoning is avoided by eating only fresh fish. Shellfish must not be eaten during dangerous seasons and red tides.

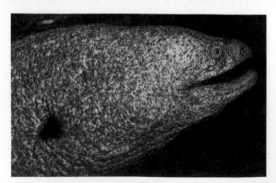

Fig. 9. Californian moray, *Gymnothorax mordax*, a potentially ciguatoxic fish. (Copyright © Prof D.A. Warrell.)

VENOMOUS MARINE INVERTEBRATES
Cnidarians (Coelenterates, Jellyfish, Portuguese-Men-o'-War, Stinging Corals, Sea Anemones, and so forth)

Cnidarian tentacles are studded with millions of stinging capsules (nematocysts) that are triggered by contact, shooting stinging hairs into the dermis and producing lines of painful, irritant weals.[13,15] Cnidarian venoms contain peptides and vasoactive amines, prostaglandins, and kinins.

Epidemiology
The notorious North Australian box jellyfish or sea wasp (*Chironex fleckeri*) and related cubomedusoids have caused some fatalities in the Australo-Indo-Pacific region. The Portuguese man-o'-war (*Physalia* spp) and the Chinese jellyfish *Stomolophus nomurai* have caused a few deaths. In northern Queensland, Florida, and the Caribbean, stings by tiny cubomedusoids such as Irukandji (*Carukia barnesi*) are sometimes fatal. Along the east coast of North America, *Chrysaora quinquecirrha* (**Fig. 10**) stings are common. In the Adriatic, there have been plagues of *Pelagia noctiluca* stings.

Prevention
Bathers must heed warning notices and keep out of the sea at times of the year when dangerous cnidarians are prevalent, or bathe in stinger-resistant enclosures. Wet suits, Lycra suits, and nylon stockings protect against nematocyst stings.

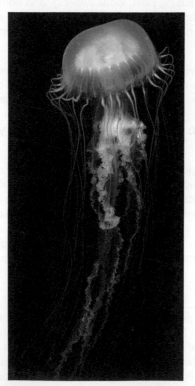

Fig. 10. Atlantic or East Coast sea nettle (*Chrysaora quinquecirrha*), a common cause of jellyfish stings along the East Coast of the United States. (Copyright © Prof D.A. Warrell.)

Clinical features

Patterns of skin weals may be diagnostic. Immediate severe pain is the commonest symptom. Chirodropids (genera *Chironex* and *Chiropsalmus*) can cause severe systemic symptoms: cough, gastrointestinal symptoms, rigors, myalgias, and profuse sweating culminating in pulmonary edema, generalized convulsions, and cardiorespiratory arrest within minutes of being stung. Irukandji syndrome consists of severe myalgia and arthralgia, anxiety, trembling, headache, piloerection, sweating, tachycardia, hypertension, and pulmonary edema starting about 30 minutes after the sting. Portuguese men-o'-war (*Physalia* species) can cause severe systemic envenoming, including intravascular hemolysis, vascular spasms leading to peripheral gangrene, and AKI.

Treatment

Victims must be rescued from the sea to prevent drowning. Commercial vinegar or 3% to 10% aqueous acetic acid solution inactivates nematocysts of *C fleckeri*, Irukandji, and other cubozoans. Adherent tentacles are shaved off the skin using a razor. Hot water treatment (see above) relieves the pain of box jellyfish and *Physalia* stings. A slurry of baking soda and water (50% w/v) is used for stings by Atlantic *Chrysaora* species. *C fleckeri* antivenom is manufactured in Australia, but its effectiveness has been questioned.

Echinodermata (Starfish and Sea Urchins)

Numerous long, sharp, projecting spines and grapples release venom when embedded in the skin, causing pain, local swelling, and sometimes systemic effects such as syncope, numbness, generalized paralysis, and cardiorespiratory arrest. Spines can penetrate bones and joints and can cause secondary infection.

Treatment

Hot water (see earlier) relieves pain. Spines should be removed after softening the skin, usually of the soles of the feet, with 2% salicylic acid ointment or acetone. No antivenoms are available. Infection by marine bacteria should be anticipated.

VENOMOUS ARTHROPODS (HYMENOPTERA: BEES, WASPS, YELLOWJACKETS, HORNETS, AND ANTS)

Allergic reactions to single hymenoptera stings are a common cause of anaphylaxis and occasional anaphylactic deaths in Western and tropical countries.[16] Bees (Apidae), wasps, yellowjackets and hornets (Vespidae), and ants (Formicidae) are responsible. Multiple stings are rare except during the recent epidemic of African killer bee attacks in the Americas, in which direct effects of massive doses of venom caused numerous fatalities. Hymenoptera venoms contain pain-producing amines, phospholipases, hyaluronidase, and polypeptide neurotoxins (apamin, melittin), which can act directly or as allergens.

Epidemiology

Each year, fewer than 5 people die from identified hymenoptera-sting anaphylaxis in England and Wales, 2 to 3 per year in Australia, and 40 to 50 per year in the United States. The prevalence of systemic allergic sting reactions is 4% in the United States. Most people who are allergic to bee venom are beekeepers or their relatives. In the United States, imported fire ants (*Solenopsis* sp) sting an estimated 2.5 million people each year, causing systemic allergic reactions in 4 per 100,000 population per year with some fatalities. In Tasmania and southern Australia, about 2% to 3% of the population are hypersensitive to jack-jumper ant (*Myrmecia pilosula*) stings, which can cause fatal anaphylaxis.

Prevention

People with a history of systemic anaphylaxis following a sting and evidence of hypersensitivity (venom-specific IgE detected by radioallergosorbent test [RAST] or skin test) should be considered for desensitization with purified venoms.[16] After 2 to 5 years of maintenance desensitization, more than 90% of subjects will remain protected against systemic reactions after stopping treatment. Desensitization is complicated by systemic reactions in 5% to 15% of patients and by local reactions in 50% of patients. Nests of aggressive hymenoptera (hornets, bees, ants) must be eradicated.

Clinical Features

Anaphylaxis

The familiar symptoms of anaphylaxis include tingling scalp, itching, flushing, dizziness, syncope, wheezing, abdominal colic (uterine colic in women), violent diarrhea, incontinence of urine and feces, tachycardia, and visual disturbances evolving rapidly within minutes of the sting. Urticaria, angioedema of the lips, gums, and tongue, a generalized redness of the skin with swelling, edema of the glottis, profound hypotension, and coma may develop. Deaths have occurred after only 2 minutes. Some people develop serum sickness a week or more after the sting. The risk of reactions is increased by β-blockers.

Diagnosis of Anaphylaxis and Venom Hypersensitivity

Raised plasma mast-cell tryptase concentrations (peak at 0.5–1.5 hours, lasting 6–8 hours) confirm the diagnosis of anaphylaxis. Type I hypersensitivity is confirmed by detecting venom-specific IgE in the serum using RAST, skin tests, or live sting challenge. Those who have suffered systemic anaphylaxis have a 50% to 60% risk of reacting to their next sting. There is no relationship between massive local reactions and the risk of systemic anaphylaxis. Children who have generalized urticaria after a sting have only a 10% chance of reacting when restung.

Treatment

Barbed bee stings must be removed immediately to prevent continuing envenoming. Vespids can sting repeatedly. Ice packs and aspirin are effective in relieving pain. Wasp stings may become infected because some species feed on rotting meat (**Fig. 11**).

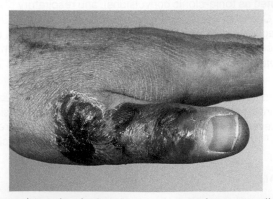

Fig. 11. Infected wasp (*Vespula* sp) sting. (Copyright © Prof D.A. Warrell.)

Massive local reactions may require histamine-H1 blockers, aspirin, nonsteroidal anti-inflammatory agents, and even corticosteroids.

Systemic anaphylaxis is treated with adrenaline/epinephrine (adults 0.5–1 mL, children 0.01 mg/kg of 0.1% [1:1000]) intramuscularly into the anterolateral thigh. Selective bronchodilators such as salbutamol are helpful if there is bronchoconstriction. A histamine-H1 blocker such as chlorphenamine maleate (adults 10 mg, children 0.2 mg/kg) can be given. Corticosteroids prevent relapses. Known hypersensitive individuals should wear an identifying tag and be trained to self-administer adrenaline using an EpiPen or similar apparatus.

SCORPIONS (SCORPIONES: BUTHIDAE, HEMISCORPIIDAE)
Epidemiology

In Arizona, 15,000 stings (mainly *Centruroides exilicauda*) are reported each year but there have been no deaths since 1968. In Mexico, deaths from *Centruroides* sp stings have decreased to 50 each year among an estimated 250,000 stings. In Brazil, there were 50 deaths among 36,000 stings by *Tityus* sp in 2005. In Tunisia there are about 40,000 stings per year, 1000 hospital admissions, and 100 deaths from *Androctonus*, *Buthus*, and *Leiurus* sp stings. In Iran, dangerous species include *Hemiscorpius lepturus*, *Androctonus* and *Buthus* sp. In Maharashtra, India, many people are stung by the red scorpion (*Hottentota tamulus*), with fatalities in both adults and children.

Prevention

Scorpions can be excluded from houses by incorporating a row of ceramic tiles into the base of the outside wall, making the doorsteps at least 20 cm high, and using residual insecticides indoors.

Clinical Features

Most stings are intensely painful. Systemic symptoms usually develop rapidly. Scorpion venoms release endogenous acetylcholine and catecholamines, producing initial cholinergic and later adrenergic symptoms. Early symptoms include vomiting, profuse sweating, piloerection, alternating bradycardia and tachycardia, abdominal colic, diarrhea, loss of sphincter control, and priapism. Later, severe life-threatening cardiorespiratory effects may appear: hypertension, shock, tachyarrhythmia and bradyarrhythmia, ECG evidence of cardiac involvement, and pulmonary edema. Neurotoxic effects such as erratic eye movements, fasciculation and muscle spasms (easily misinterpreted as tonic-clonic convulsions), and respiratory distress are seen in children stung by *Centruroides (sculpturatus) exilicauda* in Arizona. Other features are ptosis and dysphagia (*Parabuthus transvaalicus*), thrombotic strokes (*Nebo hierichonticus*), acute pancreatitis (*Tityus trinitatis*), and local necrosis, hemolysis. and AKI (*Hemiscorpius lepturus*).

Treatment

Pain responds to infiltration of local anesthetic and systemic analgesics. Antivenom is manufactured in several countries. Its effectiveness is supported by recent trials in Arizona and India.[17,18] Vasodilators such as prazosin are useful as ancillary treatment.

SPIDERS (ARANEAE)

Most spiders are venomous but few species have proved dangerous to humans.

Epidemiology

Spider bites are common in some parts of the world, but there are now few fatalities. In Brazil 19,634 bites were reported (10/100,000 population) in 2005, with only 9 deaths (0.05%). In Central and Southern America, *Loxosceles* sp are widely distributed and cause many bites. In the south and south-central United States, the brown recluse spider, *Loxosceles reclusa*, caused at least 6 deaths in the United States during the last century. Most bites occur in bedrooms while people are asleep or dressing. Black and brown widow spiders are cosmopolitan in distribution. *Loxosceles hasselti* causes up to 340 bites each year in Australia. Fatalities have been reported in Australia and the United States (*Loxosceles mactans*). Banana spiders (*Phoneutria* sp) cause bites in Latin American countries and are imported into temperate countries in bunches of bananas, causing a few bites and deaths. The highly dangerous Sydney funnel-web spider (*Atrax robustus*) and its congeners are restricted to southeastern Australia and Tasmania.

Clinical Features

Necrotic araneism

Only *Loxosceles* sp have proved capable of causing necrotic arachnidism or araneism. Bites are usually painless and unnoticed, but a burning sensation develops over several hours at the site of the bite, with swelling and development of a characteristic macular lesion, the red-white-and-blue sign, showing areas of red vasodilatation, white vasoconstriction, and blue prenecrotic cyanosis (**Fig. 12**). A blackened eschar develops, which sloughs in a few weeks, leaving a necrotic ulcer. Sometimes an entire limb or area of the face is involved. About 10% of cases have systemic symptoms

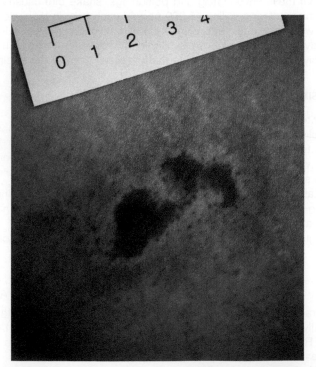

Fig. 12. Red-white-and-blue sign appearing 12 hours after a bite by a recluse spider (*Loxosceles gaucho*) in Brazil. (Copyright © Prof D.A. Warrell.)

such as fever, headaches, scarlatiniform rash, jaundice, hemoglobinemia, and hemoglobinuria resulting from intravascular hemolysis. AKI may ensue. The average case fatality is about 5%.

Neurotoxic araneism

Bites by *Latrodectus, Phoneutria*, and *Atrax* spp are immediately painful but local signs are minimal. After about 30 minutes, a pathognomonic sign, local sweating with piloerection ("gooseflesh"), appears at the bite site. There is painful regional lymphadenopathy, headache, nausea, vomiting, profuse generalized sweating, fever, tachycardia, hypertension, restlessness, irritability, psychosis, priapism, rhabdomyolysis, diffuse rash, painful muscle spasms, tremors, and rigidity involving the face and jaws (producing trismus) and abdominal muscles (simulating acute abdomen).

Treatment

Pressure immobilization (see earlier) is the recommended first-aid for funnel-web spider bites (*A robustus* and *Hadronyche* sp). Antivenoms are available for envenoming by *Latrodectus* sp, *Atrax* sp, and *Phoneutria* sp. The effectiveness of *Loxosceles* antivenoms is uncertain.[19]

SUMMARY

This article discusses the epidemiology, prevention, clinical features, first aid and medical treatment of venomous bites by snakes, lizards, and spiders; stings by fish, jellyfish, echinoderms, and insects; and poisoning by fish and molluscs, in all parts of the world. Of these envenoming and poisonings, snake bite causes the greatest burden of human suffering, killing 46,000 people each year in India alone and more than 100,000 worldwide and resulting in physical handicap in many survivors. Specific antidotes (antivenoms/antivenins) are available to treat envenoming by many of these taxa but supply and distribution is inadequate in many tropical developing countries.

USEFUL WEBSITES

http://www.toxinology.com/
http://globalcrisis.info/latestantivenom.htm
http://www.toxinfo.org/antivenoms/
http://www.who.int/bloodproducts/snake_antivenoms/en/
http://www.searo.who.int/EN/Section10/Section17.htm
http://www.afro.who.int/en/clusters-a-programmes/hss/essential-medicines/highlights/2358-whoafro-issues-guidelines-for-the-prevention-and-clinical-management-of-snakebite-in-africa.html
http://vapa.junidas.de/cgi-bin/WebObjects/vapaGuide.woa/wa/getContent?type=page&id=1

REFERENCES

1. Mohapatra B, Warrell DA, Suraweera W, et al. Snakebite mortality in India: a nationally representative mortality survey. PLoS Negl Trop Dis 2011;5(4):e1018.
2. Rahman R, Faiz MA, Selim S, et al. Annual incidence of snake bite in rural Bangladesh. PLoS Negl Trop Dis 2010;4(10):e860.
3. Warrell DA. Commissioned article: management of exotic snakebites. QJM 2009; 102(9):593–601.

4. Chappuis F, Sharma SK, Jha N, et al. Protection against snake bites by sleeping under a bed net in southeastern Nepal. Am J Trop Med Hyg 2007;77:197–9.
5. Sano-Martins IS, Fan HW, Castro SC, et al. Reliability of the simple 20 minute whole blood clotting test (WBCT20) as an indicator of low plasma fibrinogen concentration in patients envenomed by Bothrops snakes. Butantan Institute Antivenom Study Group. Toxicon 1994;32(9):1045–50.
6. Meggs WJ, Courtney C, O'Rourke D, et al. Pilot studies of pressure-immobilization bandages for rattlesnake envenomations. Clin Toxicol (Phila) 2010;48(1):61–3.
7. Tun-Pe, Aye-Aye-Myint, Khin-Aye-Han, et al. Local compression pads as a first-aid measure for victims of bites by Russell's viper (*Daboia russelii siamensis*) in Myanmar. Trans R Soc Trop Med Hyg 1995;89:293–5.
8. Saul ME, Thomas PA, Dosen PJ, et al. A pharmacological approach to first aid treatment for snakebite. Nat Med 2011;17(7):809–11.
9. de Silva HA, Pathmeswaran A, Ranasinha CD, et al. Low-dose adrenaline, promethazine, and hydrocortisone in the prevention of acute adverse reactions to antivenom following snakebite: a randomised, double-blind, placebo-controlled trial. PLoS Med 2011;8(5):e1000435.
10. Watt G, Theakston RD, Hayes CG, et al. Positive response to edrophonium in patients With neurotoxic envenoming by cobras (*Naja naja philippinensis*). A placebo-controlled study. N Engl J Med 1986;315(23):1444–8.
11. Chu ER, Weinstein SA, White J, et al. Venom ophthalmia caused by venoms of spitting elapid and other snakes: report of ten cases with review of epidemiology, clinical features, pathophysiology and management. Toxicon 2010;56:259–72.
12. Beck DD. Biology of Gila monster and beaded lizards. Berkeley (CA): University of California Press; 2005.
13. Bergbauer M, Myers RF, Kirschner M. Dangerous marine animals. London: Black; 2009.
14. Lewis RM, Poli J. Toxins in seafood. Toxicon 2010;56:107–258.
15. Williamson JA, Fenner PJ, Burnett JW, et al, editors. Venomous and poisonous marine animals: a medical and biological handbook. Sydney (New South Wales): University of New South Wales Press; 1996.
16. Müller UR. Insect venoms. Chem Immunol Allergy 2010;95:141–56.
17. Boyer LV, Theodorou AA, Berg RA, et al. Antivenom for critically ill children with neurotoxicity from scorpion stings. N Engl J Med 2009;360:2090–8.
18. Bawaskar HS, Bawaskar PH. Efficacy and safety of scorpion antivenom plus prazosin compared with prazosin alone for venomous scorpion (*Mesobuthus tamulus*) sting: randomised open label clinical trial. BMJ 2011;342:c7136.
19. Pauli I, Puka J, Gubert IC, et al. The efficacy of antivenom in loxoscelism treatment. Toxicon 2006;48:123–37.

Transplant-Associated and Blood Transfusion-Associated Tropical and Parasitic Infections

Clarisse Martins Machado, MD[a,b,*], José Eduardo Levi, PhD[a]

KEYWORDS

- Transplantation • Blood transfusion • Tropical diseases • Parasites • Transmission
- Donors

KEY POINTS

- Laboratorial and epidemiological screening is fundamental in assuring safe blood and organs for transfusion and transplantation.
- Due to the intense movement of people, animals and vegetables, tropical diseases are no longer restricted to the tropics.
- Knowledge of the life cycle of infectious agents and vectors are instrumental in promoting surveillance.
- Advanced molecular biology methods and fast communication are human weapons to prevent and fight emerging and re-emerging diseases that may threaten the blood and organ supply.

Most of the developing countries are located in tropical or subtropical regions, which have epidemiologic characteristics different from those of developed countries with temperate climates. These countries are characterized by the occurrence of endemic infections and diseases that are absent or rare in developed countries and may not be prepared to diagnose or manage them. Tourism, international commerce, and immigration are important factors for the emergence and reemergence of specific infectious diseases. Migrant populations may naturally become part of blood bank donor, transplant donor, or transplant recipient populations in destination countries and may represent an unintentional threat to blood or transplant recipients.[1] In this increasingly globalized world, the transmission of infectious diseases has no boundaries. Consequently, the interest in blood- and donor-derived disease transmission is growing globally.

The authors have nothing to disclose.
[a] Virology Laboratory, Institute of Tropical Medicine, University of São Paulo, Av. Dr Enéas de Carvalho Aguiar 470, 05403-000 São Paulo, Brazil; [b] Hematopoietic Stem Cell Transplantation Program, Amaral Carvalho Foundation, Rua Dona Silvéria 150, 17210-080 Jaú, São Paulo, Brazil
* Virology Laboratory, Institute of Tropical Medicine, University of São Paulo, Av. Dr Enéas de Carvalho Aguiar 470, 05403-000 São Paulo, Brazil.
E-mail address: clarimm@usp.br

Infect Dis Clin N Am 26 (2012) 225–241
doi:10.1016/j.idc.2012.02.008
0891-5520/12/$ – see front matter © 2012 Elsevier Inc. All rights reserved.

id.theclinics.com

Blood transfusion is an efficient mechanism to spread infectious agents in naive populations; thus several measures are taken worldwide to ensure the safety of the blood supply. However, physicians are constantly surprised by cases of transfusional transmission (TT) of new and reemergent agents. Recent waves of immigration from the South to the North took several asymptomatic carriers of tropical agents, potentially blood donors, to countries where tropical diseases are recognized exclusively in returning travelers. Cases of TT parasites, such as Trypanosoma cruzi (Chagas disease) and Plasmodium sp (malaria), in Europe and North America provoked changes in the policies for blood donor screening in these countries (discussed later). In parallel, technologies that may inactivate pathogens (pathogen reduction technologies [PRT]) by targeting nucleic acids in a nonspecific mode are in a late stage of development and in regular use for plasma and platelet units in some countries.

There are several differences among countries on the agents that require mandatory testing and the allowed assays. In limited-resource regions, testing by thick smear or antigenic rapid test is restricted to antibodies to human immunodeficiency virus (HIV), hepatitis B surface antigen (HBsAg), and malaria parasitemia. This portfolio is adopted in many African countries. Syphilis and hepatitis C virus (HCV) come next in the order of importance. Enzyme immunoassays (EIAs) for anti-Treponema pallidum antibodies are mostly used, and, possibly, the discard rate for reactive donations may be high. No case of TT syphilis has been reported in the last 15 years, even when less sensitive assays were routinely used. Donors are also screened for antibodies to human T-lymphotropic virus 1/2 (HTLV-1/2) in many countries, mainly countries in which the prevalence is significant, such as the United States, Brazil, and Japan. HCV should get the same status as HIV because it has a high prevalence among donors, and it may be an extremely harmful infection. However, anti-HCV screening is not universally performed so far. Other agents of restricted geographic occurrence are screened only locally, such as the West Nile virus (WNV) in the United States and Canada and the Q-fever agent in the Netherlands. Cytomegalovirus (CMV) antibody–negative blood is given to newborns and immunocompromised patients. Bacterial contamination is controlled in some countries, differing on the principle mentioned earlier, because testing is performed in blood products after processing, as most contamination is environmental and occurs during processing and storage. Platelets present the highest concern because they are stored at room temperature and under shaking, conditions that may foster growth of many bacterial species. Laboratory methods include automated hemoculture and other disposable rapid tests that are to be performed just before platelet release.

In the beginning of this millennium, automated nucleic acid testing (NAT) became available, and it was possible to be incorporated into the blood screening scheme. The aim of NAT introduction was to reduce the so-called window period that precedes the development of detectable antibodies in the recently infected host. HCV NAT and HIV NAT became mandatory in most developed countries, but hepatitis B virus (HBV) NAT was introduced later, and, up to 2011, this NAT was not as widespread as the NATs for HCV and HIV.

An international network for biovigilance of organ recipients would be desirable in the transplantation setting. Although national systems are already available in some countries, in many others the systems are still under development. The higher rate of incident infection transmitted by organ donors compared with that transmitted by blood donors emphasizes the need for such networks.[2] At present, the following screening tests are generally required for organ, tissue, and hematopoietic stem cell donors: anti–HIV-1/2, HIV NAT, syphilis (by either a treponemal or nontreponemal test), anti–HTLV-1/2, anti–CMV, anti–Epstein-Barr virus, anti–hepatitis B core (anti-HBc), HBsAg, anti-HCV, and HCV NAT.[3]

This article describes the epidemiologic characteristics of tropical and parasitic diseases that can be transmitted by blood and/or transplantation. **Table 1** shows the tropical and parasitic diseases with widespread transmission, epidemic activity, or high risk for infection according to the region. The diseases associated with blood and/or transplant transmission are highlighted in bold.

BACTERIAL INFECTIONS
Tuberculosis

Epidemiology
Tuberculosis (TB) is a major cause of illness and death worldwide, especially in Asia and Africa. According to the World Health Organization, in 2009, there were an estimated 9.4 million incident cases (range, 8.9 million–9.9 million) of TB globally, equivalent to 137 cases per 100,000 population. Most of the estimated number of cases occurred in Asia (55%) and Africa (30%), with smaller proportions of cases occurring in the Eastern Mediterranean region (7%), the European region (4%), and the region of the Americas (3%). India alone accounts for 21% of all TB cases worldwide, and China and India together account for 35%.[4]

The HIV pandemic has contributed to these numbers because 1.0 to 1.2 million (11%–13%) cases of TB were reported in HIV-positive people. Because the rate of cure in new cases of smear-positive TB is lower among HIV-positive patients (<40%) than among HIV-negative patients (>60%), transmission is facilitated in places where HIV infection

Table 1
Distribution of tropical and parasitic diseases according to the region

Region	Viruses	Bacteria	Parasites
Mexico, Central America	**Dengue**, hepatitis A	Leptospirosis, typhoid, and paratyphoid fever	**Leishmaniasis**
Latin America	**Dengue, yellow fever, rabies**, hepatitis A, **hepatitis B**, measles, hantavirus, other viral hemorrhagic fevers	**Tuberculosis**, leprosy, leptospirosis, plague	**Leishmaniasis, malaria, schistosomiasis, trypanosomiasis**
North Africa	Hepatitis A, **rabies**	Plague, **tuberculosis**, typhoid, and paratyphoid fever	**Leishmaniasis**
Sub-Saharan Africa	**Dengue, rabies**, hepatitis A, **hepatitis B**, yellow fever, poliomyelitis, other viral hemorrhagic fevers	Diphtheria, plague, **tuberculosis**, leprosy	**Leishmaniasis, schistosomiasis, malaria, trypanosomiasis**
Southeast Asia	**Dengue**, hepatitis A, **hepatitis B**	Leptospirosis, plague, **tuberculosis**	**Filariasis, malaria, schistosomiasis**
South Asia	**Filariasis**, hepatitis A, **rabies, hepatitis B**	Leptospirosis, plague, **tuberculosis**	**Filariasis, leishmaniasis, malaria**
East Asia	Hantavirus, hepatitis A, **hepatitis B**	Leptospirosis, plague, **tuberculosis**	—
Northern Asia	Hantavirus, hepatitis A, **hepatitis B, rabies**	Diphtheria, **tuberculosis**	—
Middle East	Hepatitis A, **hepatitis B**	**Tuberculosis**	**Leishmaniasis**

Blood- and/or transplant-transmitted infections are in bold.

is highly prevalent.[1,4] Of these HIV-positive TB cases, approximately 80% were in the African region.[4] Other immunocompromised hosts, including solid organ transplant (SOT) and hematopoietic stem cell transplant (HSCT) recipients, are also more prone to reactivation of latent *Mycobacterium tuberculosis* infection (LTBI).[5]

Transmission in transplant recipients

TB among transplant recipients may arise from reactivation of the quiescent foci of *M tuberculosis*, transmission by the graft, or contamination by actively infected persons. The risk of TB in transplant recipients is estimated to be 20 to 50 times higher than in the general population, even in developed countries,[6,7] and mortality rates vary from 20% to 40%.[8] Most reports of TB are in SOT recipients, especially after renal transplantation. The prevalence of LTBI among renal transplant recipients in North America is 0.5% to 1%, in Northern Europe is 1% to 4%, and in India and Pakistan can reach 15%.[9] In Brazil, TB is number one among the neglected tropical diseases after transplantation, with an incidence of around 1% in HSCT recipients and 2% in SOT recipients.[10,11]

Reactivation of LTBI accounts for most TB cases reported in transplant recipients and largely reflects the local incidence.[1] Graft transmission has been documented in renal, lung, and hepatic transplantation but accounts for less than 5% of all TB cases in transplant recipients. In one international study, 4% of TB infections in recipients were considered donor derived.[8] Recently, a case of donor-derived TB that resulted in the infection of 2 of the 3 transplant recipients (with 1 death) has raised the discussion regarding the need for donor TB screening with new blood tests (interferon gamma release assays [IGRAs]) to diagnose LTBI.[12]

Screening and prevention

Pretransplant evaluation of the epidemiologic risk of TB should be made for donors and recipients in countries where TB is highly prevalent. However, in the evaluation of donor eligibility, no standard assessment is conducted to determine if the potential donor is at risk of having previously undiagnosed TB or LTBI. In addition to selected laboratory testing (mentioned at the beginning of the article), the donor's medical record is reviewed for specific conditions (including known active TB), a social history is obtained with a close relative (or another person familiar with the donor), and chest radiography is performed. Although the screening process might reveal symptoms or risk factors for TB or LTBI, no further investigation or diagnostic testing is required.

LTBI can also be evaluated through the tuberculin skin test (TST), a delayed-type hypersensitivity reaction to an intracutaneous injection of antigens isolated from culture filtrate by protein precipitation. For living donors, the TST result should be interpreted as positive or negative according to the Centers for Disease Control and Prevention (CDC) guidelines for the general population.[13] However, the specificity of the TST is impaired in donors from developing countries because the delayed-type hypersensitivity reaction may indicate infection with nontuberculous mycobacteria or previous vaccination with the BCG vaccine, a live attenuated mycobacterial strain derived from *Mycobacterium bovis*. IGRAs are more specific alternatives and should be interpreted according to manufacturer instructions. If LTBI is confirmed, then active TB should be ruled out. Treatment of LTBI should be considered before organ donation, especially for recent seroconverters. Organs from potential donors, whether living or deceased, with active TB disease should not be used.[14]

Brucellosis

Epidemiology

Brucellosis is a common zoonotic disease caused by *Brucella* spp, which mainly infect cattle, swine, goats, sheep, and dogs. It can be transmitted to people via direct contact with livestock or through drinking unpasteurized milk from an infected animal. In humans, *Brucella* causes a wide range of clinical manifestations involving various body systems. The main symptom is recurrent bouts of high temperature. Therefore, it is frequently misdiagnosed as drug-resistant malaria in tropical countries.

Transmission in transplant recipients
Few cases of brucellosis have been reported after renal transplantation and as a donor-derived infection during HSCT, in endemic regions.[15] Fever, anemia, and pancytopenia are often observed and may mimic several other diseases in the immunocompromised patient. In general, the diagnosis is made by the detection of *Brucella* species in blood cultures, after extensive investigation of other causes. Consequently, complications may develop in case of delay in the diagnosis or administration of appropriate antimicrobial treatment. Fluoroquinolones, doxycycline, and streptomycin are successful therapeutic options. More recently, tigecycline was demonstrated to be safe and effective in the control of brucellosis after liver transplantation.[16]

PROTOZOAN INFECTIONS
Malaria

Epidemiology
Malaria is an acute systemic illness caused by infection with *Plasmodium falciparum*, *Plasmodium vivax*, *Plasmodium malariae*, or *Plasmodium ovale*. About 3.3 billion people, half of the world's population, are at risk of malaria. In 2010, there were an estimated 216 million episodes of malaria and nearly 655,000 deaths due to malaria, mostly among children living in Africa. People living in the poorest countries are the most vulnerable. In Africa, every 45 seconds a child dies of malaria; the disease accounts for 20% of all childhood deaths.[17]

Endemic malaria cases have been reported in Central and South America, sub-Saharan Africa, India, Southeast Asia, and part of Oceania. Awareness of *Plasmodium* species endemicity is important for early introduction of appropriate treatment. *P falciparum* is found in sub-Saharan Africa, Southeast Asia, and the Indian subcontinent as well as in South America, Haiti, the Dominican Republic, Jamaica, and areas of Oceania. *P malariae* and *P ovale* are present in sub-Saharan Africa. *P vivax* is prevalent in areas of Southeast Asia, the Indian subcontinent, and Central and South America.[18]

Malaria may be transmitted through infected blood products, by natural exposure to *Plasmodium*-infected mosquitoes in endemic regions, or via an infected organ or tissue.

Transmission through blood products
In contrast to the large number of cases of malaria transmitted through *Plasmodium*-infected mosquitoes worldwide, transmission by blood transfusion has scarcely been reported, and the majority comes from nonendemic countries. A recently published international forum report informs that only 5 TT cases were reported in the last 10 years: 2 in Italy, 2 in Brazil, and 1 in the United States.[19] This may be partially explained by the difficulty in distinguishing transmission by transfusion from vector-borne cases in endemic countries.[20] Another aspect is that malaria may be more harmful for naive patients than exposed semi-immune patients who are recipients of blood and organs in nonendemic and endemic regions, respectively.

Transmission in transplant recipients
Although not an opportunistic disease, malaria is relevant in the transplant setting because more patients either with a history of malaria or residing in an endemic malaria region are undergoing transplantation, more residents from endemic regions are being

considered as donors, and more recipients are being exposed to malaria after transplant. The washing of organ blood during the transplantation procedure may not be enough to eliminate possibly parasitized red cells within the organ, and transmission may occur. In transfusion-associated malaria, symptoms generally develop earlier (1–3 days) than if the infection is transmitted through infected cells within the organ (>1 week).[18] Plasmodium species are capable of surviving for more than 24 hours in blood at 4°C. Therefore, the cold preservation time is generally not enough to prevent transmission, especially in heart and liver transplantations, which require shorter cold preservation time (3–4 hours for heart, <12 hours for liver) than kidney transplantation (24–48 hours). The reports of malaria cases after multiorgan donation have supported the hypothesis of the graft as a source of Plasmodium in transplant recipients.[21–23]

Screening and prevention

Investigation of the epidemiologic risk for malaria is mandatory for blood and transplant donors and recipients in endemic regions. If possible, routine serologic and blood smear tests should be considered for all individuals with exposure risk. In developing countries, a past history of malaria is not a contraindication for organ or stem cell donation.

Clinicians must be aware that malaria does not always follow the typical paroxysmal or cyclic pattern in transplant recipients, and a high index of suspicion should be maintained when caring for patients with identifiable risk factors. If donors or recipients have a history of mosquito exposure in regions of P vivax or P ovale infection, clinicians should bear in mind that the parasites' exoerythrocytic schizogony in the liver makes eradication more difficult. These dormant hypnozoite forms can cause relapse up to 12 months later.

Guidelines from developed countries recommend that donors from nonendemic areas who have traveled to an area where malaria transmission occurs should be deferred from donating for 12 months after their return. Similarly, persons who have lived or are living in malaria areas should be deferred for 3 years. If these deferral times are not possible to maintain, the donor should receive empirical treatment of malaria before donation. Blood smear and immunochromatogenic tests and polymerase chain reactions (PCRs) are all inappropriate tests for evaluating asymptomatic potential donors.[24]

Chagas Disease (American Trypanosomiasis)

Epidemiology

Chagas disease is caused by T cruzi, a protozoan parasite first described by Carlos Chagas in 1909. Chagas disease is endemic in the Americas, from the south of the United States to the south of Latin America. As a consequence of the initiatives of the South and Central American countries since 1991 in the control of Chagas transmission, the disease prevalence has been reduced from the 1990 estimates of 16 to 18 million people infected to 9 to 12 million people in 2004.[25] The parasite is generally transmitted through the feces of infected triatomine insects by penetration of the parasite into the bite wound, conjunctiva, or other mucous membranes.[26] Transmission can also occur by organ transplantation, blood transfusion, from mother to child during pregnancy, and laboratory incident. More recently, some outbreaks due to the ingestion of contaminated food or drink have been reported.[27–29]

Transmission through blood products

Blood transmission is considered as the second most important method of acquiring Chagas disease. With the exception of blood derivatives, all blood components are infective. Transmission by blood transfusion was first suggested by Mazza in

Argentina in 1936, and the first cases of transfusion-associated Chagas disease were published in 1952.[30] The true number of reported cases is also underestimated because no more than 350 cases have been published.[31] In nonendemic countries, cases of transfusion-associated transmission can go undetected because acute infections are often asymptomatic and the level of awareness of Chagas disease among clinicians is low.[28] In endemic countries where mandatory screening tests have been implemented since 1991, the residual risk of infection is calculated to be around 1:200,000 units.[32]

Transmission in transplant recipients

Transplant recipients from nonendemic countries are more likely to acquire *T cruzi* infection through blood transfusion or by an infected graft, whereas infected recipients from endemic regions are at risk for reactivation of latent infection during immunosuppression. More than 7.5 million individuals are infected by *T cruzi* in endemic countries.[33]

The first strong evidence of transmission via graft was reported in Brazil in 1983. Four renal transplant recipients developed Chagas disease; all 4 had received graft from infected donors in the chronic phase of *T cruzi* infection.[34] Other series have been published, mostly from Argentina and Brazil.[35,36] In the United States, 3 cases of *T cruzi* transmission via graft were reported to the CDC in 2001. Three SOT recipients, 1 liver and 2 kidney, who received organs from the same donor developed Chagas disease.[26] In 2006, two other cases were reported in heart transplant recipients. In both cases, investigation of the source of infection showed that the blood donors tested seronegative for *T cruzi*, whereas the organ donors tested seropositive.[37]

Screening and prevention

Serologic screening of donors is routine in highly prevalent countries, and 2 positive results in different serologic tests are necessary to consider a patient infected. Hemagglutination assays, which were used as the screening method in the past, are being replaced by EIAs, which are now the standard for donor screening.

Donor/recipient pretransplant investigation of the epidemiologic risk for Chagas disease is mandatory. Risk factors for *T cruzi* infection are being part of the native population from endemic areas (continental countries of Latin America), having received blood transfusion in endemic countries, being born to mothers who are natives of endemic areas with unknown serology for Chagas disease, or having lived in an endemic area for more than a month.[33] EIAs for *T cruzi* are recommended in the case of a positive test result.[38] Donors who died of acute Chagas disease should be excluded. In the case of cardiac transplantation, the heart from a patient with chronic Chagas disease is contraindicated because of the risk of chagasic myocarditis. Similarly, the use of intestines from a donor with Chagas disease is contraindicated.[33]

In Latin America, donors chronically infected by *T cruzi* are not excluded from donation of other organs, except the heart and intestines. However, a close follow-up with serologic and parasitologic methods is strongly recommended, and immediate treatment with benznidazole for 30 to 60 days or nifurtimox for 90 to 120 days should be started if parasitemia is detected. Pretransplant treatment of infected living donors with benznidazole may be considered.[33] Based on the experience in South America, the Chagas in Transplant Working Group from the United States considered that kidneys and livers from *T cruzi*–infected donors can be transplanted with informed consent from recipients and followed up by close monitoring.[38] Surveillance includes pretransplant parasitologic studies (quantitative PCR, Strout method, direct parasitologic tests) weekly up to day 60, bimonthly between days 60 and 180, and annually thereafter.[33]

The recommendation for prophylaxis is controversial both in cardiac and other transplant recipients.[33,39] Prophylactic treatment to prevent disease reactivation should be considered in patients with chagasic cardiomyopathy who undergo cardiac transplantation from a healthy donor. In other transplant recipients, early treatment should be started if monitoring shows evidence of reactivation.

Leishmaniasis

Epidemiology
Leishmaniasis is primarily a zoonotic infection, which includes animal reservoir hosts in the transmission cycle. Anthroponotic forms of leishmaniasis have been increasingly observed as humans enter the transmission cycle of the parasite and get infected. In anthroponotic forms, man is the sole source of infection for the vector.[11] The protozoan is transmitted to humans through the bite of an infected female mosquito from the genus *Phlebotomus* (in the Old World) or *Lutzomyia* (in the New World). However, incidental transmission through blood transfusions or needle sharing among intravenous drug addicts has also been described.[40]

Leishmaniasis is prevalent in 4 continents and considered endemic in 88 countries, of which 72 are developing countries: 90% of all visceral leishmaniasis (VL) cases occur in Bangladesh, Brazil, India, Nepal, and Sudan; 90% of mucocutaneous leishmaniasis cases occur in Bolivia, Brazil, and Peru; and 90% of cutaneous leishmaniasis cases occur in Afghanistan, Brazil, Iran, Peru, Saudi Arabia, and Syria.[41] An estimated 12 million people worldwide are presently infected, with 1 to 2 million estimated new cases occurring every year.

Transmission through blood products
TT of VL with clinical features and outcomes similar to those of the natural infection has been described in endemic and nonendemic areas.[42] In a recent study, *Leishmania* DNA was found in up to 36% of asymptomatic blood donors who tested positive for anti-*Leishmania* antibodies, and, therefore, a theoretical risk of TT VL is present.[43]

Transmission in transplant recipients
More than 100 cases of leishmaniasis have been described in transplant recipients. VL is the most frequently observed clinical presentation. Most cases occurred in SOT recipients, mainly kidney and liver, with few cases reported in HSCT recipients.[11] The geographic distribution of leishmaniasis cases among transplant recipients reflects the endemic areas of human leishmaniasis disease and the number of transplantations performed. More than two-thirds of the reported cases are from Spain, Italy, and France.[44]

In transplant recipients, leishmaniasis may occur due to reactivation of latent infection in a previously infected recipient or due to de novo infection in transplant recipients living in or traveling to areas of endemicity, by blood transfusion, or via an infected graft.[45] This route of transmission is rare and more likely to occur in organs that form part of the reticuloendothelial system, such as the liver.

Screening and prevention
At present, routine serologic screening of organ donors from endemic countries is not recommended. If a donor is known to be positive for leishmaniasis, monitoring of the recipient in the posttransplant period is advised. In suspected cases, serologic tests and direct detection of *Leishmania* amastigotes in bone marrow biopsy samples should be performed. Fluorescent antibody technique or enzyme-linked immunosorbent assay should be used, with Western blot confirmation.[45]

VIRAL INFECTIONS
HIV Infection

Epidemiology

HIV is a zoonosis that originated from simian viruses and transmitted to man probably in the beginning of the twentieth century in Africa. Urbanization favored the adaptation of these viruses to the human host, with sexual transmission being the main route of spread. From Africa, HIV reached several countries, including the United States where the first AIDS case was described in the 1980s. It has been estimated that there are approximately 33 million persons infected worldwide, the majority in Africa. HIV-1 is responsible for more than 95% of the cases and is present in all countries.

Transmission through blood products

Transmission through blood transfusion became evident by the large number of infected individuals among persons exposed to blood products. In the United States, the risk decreased from 1:100 units before any test was available to 1:1,500,000 units after NAT was introduced.[46] Thousands of TT cases occurred worldwide, with incidence and AIDS-related mortality dramatically affecting patients demanding multiple transfusions or constant use of plasma products, such as those with hemophilia. Fear of TT HIV infection and the enormous impact on the society were the driving forces that led to the current level of safety, achieved by many technological developments and massive investments in the blood industry.

Transmission in transplant recipients

The first report of HIV infection transmitted by organ transplantation was in 1989.[47] Other cases were extensively documented, forcing donor testing to be mandatory in most countries.[3] Since laboratory screening for HIV infection became available in 1985, only 1 case of HIV transmission through organ transplantation was documented in the United States, emphasizing the success of the initiative.

Screening and prevention

The fourth-generation antibody tests, which are able to detect both anti-HIV antibodies and the presence of the p24 capsid antigen in a conjugated format, provide a high degree of safety to organs available for transplantation. However, they require obtaining plasma or serum from donors, which may not be possible from cadaveric donors. Because a single organ donor may infect several recipients, all guidelines strongly recommend using organs exclusively from negative donors. NAT also contributes to reducing the window period and increasing protection for the transplant recipient. After the introduction of NAT, the risk of TT of HBV, HCV, and HIV in the United States was 1:600, 1:1149, and 1:1467, respectively.[48] Nevertheless, the additional yield obtained by NAT over a fourth EIA is minimal and becomes significant only in regions where HIV prevalence and incidence are high, such as in South Africa.[49]

However, the risk of transmission through organ transplantation must be balanced against the risk of recipients dying while waiting for an organ. Due to organ shortage and because organ transplantation is often lifesaving, organs from donors with elevated risk of HIV infection may be accepted (with informed consent from the recipient) whenever the benefit of transplantation is considered to outweigh the risk of potential disease transmission.[50] Recipients of organs from increased-risk donors are recommended to undergo testing 1, 3, and 12 months after transplantation.[51]

Hepatitis B

Epidemiology

HBV is a small DNA virus, with efficient transmission by blood and sexual contact. It is prevalent globally, with an estimated 370 million carriers. Infection in adults is relatively harmless, in that 95% of the exposed population clear it without any symptoms. When it becomes chronic, infection may lead to liver inflammation, cirrhosis, and hepatocellular carcinoma. A vaccine that was developed and introduced in the 1990s led to a reduction in the prevalence of infection among vaccinees, which is observed nowadays as these vacinees are becoming young adults and being sexually exposed. However, liver failure caused by HBV is still an important indication for transplantation.

Transmission through blood products

Before the introduction of HBsAg testing for blood donors, TT HBV was observed in approximately 6% of patients with multiple transfusions. Improvement of this test and further introduction of the anti-HBc test significantly decreased this rate. However, HBV is still the most frequently transmitted viral infection, and several cases of transmission continue to be reported in countries of low and high endemicity,[52] and it may have an aggressive course in immunocompromised hosts.[53]

Transmission in transplant recipients

HBV transmission was reported from the transplantation of not only organs such as the kidney and liver but also the cornea and bone marrow. Because the presence of HBV is an important indication for liver transplants, in certain circumstances it is difficult to distinguish a new infection on the liver graft from a reactivation of the recipient's previous infection. Without any prophylaxis, in almost all cases, HBV-infected recipients present recurrence after transplantation. The availability of high-titer anti–hepatitis B surface immunoglobulins and oral antiviral drugs, such as lamivudine, greatly reduced the incidence of HBV-related posttransplantation morbidities.

Screening and prevention

Anti-HBc is a marker of exposure, whereas HBsAg is a marker of virus replication, precluding donation of blood and organs by donors reactive for the latter. Due to organ scarcity, it is acceptable to transplant organs when both the donor and the recipient are reactive for anti-HBc, and, in some centers, HbsAg-positive organs are transplanted into recipients with anti-HBsAg titers that are considered to be protective, that is, more than 100 IU/L. However, this situation is associated with a worse prognosis and frequent reactivation of HBV, leading to graft loss. In endemic countries, such as Italy, Greece, China, and Taiwan, blood donors are screened by the HBsAg test because the prevalence of a high anti-HBc titer would considerably affect the pool of available donors. Other countries such as the United States, Germany, and Brazil use both HBV markers for screening. More recently, NAT was extended to HBV-DNA and incorporated in a multiplex format to HCV and HIV NAT platforms. NAT not only identifies donors on the HBV window period but also interdicts donations regarded as having occult B infection (OBI), thus deeming individuals negative for HBsAg but harboring HBV-DNA as potentially infectious. OBI is common in areas where HBV is endemic and is responsible for the few transfusional cases verified before the introduction of NAT. The current risk of TT HBV in the United States, where 3 parallel tests are performed (NAT, anti-HBc, and HBsAg), is estimated as greater than 1:500,000. Whenever possible, NAT of organ donors should be accomplished because this group usually presents a higher risk for infectious markers.[54]

Hepatitis C

Epidemiology

HCV is an RNA virus belonging to the Flaviviridae family. It is transmitted by contact with blood, and, in contrast to other members of the Flaviviridae family, HCV transmission to humans by arthropod vectors was never reported. HCV was first cloned from the plasma of individuals experiencing posttransfusion hepatitis not associated with hepatits A viruses (HAVs) or HBVs. After HCV was cloned and characterized in 1989, a laboratorial tool for identification of infected patients was rapidly developed and used in epidemiologic studies and for screening blood and organ donors.[55]

It is estimated that approximately 2% of the world population are carriers of HCV.[56] A population-based survey has shown that the true prevalence is 1.42% in the United States. Egypt has the highest prevalence (15%–20%), and this has been attributed to massive spread of this virus during campaigns for the treatment of schistosomiasis along the Nile River from 1961 to 1986.[57]

Transmission through blood products

HCV was identified in the search for a cause of hepatitis that is frequently observed in transfusion recipients in whom HBV and HAV infections were ruled out by laboratory tests. Before anti-HCV tests were made available in 1990, the so-called non-A non-B hepatitis had an incidence greater than 10% in patients with multiple transfusions. Nowadays, the risk is about 1 in 1,000,000 transfused units when NAT and antibody testing are performed.[58]

Transmission in transplant recipients

To date, HCV is the main cause for the failure of kidney transplantation, and the use of organs from HCV-positive donors is acceptable and common, mainly for kidney recipients whose anti-HCV test result is also positive. However, HCV and HIV cotransmissions have also been observed in HCV-negative recipients, presumably by a donor in the window period.[50] Although the use of NAT could have prevented such cases, its use is not recommended because it may cause delay in transplantation and increase organ shortage, which strongly contrasts the policies on blood transfusion.

Screening and prevention

Detection of antibodies to several HCV antigens in the EIA format is the test of choice for screening blood and organ donors. At present, these EIAs are in their fourth generation, which, similar to the anti-HIV assay, allows the simultaneous detection of both antibodies and HCV core antigen. A difficulty associated with excluding donors at risk for HCV infection by predonation interviewing is that up to 50% of the infected donors do not report any obvious source of transmission (eg, use of intravenous drug, previous transfusion, needle sharing), and hence prevention of TT HCV infection largely relies on laboratory testing. Because of the longer time to seroconversion, approximately 90 days, HCV was the first agent to be targeted by NAT. The yield of NAT-only donors worldwide is about 1:250,000 donations, with important regional variations.[59]

Arbovirus

Epidemiology

Arboviruses are a heterogeneous group of agents transmitted to humans by arthropods, most significantly mosquitoes and ticks. By feeding on human blood, several species of female mosquitoes transmit the pathogens present in their digestive system to the individual from whom blood is sucked. *Aedes aegypti* and *Aedes albopictus* have adapted to living close to humans by reproducing in water accumulated near human habitats. Being spread worldwide, dengue is the most important human-arthropod–borne viral disease. Autochthonous cases have been described from the United States (Florida) to Argentina, and there is no vaccine available. At present, the incidence has been estimated at more than 50 million cases globally and is rising every year, mainly in the Americas.

There are 4 dengue serotypes. Infection by one serotype provides lifelong immunity against that serotype but only partial and transient protection against subsequent infection by the other 3 serotypes. There is compelling evidence that secondary and tertiary dengue infections tend to be more severe than primary dengue infection. After being bitten by an infected mosquito, symptoms develop in approximately 7 to 10 days, lasting for a maximum of 15 days.

Transmission through blood products

The contrast between the huge number of cases of dengue fever in endemic countries and the rare reports of transfusion-transmitted dengue is astonishing. Only 3 well-documented episodes of dengue virus transmission by blood transfusion, and only 1 of them resulting in clinically evident disease (dengue hemorrhagic fever) in the recipient, have been reported so far,[60] much less than what would be expected from the prevalence projected from blood donors, although transient asymptomatic dengue viremia is a potential risk to the blood supply. In a recent publication, dengue viremia was detected in 0.04% and 0.30% of asymptomatic blood donors from Brazil and Honduras, respectively.[61] Because recipients are not systematically investigated, the detection of transfusion/organ transmission occurs only when they present with overt symptoms. Further studies are needed to establish the rates of TT by viremic donations and the clinical consequences in recipients.

Transmission in transplant recipients

The transmission of dengue in transplant recipients living or traveling to endemic areas is, by far, via a mosquito bite. In most of the published cases, dengue was acquired by vector transmission.[11] Dengue transmission via graft has also been reported in HSCT and renal transplant recipients.[62–64] The disease has certainly been underdiagnosed in transplant populations from endemic areas because most of the cases are mild and present as a flulike syndrome. Consequently, the actual incidence, morbidity, and mortality associated with dengue and its complications are difficult to estimate.

Screening and prevention

Patients who had dengue are eligible for blood and organ donation after recovery, when development of IgM and IgG indicates virus clearance. The risk of transmission by blood and organ donation stems from asymptomatic hosts and the short incubation period preceding viremia/fever. It has been observed that for each case of dengue fever, there are 2 other asymptomatic infected cases. Not unexpectedly, dengue RNA has been detected among blood donors in endemic areas.[64] So far there are no screening tests validated for blood and organ donation. Testing strategies, in analogy to the WNV, belonging to the Flaviviridae family, include NATs or antigenic assays with high sensitivity.

Rabies

Epidemiology

Rabies is a zoonotic viral disease, which infects domestic and wild animals. It is distributed worldwide, but few countries are free of rabies: Japan, New Zealand, Sweden, Norway, Greece, Portugal, Barbados, Fiji, Seychelles, Maldives, Uruguay, and Chile. Rabies is most prevalent in developing countries and is certainly underreported.

Several countries that are considered endemic for canine rabies (among them India and Pakistan) do not include rabies among notifiable diseases, and hence the actual incidence is unknown.

Dog bites are the most frequent mode of transmission in most countries in Africa, Asia, Latin America, and the Middle East. In contrast, in North America, most documented human rabies deaths occurred as a result of infection from the bat rabies virus.[65] The contact of infected saliva with scratches, licks on broken skin, and mucous membranes may also cause rabies.[66] Human-to-human transmission occurs almost exclusively as a result of organ or tissue transplantation.

The rabies virus causes acute viral encephalomyelitis, which is virtually 100% fatal. The virus may remain latent near the inoculation site, then replicate in muscle or dermal cells (in the case of some bat variants).[67] Around 55,000 rabies deaths occur annually and are generally associated with dog bites. Bat rabies variants may cause clinical manifestations different from what is seen in humans infected with canine rabies.

Rabies in transplant recipients
Human-to-human transmission of rabies has occurred in 16 organ and tissue transplant recipients (8 corneas, 7 solid organs, 1 vascular tissue). The 16 cases occurred in 6 countries: 5 in the United States, 4 in Germany, 2 in Thailand, 2 in India, 2 in Iran, and 1 in France.[67,68] In all cases, the donors died of an illness compatible with rabies, even though the diagnosis was only suspected when the recipients died of rabies.[68] These cases illustrate how easily the diagnosis of rabies may be missed if a clear investigation of rabies exposure is not done. In the SOT cases, the donors had a recent history of bat and dog bites, which were not elicited or considered important. Because bat teeth are very fine, bat bites and bat-inflicted scratch marks may be undetectable and the epidemiologic risk underestimated. In the United States and Canada, the incidence of bat-variant rabies cases increased from 2.2 cases per billion person-years from 1950 to 1989 to 6.7 cases per billion person-years from 1990 to 2007.[65]

Screening and prevention
A detailed history of contact with bats should be obtained from the organ donors' relatives and friends. In the absence of a clear history, physical signs, and reliably performed rabies diagnostic tests, the safest strategy is to exclude any donor with neurologic signs and symptoms of unknown cause. In the case of exposure (suspected history or rabies diagnosed postmortem in the donor), postexposure prophylaxis with human rabies immunoglobulin should be immediately started (20 IU/kg), as well as the first dose of rabies vaccine. Additional doses should then be administered on days 3, 7, 14, and 28 after the first dose. The vaccination should always be administered intramuscularly in the deltoid area (adults) or in the anterolateral aspect of the thigh (children).[68]

SUMMARY

In the previous century, the discovery and successful introduction of penicillin and further development of antibiotic therapy led the medical community to predict that infectious diseases would decline as a leading cause of death worldwide, giving place to cancer and circulatory illnesses. Surprisingly, in 2012, infectious diseases, mainly malaria, continue to kill thousands and affect millions around the world. Chaotic urbanization, waste accumulation, global warming, tourism, and human migrations have all contributed to the dissemination of infectious agents and associated vectors. Autochthonous dengue cases in the United States and France and the chikungunya outbreak in Italy illustrate this new scenario of the diseases that were previously named tropical.

As long as reliance on humans as donors of blood and tissues for transplantation continues, issues with transmissible agents and the fact that several agents are no more restricted to the tropics have to be dealt with. Technological advances in molecular diagnostics and vaccine production provide tools for active surveillance and quick response, as seen recently for severe acute respiratory syndrome and influenza H1N1 threats when appropriate measures avoided potential pandemics of these lethal agents. Permanent research and active communication is the effective answer, and the authors hope to give a small contribution with this article.

REFERENCES

1. Machado CM. Transplant infections in developing countries. In: Bowden RA, Ljungman P, Snydman DR, editors. Transplant infections. 3rd edition. Philadelphia: Lippincott Williams and Wilkins; 2010. p. 90–103.
2. Zou S, Dodd RY, Stramer SL, et al. Probability of viremia with HBV, HCV, HIV, and HTLV among tissue donors in the United States. N Engl J Med 2004;351(8): 751–9.
3. Morris MI, Fischer SA, Ison MG. Infections transmitted by transplantation. Infect Dis Clin North Am 2010;24(2):497–514.
4. World Health Organization. Global tuberculosis control. Geneva: World Health Organization; 2011. Available at: http://www.who.int/tb/publications/global_report/en/index.html. Accessed February 29, 2012.
5. Rose DN. Benefits of screening for latent Mycobacterium tuberculosis infection. Arch Intern Med 2000;160(10):1513–21.
6. Aguado JM, Herrero JA, Gavalda J, et al. Clinical presentation and outcome of tuberculosis in kidney, liver, and heart transplant recipients in Spain. Spanish Transplantation Infection Study Group, GESITRA. Transplantation 1997;63(9): 1278–86.
7. Munoz P, Rodriguez C, Bouza E. Mycobacterium tuberculosis infection in recipients of solid organ transplants. Clin Infect Dis 2005;40(4):581–7.
8. Singh N, Paterson DL. Mycobacterium tuberculosis infection in solid-organ transplant recipients: impact and implications for management. Clin Infect Dis 1998; 27(5):1266–77.
9. Koseoglu F, Emiroglu R, Karakayali H, et al. Prevalence of mycobacterial infection in solid organ transplant recipients. Transplant Proc 2001;33(1–2):1782–4.
10. Batista MV, Pierrotti LC, Abdala E, et al. Endemic and opportunistic infections in Brazilian solid organ transplant recipients. Trop Med Int Health 2011;16(9): 1134–42.
11. Machado CM, Martins TC, Colturato I, et al. Epidemiology of neglected tropical diseases in transplant recipients. Review of the literature and experience of a Brazilian HSCT center. Rev Inst Med Trop Sao Paulo 2009;51(6):309–24.
12. Centers for Disease Control and Prevention (CDC). Transplantation-transmitted tuberculosis—Oklahoma and Texas, 2007. MMWR Morb Mortal Wkly Rep 2008; 57(13):333–6.
13. Targeted tuberculin testing and treatment of latent tuberculosis infection: this official statement of the American Thoracic Society was adopted by the ATS Board of Directors, July 1999. This is a joint statement of the American Thoracic Society (ATS) and the Centers for Disease Control and Prevention (CDC). This statement was endorsed by the Council of the Infectious Diseases Society of America

(IDSA), September 1999, and the sections of this statement as it relates to infants and children were endorsed by the American Academy of Pediatrics (AAP), August 1999. Am J Respir Crit Care Med 2000;161(4 Pt 2):S221–47.

14. Subramanian A, Dorman S. Mycobacterium tuberculosis in solid organ transplant recipients. Am J Transplant 2009;9(Suppl 4):S57–62.

15. Kotton CN. Zoonoses in solid-organ and hematopoietic stem cell transplant recipients. Clin Infect Dis 2007;44(6):857–66.

16. Al-Anazi KA, Jafar SA, Al-Jasser AM, et al. Brucella bacteremia in a recipient of an allogeneic hematopoietic stem cell transplant: a case report. Cases J 2009;2(1):91.

17. Aregawi M, Cibulskis R, Lynch M, et al. World Malaria Report 2011. Available at: http://www.who.int/malaria/world_malaria_report_2011/9789241564403_eng.pdf. Accessed April 3, 2012.

18. Martin-Davila P, Fortun J, Lopez-Velez R, et al. Transmission of tropical and geographically restricted infections during solid-organ transplantation. Clin Microbiol Rev 2008;21(1):60–96.

19. Reesink HW, Panzer S, Wendel S, et al. The use of malaria antibody tests in the prevention of transfusion-transmitted malaria. Vox Sang 2010;98(3 Pt 2): 468–78.

20. Owusu-Ofori AK, Parry C, Bates I. Transfusion-transmitted malaria in countries where malaria is endemic: a review of the literature from sub-Saharan Africa. Clin Infect Dis 2010;51(10):1192–8.

21. Chiche L, Lesage A, Duhamel C, et al. Posttransplant malaria: first case of transmission of Plasmodium falciparum from a white multiorgan donor to four recipients. Transplantation 2003;75(1):166–8.

22. Fischer L, Sterneck M, Claus M, et al. Transmission of malaria tertiana by multiorgan donation. Clin Transplant 1999;13(6):491–5.

23. Menichetti F, Bindi ML, Tascini C, et al. Fever, mental impairment, acute anemia, and renal failure in patient undergoing orthotopic liver transplantation: posttransplantation malaria. Liver Transpl 2006;12(4):674–6.

24. Tomblyn M, Chiller T, Einsele H, et al. Guidelines for preventing infectious complications among hematopoietic cell transplantation recipients: a global perspective. Biol Blood Marrow Transplant 2009;15(10):1143–238.

25. Schofield CJ, Jannin J, Salvatella R. The future of Chagas disease control. Trends Parasitol 2006;22(12):583–8.

26. Bern C, Montgomery SP, Herwaldt BL, et al. Evaluation and treatment of chagas disease in the United States: a systematic review. JAMA 2007;298(18):2171–81.

27. Centers for Disease Control and Prevention (CDC). Chagas disease after organ transplantation—Los Angeles, California, 2006. MMWR Morb Mortal Wkly Rep 2006;55(29):798–800.

28. Centers for Disease Control and Prevention (CDC). Blood donor screening for chagas disease—United States, 2006–2007. MMWR Morb Mortal Wkly Rep 2007;56(7): 141–3.

29. Dias JP, Bastos C, Araujo E, et al. Acute Chagas disease outbreak associated with oral transmission. Rev Soc Bras Med Trop 2008;41(3):296–300.

30. Freitas JLP, Amato V, Sonntag R, et al. Primeiras verificacoes de transmissao acidental da molestia de Chagas ao homem por transfusao de sangue. Rev Paul Med 1952;40:36–40 [in Portuguese].

31. Wendel S. Transfusion transmitted Chagas disease: is it really under control? Acta Trop 2010;115(1–2):28–34.

32. Schmunis GA, Cruz JR. Safety of the blood supply in Latin America. Clin Microbiol Rev 2005;18(1):12–29.

33. Pinazo MJ, Miranda B, Rodriguez-Villar C, et al. Recommendations for management of Chagas disease in organ and hematopoietic tissue transplantation programs in nonendemic areas. Transplant Rev (Orlando) 2011;25(3):91–101.
34. Chocair PR, Sabbaga E, Amato Neto V, et al. Kidney transplantation: a new way of transmitting chagas disease. Rev Inst Med Trop Sao Paulo 1981;23(6):280–2 [in Portuguese].
35. Bacal F, Silva CP, Pires PV, et al. Transplantation for Chagas' disease: an overview of immunosuppression and reactivation in the last two decades. Clin Transplant 2010;24(2):E29–34.
36. D'Albuquerque LA, Gonzalez AM, Filho HL, et al. Liver transplantation from deceased donors serologically positive for Chagas disease. Am J Transplant 2007;7(3):680–4.
37. From the Centers for Disease Control and Prevention. Chagas disease after organ transplantation—United States, 2001. JAMA 2002;287(14):1795–6.
38. Chin-Hong PV, Schwartz BS, Bern C, et al. Screening and treatment of chagas disease in organ transplant recipients in the United States: recommendations from the chagas in transplant working group. Am J Transplant 2011;11(4):672–80.
39. Bocchi EA, Fiorelli A. The paradox of survival results after heart transplantation for cardiomyopathy caused by Trypanosoma cruzi. First Guidelines Group for Heart Transplantation of the Brazilian Society of Cardiology. Ann Thorac Surg 2001; 71(6):1833–8.
40. Cruz I, Morales MA, Noguer I, et al. Leishmania in discarded syringes from intravenous drug users. Lancet 2002;359(9312):1124–5.
41. WHO Expert Committee on the Control of Leishmaniases. Control of the Leishmaniases - WHO Technical Series (949). Geneva: World Health Organization; 2010. Available at: http://new.paho.org/hq/index.php?option=com_docman&task=doc_view&gid=16971&Itemid=. Accessed February 29, 2012.
42. Dey A, Singh S. Transfusion transmitted leishmaniasis: a case report and review of literature. Indian J Med Microbiol 2006;24(3):165–70.
43. Scarlata F, Vitale F, Saporito L, et al. Asymptomatic Leishmania infantum/chagasi infection in blood donors of western Sicily. Trans R Soc Trop Med Hyg 2008; 102(4):394–6.
44. Antinori S, Cascio A, Parravicini C, et al. Leishmaniasis among organ transplant recipients. Lancet Infect Dis 2008;8(3):191–9.
45. Basset D, Faraut F, Marty P, et al. Visceral leishmaniasis in organ transplant recipients: 11 new cases and a review of the literature. Microbes Infect 2005;7(13): 1370–5.
46. Zou S, Stramer SL, Dodd RY. Donor testing and risk: current prevalence, incidence, and residual risk of transfusion-transmissible agents in US allogeneic donations. Transfus Med Rev 2011;26(2):119–28.
47. Quarto M, Germinario C, Fontana A, et al. HIV transmission through kidney transplantation from a living related donor. N Engl J Med 1989;320(26):1754.
48. Stramer SL, Wend U, Candotti D, et al. Nucleic acid testing to detect HBV infection in blood donors. N Engl J Med 2011;364(3):236–47.
49. Vermeulen M, Lelie N, Sykes W, et al. Impact of individual-donation nucleic acid testing on risk of human immunodeficiency virus, hepatitis B virus, and hepatitis C virus transmission by blood transfusion in South Africa. Transfusion 2009;49(6): 1115–25.
50. Ison MG, Llata E, Conover CS, et al. Transmission of human immunodeficiency virus and hepatitis C virus from an organ donor to four transplant recipients. Am J Transplant 2011;11(6):1218–25.

51. Humar A, Morris M, Blumberg E, et al. Nucleic acid testing (NAT) of organ donors: is the 'best' test the right test? A consensus conference report. Am J Transplant 2010;10(4):889–99.
52. Candotti D, Allain JP. Transfusion-transmitted hepatitis B virus infection. J Hepatol 2009;51(4):798–809.
53. Gerlich WH, Wagner FF, Chudy M, et al. HBsAg non-reactive HBV infection in blood donors: transmission and pathogenicity. J Med Virol 2011;79:S32–6.
54. Pruss A, Caspari G, Kruger DH, et al. Tissue donation and virus safety: more nucleic acid amplification testing is needed. Transpl Infect Dis 2010;12(5):375–86.
55. Choo QL, Kuo G, Weiner AJ, et al. Isolation of a cDNA clone derived from a blood-borne non-A, non-B viral hepatitis genome. Science 1989;244:359–62.
56. Negro F, Alberti A. The global health burden of hepatitis C virus infection. Liver Int 2011;31(Suppl 2):1–3.
57. Frank C, Mohamed MK, Strickland GT, et al. The role of parenteral antischistosomal therapy in the spread of hepatitis C virus in Egypt. Lancet 2000;355(9207): 887–91.
58. Alter HJ, Klein HG. The hazards of blood transfusion in historical perspective. Blood 2008;112(7):2617–26.
59. Roth WK, Busch MP, Schuller A, et al. International survey on NAT testing of blood donations: expanding implementation and yield from 1999 to 2009. Vox Sang 2012;102(1):82–90.
60. Levi JE. Arboviruses and transfusion transmitted infectious diseases. ISBT Sci Ser 2011;6(1):116–8.
61. Linnen JM, Vinelli E, Sabino EC, et al. Dengue viremia in blood donors from Honduras, Brazil, and Australia. Transfusion 2008;48(7):1355–62.
62. Rigau-Perez JG, Vorndam AV, Clark GG. The dengue and dengue hemorrhagic fever epidemic in Puerto Rico, 1994–1995. Am J Trop Med Hyg 2001;64(1–2): 67–74.
63. Tan FL, Loh DL, Prabhakaran K, et al. Dengue haemorrhagic fever after living donor renal transplantation. Nephrol Dial Transplant 2005;20(2):447–8.
64. Wiwanitkit V. Unusual mode of transmission of dengue. J Infect Dev Ctries 2010; 4(1):51–4.
65. De SG, Dallaire F, Cote M, et al. Bat rabies in the United States and Canada from 1950 through 2007: human cases with and without bat contact. Clin Infect Dis 2008;46(9):1329–37.
66. Rupprecht CE, Hanlon CA, Hemachudha T. Rabies re-examined. Lancet Infect Dis 2002;2(6):327–43.
67. Bronnert J, Wilde H, Tepsumethanon V, et al. Organ transplantations and rabies transmission. J Travel Med 2007;14(3):177–80.
68. Manning SE, Rupprecht CE, Fishbein D, et al. Human rabies prevention—United States, 2008: recommendations of the Advisory Committee on Immunization Practices. MMWR Recomm Rep 2008;57(RR-3):1–28.

Malaria: An Update for Physicians

Behzad Nadjm, MB ChB, MD, DTM&H*,
Ron H. Behrens, MB ChB, MD, FRCP

KEYWORDS

- Malaria • *Plasmodium* • Travel • Antimalarials

KEY POINTS

- Malaria continues to be the most important human protozoal infection worldwide, directly causing over 2000 deaths every day and causing increased susceptibility to bacterial infection.
- Artemisins, taken orally in combination with other antimalarials in non-severe malaria and administered intravenously for severe malaria have become the gold standard treatment for P falciparum malaria.
- The priorities in the management of imported malaria are in prevention, early recognition and early treatment.
- The priorities in management of falciparum malaria globally are prevention of the development of full artemisinin resistance and ensuring that appropriate treatments are available to all who need them.

INTRODUCTION AND HISTORICAL PERSPECTIVE

Malaria is caused by infection with protozoan parasites of the *Plasmodium* genus, transmitted to humans by female anopheline mosquitoes. Plasmodia have adapted to a wide variety of vertebrate hosts ranging from reptiles to mammals, although with 1 notable exception, human malaria is not a zoonosis. Infections likely to represent malaria have been described since mankind began to record its experiences. The earliest accurate description of human malaria in European literature has been attributed to Celsus (25 BC TO AD 54), who described tertian and quartan periodicity of fevers in his treatise *De Medicina*. Five species are now recognized as agents of human malaria (**Table 1**), although most infections are caused by 2: *Plasmodium falciparum* and *Plasmodium vivax*. Worldwide, there are estimated to be several hundred million infections with malaria every year and the historical burden of infection has helped to shape the human genome through evolutionary pressure on genes involved in erythrocyte metabolism and structure.[1] Malaria continues to kill more than 2000 people every

BN has no conflicts of interest to declare. RHB received funds from Sigma-Tau for contributing to their advisory board.
Department of Clinical Research, London School of Hygiene & Tropical Medicine, Keppel Street, London WC1E 7HT, UK
* Corresponding author.
E-mail address: behzad.nadjm@lshtm.ac.uk

Infect Dis Clin N Am 26 (2012) 243–259
doi:10.1016/j.idc.2012.03.010
0891-5520/12/$ – see front matter © 2012 Elsevier Inc. All rights reserved.

Table 1
The human malaria species

Species	Distribution	Clinical/Pathologic Details
Plasmodium falciparum	Widespread in tropics	Causes the most fatalities Pronounced rosetting and sequestration
Plasmodium vivax	Widespread in tropics and subtropics except West Africa	Relapses caused by hepatic hypnozoites Requires RBC Duffy antigen for entry into cells
Plasmodium ovale	Patchy in West Africa and southwest Pacific	Relapses caused by hepatic hypnozoites
Plasmodium malariae	Patchy, worldwide	Late recrudescence and chronic infections Nephrotic syndrome (rarely)
Plasmodium knowlesi	Malaysia, Indonesia and other southeast Asia	Zoonosis (macaque monkeys primary hosts) Severe disease

Abbreviation: RBC, red blood cell.

day,[2] with strong evidence emerging that it is also indirectly responsible for more than half of all cases of invasive bacterial disease in high-transmission settings.[3]

Malaria was once widespread, with ongoing transmission in the southern United States and the Mediterranean rim within the last 100 years. The Centers for Disease Control and Prevention (CDC) is located in Atlanta, Georgia, because of the high prevalence of malaria in the Mississippi basin at the time of its inception. However, by 1951, malaria was eliminated from the United States and the Global Malaria Eradication Campaign, initiated in 1955 by the Global Health Assembly, succeeded in eliminating transmission from several other countries, although not in sub-Saharan Africa or south Asia.[4]

EPIDEMIOLOGY

The current distribution of malaria covers the tropics and large parts of the subtropics (**Fig. 1**). World Health Organization (WHO) estimates of malaria deaths worldwide

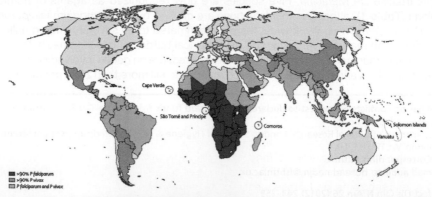

Fig. 1. Worldwide distribution of malaria. (*From* Feachem RG, Phillips AA, Hwang J, et al. Shrinking the malaria map: progress and prospects. Lancet 2010;376(9752):1570; with permission.)

decreased from 1 million in 2000 to more than 700,000 in 2009, with an estimated 756 million people at risk of the disease.[2] In line with these WHO data, largely derived from data supplied by National Malaria Control Programs, a summary of recent peer-reviewed publications also points to substantial reductions in malaria cases in many countries in sub-Saharan Africa, although there are difficulties in attributing this to control measures.[5] However, there remain arguments about the accuracy of such estimates, with a recent retrospective study into malaria deaths in India suggesting that the WHO estimate for the years studied was an underestimate by a factor of 10.[6]

In the United States, the number of imported cases of malaria reported remained static between 2005 and 2009 (the last year with data available) at around 1500 cases. In 2009, of infections in which a species was identified, 74% were P falciparum and 18% P vivax, which represents a decline in the proportion of cases diagnosed with P vivax and a corresponding increase in those diagnosed with P falciparum since 2007.[7] In the United Kingdom, there were 1762 cases reported in 2010, with 70% of cases caused by P falciparum.[8] A similar reduction in the proportion of imported malaria cases caused by P vivax occurred in the United Kingdom between 1987 and 2006.[9]

It is increasingly recognized that there is marked variation in malaria transmission within many high-transmission regions, with foci of high transmission and lower transmission in neighboring areas.[10–13] This variation has potential consequences for malaria control, local treatment protocols, and risk assessment for international travelers. The emergence of a new human plasmodia species, *Plasmodium knowlesi*, as a zoonosis and significant cause of infection in parts of southeast Asia has attracted significant attention.[14,15] There may be further discoveries of zoonotic malaria as molecular techniques become more widespread.

PATHOGENESIS

The primary route of infection for all plasmodia infections is through the bite of a female anopheline mosquito. Less common routes of infection include blood transfusion of parasitized erythrocytes and congenital transmission. Following the bite of an infected mosquito, plasmodia sporozoites enter the subcutaneous tissue of the skin and migrate to local capillaries and lymphatics before passing to the liver, where they invade hepatocytes and develop into merozoites via a process of asexual reproduction known as hepatic schizogeny. After a period of at least 7 days, and often longer, infected hepatocytes release tens of thousands of merozoites that each invade an erythrocyte. Having invaded an erythrocyte, each merozoite either undergoes a further round of asexual reproduction (erythrocytic schizogeny) or develops into the sexual form of the malaria parasite (male and female gametocytes) (**Fig. 2**). Symptoms occur with the release of parasite toxins following the development of the blood stage of disease and are associated with asexual parasitemia.[16] Gametocytes are not thought to cause symptoms, but are taken up by mosquitoes and involved in the sexual reproductive cycle within the mosquito gut.

Relapsing Malaria: P vivax and Plasmodium ovale

Unlike other human plasmodia, P vivax and *Plasmodium ovale* infections are characterized by relapses related to hepatic hypnozoites. A proportion of hepatocytes, infected by sporozoites from a mosquito bite, develop into dormant hypnozoites rather than into actively dividing schizonts.[16] Later development of these hypnozoites into hepatic schizonts, and subsequent rupture, with the release of merozoites into the bloodstream, account for the observed relapses. Multiple, frequent relapses are characteristic of infections acquired in the tropics, whereas infections acquired in

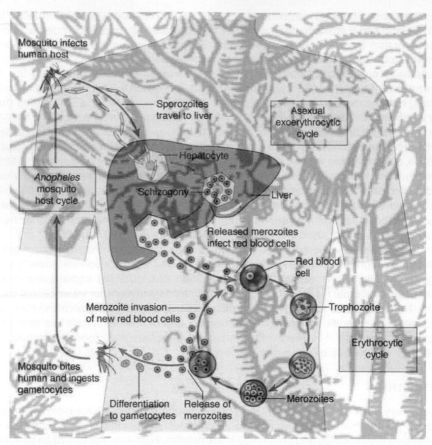

Fig. 2. The lifecycle of *Plasmodium falciparum* in the human body. (*From* Actor JA. Elsevier's Integrated Review: Immunology and Microbiology. 2nd edition. Philadelphia: Elsevier; 2012; with permission.)

temperate regions have less frequent relapses, often occurring some months after the initial infection. Despite attractive theories concerning adaptation to seasons or response to anopheline bites, the determinants of malaria relapse, like much of the biology of the hypnozoite, remain to a large degree a mystery and must be a priority for future research.[17,18] Although many theories have been espoused concerning the determinants of malaria relapse, a compelling explanation proposed recently is that febrile illness (notably *P falciparum* infection) activates latent hypnozoites.[19] Given the recent data suggesting that liver-stage infection in mice is suppressed by acute *Plasmodium* infection through the hormone hepcidin,[20] it may be that changes in hepcidin also play a role in hypnozoite activation.

Plasmodium malariae is not associated with relapse but can cause chronic, low-grade infections that persist for years, often at levels that are less than the limits of detection by light microscopy.[21]

Pathogenesis of Severe Malaria

The nature of the pathophysiologic changes that result in severe malaria have not been completely resolved. *P falciparum* is able to invade erythrocytes of all ages, a characteristic it shares with *P knowlesi*,[14] whereas *P vivax* and *P ovale* invade only young cells and *P malariae* older cells. This ability may contribute to the higher parasitemia seen in infections with *P falciparum* and *P knowlesi*, with the subsequent increase in virulence observed. Erythrocytes infected by midstage to late-stage *P falciparum* (trophozoites and schizonts) express the parasite-derived *P falciparum* erythrocyte membrane protein 1 (PfEMP1), which mediates both adherence to vascular endothelium (sequestration) and binding uninfected erythrocytes (rosetting).[16] Together with a reduction in the deformability of both infected and uninfected erythrocytes, rosetting and sequestration result in alterations in microvascular blood flow that are a key factor in development of severe falciparum disease.[22] Both rosetting and sequestration seem to occur at reduced magnitude in non-falciparum malaria,[23] and red cell deformability may be increased in erythrocytes infected with *P vivax*.[24] Although it is tempting to blame the pathogenesis of severe falciparum malaria entirely on microcirculatory disturbance, it is likely that multiple factors are involved, including dyserythropoiesis, erythrocyte hemolysis, and both local and systemic cytokine effects.[16]

CLINICAL FEATURES

In European and North America, more than 95% of malaria infections occur in travelers, often within the first month of return.[25] Delay in developing illness has been associated with the use of appropriate antimalarial prophylaxis, and clinicians seeing returning travelers should be aware of this possibility.[26] Presentation is nonspecific and may mimic other diseases including influenza, septicemia, gastroenteritis, and viral syndromes. A high index of suspicion is required, usually triggered by a travel history. Long delays and misdiagnosis in the management of malaria have been reported from studies in Europe[27] and North America,[28,29] highlighting the critical importance of a travel history in all patients presenting with fever or history of fever.

If a travel history is unavailable, factors that may suggest malaria include splenomegaly, fever without localizing signs, thrombocytopenia, hyperbilirubinemia and a normal peripheral blood leukocyte count.[30] A recordable fever may be absent on presentation in around one-third of patients. Because falciparum malaria can progress rapidly if untreated, it is recommended that family physicians refer all suspected cases of malaria to a facility that can provide a rapid diagnosis and instigate treatment without delay.

In highly endemic countries, where infection in childhood is common and repeated infection results in an immune tolerance of malaria parasitemia, differentiating malaria from bacterial disease can be difficult. In these settings, coinfection is common, often making treatment of both necessary.[31–33]

Severe Malaria

The WHO defines severe malaria by the presence of any 1 of several clinical or laboratory criteria in a patient with *P falciparum* asexual parasitemia and no other obvious cause (**Box 1**).[34] Even in trial conditions, the mortality among children with severe malaria in sub-Saharan Africa is between 10% and 15%, and in adults in Asia 15% to 20%,[35,36] whereas the mortality among adult admissions to intensive care in European centers has been reported as 8% to 10%.[37,38]

Severe non-falciparum malaria does occur, and in some specific locations in Asia it is increasingly being recognized as a major cause of severe malaria.[14,15,39] Among returning travelers to the United States in 2009, non-falciparum malaria accounted for 14% of cases presenting with signs of severe disease, although this figure was lower in European data.[7,40] Case fatality rates for non-falciparum malaria are much lower in all settings.

Box 1
Criteria for severe malaria (WHO 2010)

Clinical

Impaired consciousness or unrousable coma

Prostration (inability to walk/sit/feed)

Multiple convulsions

Respiratory distress/acidotic breathing

Circulatory shock

Jaundice with other vital organ dysfunction

Abnormal bleeding

Hemoglobinuria

Laboratory

Metabolic acidosis (plasma bicarbonate <15 mmol/L or lactate >5 mmol/L)

Hypoglycemia

Severe anemia (hemoglobin <5 g/dL or packed cell volume <15%)

Hemoglobinuria

Renal impairment (serum creatinine >265 μmol/L)

Hyperparasitemia (>2%)

DIAGNOSIS

Once malaria is suspected, it is usually straightforward to diagnose. Commonly used diagnostics include thick and thin Giemsa-stained blood smears and immuno-chromatographic rapid diagnostic tests (RDTs) of malaria antigens, both of which are in widespread use.[41,42] In expert centers, light microscopy can detect as few as 50 parasites/μL (approx 0.001%), increasing to around 500/μL in routine settings. Sensitivity for RDTs decreases with parasitemias less than 100/μL for *P falciparum*, with lower sensitivity for non-falciparum malaria.[43] RDTs have several drawbacks; they are unable to provide a quantification of parasitemia, they perform poorly with non-falciparum malaria, and tests based on the detection of histidine rich protein 2 (HRP2) may remain positive for several weeks after malaria has been treated.

Diagnosis needs to be prompt to enable immediate treatment of falciparum disease, which can progress rapidly if untreated.[44] Despite the ability to detect parasites at a lower density than either light microscopy or RDTs, PCR-based techniques are of little use in the routine diagnosis of malaria because, in most settings, operational issues result in an unacceptable delay in providing results. Polymerase chain reaction (PCR) may have a role as the second-line test of choice for difficult cases and situations in which low parasitemia infection is suspected (eg, suppression with antimalarial chemoprophylaxis, *P malariae* infection).[45] Attempts to develop a simple PCR-based assay for use in endemic areas are continuing.[46]

MANAGEMENT

The management of malaria depends on the species involved. If there is doubt or difficulty identifying the infecting species, management should be as for *P falciparum* infection while clarification as to the infecting organism is sought (a separate thick and thin blood slide should be sent to the local reference laboratory, ideally accompanied by ethylenediamine tetraacetic acid (EDTA) blood in case PCR is required). In all cases, management should be undertaken in conjunction with a physician experienced in dealing with malaria.

Drug therapy for malaria has been transformed by the introduction of artemisinin-containing combination therapies (ACTs). Although their mechanism of action remains uncertain, artemisinins act on almost all stages of the *Plasmodium* erythrocytic cycle, causing rapid falls in parasitemia. In addition, by killing the early ring forms, artemisinin derivatives are able to prevent the development of the more mature trophozoites and schizonts that sequester and cause severe disease.[47] Globally, the main challenges in the treatment of malaria are delivering these lifesaving drugs to the poor and vulnerable at greatest risk and ensuring that resistance is contained.[48]

Falciparum Malaria

P falciparum infection is categorized as severe or nonsevere (also known as complicated and uncomplicated) malaria. This categorization is based on the presence of at least 1 of the WHO severe malaria criteria (see **Box 1**). These criteria were developed and validated in studies largely of African children and Asian adults with positive slides for *P falciparum*. However, there have subsequently been several studies that have described the use of these criteria in the context of managing malaria in patients returning to a resource-rich setting from a visit to an endemic setting (imported malaria).[27,37,38,49–55]

Nonsevere Falciparum Malaria

Drug treatment

Recommendations on the treatment of nonsevere malaria vary from country to country. Both CDC and UK guidelines suggest that treatment should not be started until there has been a laboratory-confirmed diagnosis, except in exceptional circumstances.[44,56] Treatment should be started urgently once falciparum malaria has been diagnosed, with priority given to starting some form of treatment rather than the precise choice of treatment. A preferred, but not immediately available, treatment can always be substituted after a less ideal, but available, treatment has been begun.

The WHO recommends that ACTs are the first-line treatments for uncomplicated falciparum malaria. Five ACTs are recommended by the WHO (**Table 2**), the choice depending on local availability and, in some cases, resistance to the nonartemisinin component.[34] The CDC still recommends chloroquine for disease acquired in regions where falciparum is chloroquine sensitive. For disease acquired in areas of known chloroquine resistance or where resistance is unknown, CDC suggest a choice of atovaquone-proguanil (Malarone), artemether-lumefantrine (Coartem), or quinine plus doxycycline/tetracycline/clindamycin, with mefloquine only when the other options cannot be used.[56] UK guidelines recommend that chloroquine should no longer be used for the management of falciparum malaria and are similar to the CDC guidelines for the management of malaria from chloroquine-resistant areas.[44] Treatments for nonsevere falciparum malaria recommended by CDC and UK guidelines are shown in **Table 3**.

Admission to hospital of imported nonsevere falciparum malaria

CDC and UK guidelines suggest that all patients with falciparum malaria should be admitted to monitor response to treatment and observe for progression of disease severity.[44,56] The basis of these recommendations is the significant mortality among young, previously fit patients and the observation that patients can rapidly deteriorate despite initially presenting with less severe disease.[57] There has been increasing interest in the question of whether a subgroup of patients can be treated as outpatients

Table 2
ACTs recommended by WHO

Drug	Area Malaria Acquired			Comments
	Africa	East Asia	Other	
Artemether/lumefantrine	+	+	+	Should be taken after a meal containing fat to aid absorption
Artesunate/amodiaquine	+/−	−	+	Resistance to amodiaquine component reported, limiting use in East Africa
Artesunate/mefloquine	+	+	+	Increased dysphoria, sleep disturbance, nausea, and vomiting reported in trials. Widely used in southeast Asia for resistant *P falciparum*
Artesunate/sulfadoxine-pyrimethamine	+/−	−	+	Resistance to sulfadoxine-pyrimethamine component reported, limiting use in East Africa
Dihydroartemisinin/piperaquine	+	+	+	Widely used in southeast Asia for resistant *P falciparum*

for nonsevere falciparum malaria. Several case series have been cited in defense of this policy.[50,51,55,58] Together, these series describe 400 adults treated as outpatients and claim to show no adverse outcomes, although a small proportion (13/400, 3.25%) of patients required admission after therapy had been started. These series were in

Table 3
Drugs recommended by UK and CDC guidelines for the treatment of nonsevere falciparum malaria

Drug	Dose (60 kg Adult)	Comments
Artemether-lumefantrine	4 tablets at 0, 8, 24, 36, 48, and 60 h	WHO first-line treatment in adults, children, and pregnancy after the first trimester. Should be taken after fatty meal
Atovaquone-proguanil (Malarone)	4 tablets once a day for 3 d	May cause diarrhea and vomiting
Quinine	600 mg every 8 h for 5–7 d With Doxycycline 200 mg once a day for 7 d Or Clindamycin 450 mg 3 times a day for 7 d	Often causes reversible tinnitus and deafness. Itch in dark-skinned patients. Not in children or pregnancy. May cause gastritis. Choice in pregnancy and children <12 y
Chloroquine	600 mg base followed by 300 mg at 6, 24, 48 h	Not in UK guidelines. Only if acquired in chloroquine-sensitive region (CDC guideline)
Hydroxychloroquine	620 mg base followed by 310 mg at 6, 24, 48 h	Not in UK guidelines. Only if acquired in chloroquine-sensitive region (CDC guideline)

a variety of settings, although all are likely to have occurred where there was significant expertise in slide reading and the management of malaria. Consequently these studies may not be representative of many of the settings where infection is being treated. None of these studies involved the use of ACTs, which should result in faster parasite clearance and are better tolerated than older drugs such as quinine.[59,60] Given these difficulties in interpreting the current data, we think that outpatient management of falciparum malaria should only be considered in selected individuals in centers with experience of managing the disease, ideally as part of prospective studies or randomized trials.

Severe Falciparum Malaria

Drug treatment

Two large-scale trials in southeast Asia and Africa have shown the superiority of artesunate compared with quinine for the treatment of severe malaria.[35,36] A recent Cochrane review showed a 39% (95% confidence interval [CI] 25%–50%) reduction in the risk of death when an adult with severe malaria was treated with artesunate rather than quinine, with a 24% (95% CI 10%–35%) reduction in children.[61] Although these studies have made it imperative to deploy artesunate as the first-line antimalarial for severe malaria in endemic regions, some remain concerned about the use of artesunate for the treatment of severe imported malaria.[62] These concerns focus on the unblinded nature of the trials, the extrapolation of results from endemic countries to nonendemic countries, and the lack of an approved product. In addition, recent studies have shown previously unforeseen adverse effects, with neutropenia occurring in both African children coinfected with human immunodeficiency virus (HIV) and receiving oral artesunate-amodiaquine[63] and in Cambodian adults treated with high doses of artesunate monotherapy.[64] A retrospective analysis of travelers treated for severe malaria with intravenous artesunate has highlighted severe and unexplained late hemolysis occurring up to 3.5 weeks after cessation of artesunate.[65] Despite these concerns the data clearly indicate the superiority of artesunate for the treatment of severe malaria, there is therefore a need for a robust reporting system to record potential adverse events as artesunate is more extensively prescribed. An approved preparation of intravenous artesunate is likely to be available by the end of 2012.

As a result of the concerns described earlier, although largely resulting from the lack of a fully approved formulation of artesunate, many guidelines outside endemic areas do not endorse artesunate as the first-line antimalarial for severe disease. Notable approaches to this predicament have been made in Australia, where supplies of artesunate are sourced from Guilin Pharmaceuticals in China, batch tested for purity, stability, and sterility, and distributed to hospitals across the country and in the United States, where the CDC have arranged to provide artesunate sourced from the Walter Reed Army Institute of Research as an investigational drug.

Drugs recommended by CDC and UK guidelines for the treatment of severe falciparum malaria are shown in **Table 4**. Of critical importance in managing severe malaria is to urgently administer one of these treatments. It is important to follow quinine or artesunate therapy with a second antimalarial, once the patient is able to tolerate oral medications, to clear residual parasitemia and prevent recrudescence.

Supportive care

Severe malaria is a life-threatening condition and should be managed in an appropriate setting. Supportive care is similar to that for other severe infections, although direct evidence for goal-directed therapy in severe malaria as recommended for severe sepsis[66] is lacking and there is some uncertainty about the fluid management of severe malaria. One large randomized controlled trial of fluid bolus in African

Table 4
Drugs recommended by UK and CDC guidelines for the treatment of severe falciparum malaria from non–chloroquine-sensitive sites

Drug	Dose (Adult)	Comments
Artesunate	2.4 mg/kg IV at time 0, 12, 24, and every 24 h Until able to take oral medication (minimum 3 doses)	Avoid in first trimester Unlicensed drug, in the United States, contact CDC for supply Follow-on therapy with a full course of any appropriate drug from **Table 3**
Quinidine gluconate	6.25 mg base/kg (=10 mg salt/kg) loading dose IV over 1–2 h, then 0.0125 mg base/kg/min (=0.02 mg salt/kg/min) continuous infusion for at least 24 h or 15 mg base/kg (=24 mg salt/kg) loading dose IV infused over 4 h, followed by 7.5 mg base/kg (=12 mg salt/kg) infused over 4 hours every 8 hours, starting 8 h after the loading dose Until parasite density <1% and patient can take oral medication, complete treatment with oral quinine, dose as nonsevere malaria	Not in United Kingdom Risk of arrhythmia and hypotension Risk of hypoglycemia Quinidine/quinine course = 7 d in southeast Asia and 3 d in Africa or South America Follow-on or overlapping therapy with a full course of any appropriate drug from **Table 3**
Quinine dihydrochloride	20 mg/kg loading dose IV over 4 h followed by 10 mg/kg IV infusion every 8 h Dosing interval should be reduced to 12 hourly if IV therapy continuing for more than 48 h Until patient can tolerate oral therapy Minimum of 5 d quinine (given IV or oral) recommended (unless Coartem used as follow-on)	Avoid loading dose if quinine or mefloquine administered within 12hrs Risk of arrhythmia and hypotension Risk of hypoglycemia Reversible tinnitus and deafness common. Itch in dark-skinned patients Choice in first trimester Follow-on or overlapping therapy with a full course of any appropriate drug from **Table 3**

Abbreviation: IV, intravenous.

children with severe infection and signs of poor perfusion found a significant increase in mortality associated with fluid bolus therapy.[67] Around 60% of these children had infection with *P falciparum*, and results in this subgroup were similar to those without malaria. Although it would be a mistake to extrapolate such results to other settings where better resources allow for more intensive monitoring and intervention, proposed UK guidelines in children may need review in the light of this evidence.[68] UK guidelines for management of adults with severe malaria suggest monitoring of central venous pressure with the aim of maintaining perfusion with a right atrial pressure less than 10 cm H_2O, whereas WHO guidelines suggest a central venous pressure of 0 to 5 cm H_2O as a target, in the belief that this may help to avoid ARDS.[34,44] However, recent data are challenging the usefulness of such targets and questioning whether they achieve improvements in microvascular flow, although it is still advised that over-zealous fluid resuscitation should be avoided.[69,70]

Although bacterial coinfection in severe imported malaria is thought to be un-common, a European case series identified community-acquired infection in 30/400 (7.5%) admissions to an intensive care unit with severe malaria, including 10 cases of bacteremia and 13 cases of pneumonia.[38] Blood culture should be performed in all patients presenting with severe malaria and there should be a low threshold for broad-spectrum antibiotics. Further data describing the prevalence of community-acquired bacteremia associated with imported malaria are needed.

Both quinine and quinidine can induce hyperinsulinemic hypoglycemia, a complication significantly less common with artesunate therapy.[35,36,61] Close blood glucose moni-toring should be in place for all patients with severe malaria. Quinine and quinidine can both cause lethal hypotension if given rapidly because of their α-blocking activity, neces-sitating administration by controlled infusion. Both quinine and quinidine prolong the QRS complex and the QT interval, although the effect on the QT interval is about 4 times as severe for quinidine.[71] All patients receiving parenteral quinidine should have contin-uous cardiac monitoring.[56] Older patients and those with preexisting cardiac disease receiving parenteral quinine therapy should have continuous cardiac monitoring.[44]

Adjunctive treatments

Many adjunctive therapies to reduce mortality in malaria have been trialed, including dexamethasone, anti–tumor necrosis factor-α antibodies, pentoxifylline, deferrox-amine, N-acetylcysteine, heparin, aspirin, and mannitol.[72] There is no evidence that any of these therapies is effective in reducing mortality.

Intravenous artesunate therapy, with its rapid reduction in circulating parasitemia, may render exchange blood transfusion (EBT) or erythrocytapheresis unnecessary.[44] CDC guidelines currently recommend EBT be considered if parasitemia is greater than 10%, or cerebral malaria, ARDS, or renal complications exist.[56] UK guidelines are more stringent, suggesting EBT if parasitemia is greater than 30% or greater than 10% with other manifestations of severe disease.[44] Robust evidence supporting the use of EBT is lacking,[73] although there have been numerous case reports and case series of its effective use.

Non-Falciparum Malaria

The management of vivax and ovale malaria is divided into management of the acute fever, and management of hypnozoites to prevent relapses. P malariae and P knowlesi have no hypnozoite stage, and treatment targeted at the acute illness is sufficient.

If there is doubt as to the infecting species, treatment of the acute illness should be as for falciparum malaria (see **Table 3**); following expert review of the blood film, treat-ment of hypnozoites can be administered at a later date if necessary.

The recommended treatment of acute non-falciparum malaria is chloroquine, usually given as 600 mg base initially, followed by 300 mg 6 to 8 hours later and 300 mg on days 2 and 3.[44,56] With severe disease and a lack of injectable chloroquine, quinine, quini-dine, or artesunate can be used at doses as for severe falciparum malaria.

The only drugs currently licensed for the prevention of relapse are based on the 8-aminoquinoline primaquine. Both primaquine and a related compound, tafenoquine, can cause severe hemolysis in patients with glucose-6 phosphate dehydrogenase (G6PD) deficiency and patients should be tested for this deficiency before primaquine therapy. The genetics of G6PD deficiency are complex and primaquine-related hemo-lysis is variable within this condition. If hemolysis is likely to be clinically significant, there are several possible approaches to treatment to prevent relapse. First, chloroquine can be prescribed at a weekly prophylactic dose for 6 months to cover the period of highest risk of relapse, or, second, a treatment course of chloroquine can be issued with the advice to start therapy if a fever is detected. Third, a prophylactic course could be provided for use during periods in which a clinical episode of malaria would be most disadvantageous.

Personal Prevention and Chemoprophylaxis

A combination of measures is necessary to prevent malaria and reduce morbidity in travelers. These measures include awareness of malaria risk, the use of bite-avoidance measures, using chemoprophylaxis, and seeking an early diagnosis, which is remembered through the mnemonic ABCD.

The malaria risk to travelers is usually defined by national or international guidelines, and preventative policy is based on a combination of rate of infection or transmission intensity of malaria, species of malaria, and geographic distribution, including altitude and seasonality. The risk of acquisition of an infection has, until recently, been a consensus opinion of policy makers based on local population malaria. More recently, the incidence in travelers has allowed more precise estimates to be defined; for the average traveler to Vietnam, Thailand, Cambodia, and China, the risk of all malaria is less than or equal to 1 case per 100,000 visits, and, for all travelers to West Africa, the risk is 169 and for East Africa (Kenya) 7 per 100,000 visits.[74,75] The risk depends on the reason for travel, and individuals who visit friends and relatives (VFR) have a 3-times higher malaria incidence than travelers visiting for other reasons.[74] The reliance on prescribing chemoprophylaxis for the prevention of malaria is based on the unreliable use of personal bite prevention measures related to incorrect health beliefs and low adherence to advice. Most VFR travelers who develop malaria have not sought advice or used malaria chemoprophylaxis during their travel.

Malaria chemoprophylaxis is the use of antimalarial medication to prevent the symptoms of malaria. Regimens may act as causal prophylactics, in which the drug acts on the parasite in the liver tissue, for example atovaquone-proguanil and primaquine, or as suppressive prophylactics acting on blood-destroying erythrocytic parasites; these include mefloquine, proguanil, chloroquine, and doxycycline, or both.

For regions in which chloroquine-resistant *P falciparum* is the predominant species, the regimens recommended by most policy groups are either atovaquone-proguanil (Malarone) doxycycline, or mefloquine. The choice of regimen depends on several variables, which include adverse event profile, and, in particular, the reputation of the regimen held by the traveler, duration of travel, and prior medical problems. Cost and simplicity of a regimen have a bearing on final choice, as does the health advisor's preference of drug. Efficacy as a schizonticidal agent is similar for the 3 regimens, but effectiveness as a combination of efficacy and adherence may be different. The mild to moderate adverse event profiles of the 3 regimens are similar, with 45% of chloroquine and proguanil users, 42% of mefloquine users, 33% of doxycycline users, and 32% of atovaquone/proguanil users reporting mild to moderate problems. Significant adverse events (that interfered with daily activity) were reported in 11% of mefloquine users, 12% of chloroquine plus proguanil users, 6% of doxycycline users, and 7% of atovaquone and proguanil users. Neuropsychiatric events were reported in as many as 42% of mefloquine users and 30% of atovaquone and proguanil users, respectively, during blinded use of chemoprophylaxis.[76,77] Incidence of serious adverse events requiring hospitalization are not well understood but are important where the risk of malaria is low, and may be an important cause of morbidity when used in settings with low malaria prevalence.

Bite Prevention

The 2 major strategies used to prevent bites are the application of topical repellents and barrier methods to reduce contact with biting arthropods. Deet (diethyltoluamide) is the best broad-spectrum repellent available with an extensive safety history and is a compound with which newer repellents are compared in reducing nuisance bites from arthropods. Icaridin (2-(2-hydroxyethyl)-piperidinecarboxylic acid 1-methyl ester) and PMD (p-methane 3,8-diol) are reasonable alternatives to Deet for those visiting areas where arthropod-borne diseases are endemic. IR3535 (ethyl butylacetylamino-propionate) has lower efficacy against anopheles mosquitoes and should not be advised for areas where malaria is endemic. The higher concentrations of active repellent results in longer duration of activity but Deet concentrations of more than 50% have little added benefit.

The use and benefit of insecticide-treated mosquito nets is clear and should be advised for all travelers visiting endemic areas where there is a risk from biting arthropods when asleep. The usefulness of electric insecticide vaporizers, essential oil candles, and burning cardboard to reduce bites from arthropods has some benefits but the benefit of knockdown insecticide sprays is minimal.[78]

EARLY DIAGNOSIS

Many malaria deaths in travelers result from a delay in diagnosis of malaria. The reasons for the delay are multifactorial. Education on preventing delay in seeking medical help for malaria must be provided at the pretravel consultation. Preventing delays in recognizing and testing for malaria at the first medical contact requires educating physicians and other health professionals on appreciating the symptoms and signs of malaria.

MALARIA AND PREGNANCY

In highly endemic areas where immunity to severe disease is acquired in childhood, malaria may account for up to one-half of all low birth weight babies and one-quarter of severe maternal anemia.[79] In this context, severe disease is confined largely to primigravidas, and pregnant women coinfected with HIV. Malaria in the multigravida pregnancy can present insidiously with little sign of the infection other than anemia and fetal growth retardation. In contrast, all pregnant women from nonendemic settings are at increased risk of severe malaria and potentially severe consequences for them and their pregnancy. Consequently a low threshold for admission should be applied to pregnant women returning with fever from regions where malaria is endemic, and pregnancy itself is considered by many as a criteria for intravenous therapy if falciparum malaria is diagnosed. Obstetric advice should be sought early in such cases and patients should be monitored closely for hypoglycemia, which is common in this context. Artesunate and artemisinin combination therapies should be avoided if possible in the first trimester of pregnancy. Women who are pregnant when traveling to areas where malaria is endemic should be advised of the increased disease severity and encouraged not to travel. Mefloquine chemoprophylaxis has been used in pregnant travelers and no unexpected outcomes to pregnancy have been reported when used during pregnancy.

SUMMARY

Despite efforts to control malaria, it continues to claim the lives of more than 2000 people every day and remains the most important human parasitic disease. The development of artemisinin combination therapies for nonsevere malaria and parenteral artesunate for severe malaria represent the most important advances in antimalarial therapeutics. Progress in reducing global mortality depends on ensuring that such treatments reach those most in need. These drugs also offer the clearest therapeutic advance in managing imported malaria, although the greatest benefits available are in prevention, early recognition, and early treatment.

REFERENCES

1. Carter R, Mendis KN. Evolutionary and historical aspects of the burden of malaria. Clin Microbiol Rev 2002;15(4):564.
2. World Health Organization. World malaria report 2010. World Health Organization. Geneva (Switzerland): WHO Press; 2010.
3. Scott JA, Berkley JA, Mwangi I, et al. Relation between falciparum malaria and bacteraemia in Kenyan children: a population-based, case-control study and a longitudinal study. Lancet 2011;6736(11):1–8.
4. Anon. Elimination of malaria in the United States (1947–1951). Available at: http://www.cdc.gov/malaria/about/history/elimination_us.html. Accessed September 2, 2011.
5. O'Meara WP, Mangeni JN, Steketee R, et al. Changes in the burden of malaria in sub Saharan Africa. Lancet Infect Dis 2010;10(8):545–55.
6. Dhingra N, Jha P, Sharma VP, et al. Adult and child malaria mortality in India: a nationally representative mortality survey. Lancet 2010;376(9754):1768–74.
7. Mali S, Tan KR, Arguin PM. Malaria surveillance–United States, 2009. MMWR Surveill Summ 2011;60(3):1–15.
8. Health Protection Agency. Malaria imported into the United Kingdom in 2010: implications for those advising travellers. Health Protection Report. 2011;5(17). Available at: http://www.hpa.org.uk/hpr/archives/2011/hpr1711.pdf. Accessed September 11, 2011.
9. Smith AD, Bradley DJ, et al. Imported malaria and high risk groups: observational study using UK surveillance data 1987-2006. BMJ 2008;337:a120.
10. Bejon P, Williams TN, Liljander A, et al. Stable and unstable malaria hotspots in longitudinal cohort studies in Kenya. PLoS Med 2010;7(7):e1000304.
11. Woolhouse ME. Heterogeneities in the transmission of infectious agents: implications for the design of control programs. Proc Natl Acad Sci U S A 1997;94(1):338–42.
12. Kreuels B, Kobbe R, Adjei S, et al. Spatial variation of malaria incidence in young children from a geographically homogeneous area with high endemicity. J Infect Dis 2008;197(1):85–93.
13. Bousema T, Drakeley C, Gesase S, et al. Identification of hot spots of malaria transmission for targeted malaria control. J Infect Dis 2010;201(11):1764–74.
14. Kantele A, Jokiranta TS. Review of cases with the emerging fifth human malaria parasite, Plasmodium knowlesi. Clin Infect Dis 2011;52(11):1356–62.
15. Daneshvar C, Davis TM, Cox-Singh J, et al. Clinical and laboratory features of human Plasmodium knowlesi infection. Clin Infect Dis 2009;49(6):852–60.
16. Miller LH, Baruch DI, Marsh K, et al. The pathogenic basis of malaria. Nature 2002;415(6872):673–9.
17. Hulden L, Hulden L. Activation of the hypnozoite: a part of Plasmodium vivax life cycle and survival. Malar J 2011;10(1):90.
18. Wells TN, Burrows JN, Baird JK. Targeting the hypnozoite reservoir of Plasmodium vivax: the hidden obstacle to malaria elimination. Trends Parasitol 2010; 26(3):145–51.

19. White NJ. Determinants of relapse periodicity in *Plasmodium vivax* malaria. Malar J 2011;10:297.
20. Portugal S, Carret C, Recker M, et al. Host-mediated regulation of superinfection in malaria. Nat Med 2011;17(6):732–7.
21. Mueller I, Zimmerman PA, Reeder JC. *Plasmodium malariae* and *Plasmodium ovale*-the "bashful" malaria parasites. Trends Parasitol 2007;23(6):278–83.
22. Dondorp AM, Kager PA, Vreeken J, et al. Abnormal blood flow and red blood cell deformability in severe malaria. Parasitol Today 2000;16(6):228–32.
23. Anstey NM, Russell B, Yeo TW, et al. The pathophysiology of vivax malaria. Trends Parasitol 2009;25(5):220–7.
24. Handayani S, Chiu DT, Tjitra E, et al. High deformability of *Plasmodium vivax*-infected red blood cells under microfluidic conditions. J Infect Dis 2009;199(3): 445–50.
25. Nic Fhogartaigh C, Hughes H, Armstrong M, et al. Falciparum malaria as a cause of fever in adult travellers returning to the United Kingdom: observational study of risk by geographical area. QJM 2008;101(8):649–56.
26. Schwartz E, Parise M, Kozarsky P, et al. Delayed onset of malaria–implications for chemoprophylaxis in travelers. N Engl J Med 2003;349(16):1510–6.
27. Ladhani S, Aibara RJ, Riordan FA, et al. Imported malaria in children: a review of clinical studies. Lancet Infect Dis 2007;7:349–57.
28. Kain KC, Harrington MA, Tennyson S, et al. Imported malaria: prospective analysis of problems in diagnosis and management. Clin Infect Dis 1998;27(1):142–9.
29. Kyriacou DN, Spira AM, Talan DA, et al. Emergency department presentation and misdiagnosis of imported falciparum malaria. Ann Emerg Med 1996;27(6):696–9.
30. D'Acremont V, Landry P, Mueller I, et al. Clinical and laboratory predictors of imported malaria in an outpatient setting: an aid to medical decision making in returning travelers with fever. Am J Trop Med Hyg 2002;66(5):481–6.
31. Bassat Q, Guinovart C, Sigaúque B, et al. Severe malaria and concomitant bacteraemia in children admitted to a rural Mozambican hospital. Trop Med Int Health 2009;14(9):1011–9.
32. Berkley J, Mwarumba S, Bramham K, et al. Bacteraemia complicating severe malaria in children. Trans R Soc Trop Med Hyg 1999;93(3):283–6.
33. Nadjm B, Amos B, Mtove G, et al. WHO guidelines for antimicrobial treatment in children admitted to hospital in an area of intense *Plasmodium falciparum* transmission: prospective study. BMJ 2010;340:c1350.
34. Guidelines for the treatment of malaria. Geneva (Switzerland): WHO; 2010.
35. Dondorp A, Nosten F, Stepniewska K, et al. Artesunate versus quinine for treatment of severe falciparum malaria: a randomised trial. Lancet 2005;366(9487):717–25.
36. Dondorp AM, Fanello CI, Hendriksen IC, et al. Artesunate versus quinine in the treatment of severe falciparum malaria in African children (AQUAMAT): an open-label, randomised trial. Lancet 2010;376(9753):1647–57.
37. Phillips A, Bassett P, Zeki S, et al. Risk factors for severe disease in adults with falciparum malaria. Clin Infect Dis 2009;48(7):871–8.
38. Bruneel F, Tubach F, Corne P, et al. Severe imported falciparum malaria: a cohort study in 400 critically ill adults. PloS One 2010;5(10):e13236.
39. Tjitra E, Anstey NM, Sugiarto P, et al. Multidrug-resistant *Plasmodium vivax* associated with severe and fatal malaria: a prospective study in Papua, Indonesia. PLoS Med 2008;5(6):e128.
40. Mühlberger N, Jelinek T, Gascon J, et al. Epidemiology and clinical features of vivax malaria imported to Europe: sentinel surveillance data from TropNetEurop. Malar J 2004;3:5.

41. Chilton D, Malik AN, Armstrong M, et al. Use of rapid diagnostic tests for diagnosis of malaria in the UK. J Clin Pathol 2006;59(8):862–6.
42. Stauffer WM, Cartwright CP, Olson DA, et al. Diagnostic performance of rapid diagnostic tests versus blood smears for malaria in US clinical practice. Clin Infect Dis 2009;49(6):908–13.
43. Moody A. Rapid diagnostic tests for malaria parasites. Clin Microbiol Rev 2002; 15(1):66–78.
44. Lalloo DG, Shingadia D, Pasvol G, et al. UK malaria treatment guidelines. J Infect 2007;54(2):111–21.
45. Berry A, Benoit-Vical F, Fabre R, et al. PCR-based methods to the diagnosis of imported malaria. Parasite 2008;15:484.
46. Poon LL, Wong BW, Ma EH, et al. Sensitive and inexpensive molecular test for falciparum malaria: detecting Plasmodium falciparum DNA directly from heat-treated blood by loop-mediated isothermal amplification. Clin Chem 2006; 52(2):303–6.
47. White NJ. Qinghaosu (artemisinin): the price of success. Science 2008;320(5874): 330–4.
48. Dondorp AM, Fairhurst RM, Slutsker L, et al. The threat of artemisinin-resistant malaria. N Engl J Med 2011;365(12):1073–5.
49. Briand V, Bouchaud O, Tourret J, et al. Hospitalization criteria in imported falciparum malaria. J Travel Med 2007;14(5):306–11.
50. Bottieau E, Clerinx J, Colebunders R, et al. Selective ambulatory management of imported falciparum malaria: a 5-year prospective study. Eur J Clin Microbiol Infect Dis 2007;26(3):181–8.
51. Chih DT, Heath CH, Murray RJ, et al. Outpatient treatment of malaria in recently arrived African migrants. Med J Aust 2006;185(11):598–601.
52. Cherian S, Burgner D. Selective ambulatory management of Plasmodium falciparum malaria in paediatric refugees. Arch Dis Child 2007;92(11):983–6.
53. Jennings RM, DE Souza JB, Todd JE, et al. Imported Plasmodium falciparum malaria: are patients originating from disease-endemic areas less likely to develop severe disease? A prospective, observational study. Am J Trop Med Hyg 2006; 75(6):1195–9.
54. Miura T, Kimura M, Koibuchi T, et al. Clinical characteristics of imported malaria in Japan: analysis at a referral hospital. Am J Trop Med Hyg 2005;73(3): 599–603.
55. Melzer M, Lacey S, Rait G. The case for outpatient treatment of Plasmodium falciparum malaria in a selected UK immigrant population. J Infect 2009;59(4): 259–63.
56. CDC. Malaria treatment (United States). Available at: http://www.cdc.gov/malaria/diagnosis_treatment/treatment.html. Accessed September 18, 2011.
57. Moore DA, Jennings RM, Doherty TF, et al. Assessing the severity of malaria. BMJ 2003;326:808–9.
58. D'Acremont V, Landry P, Darioli R, et al. Treatment of imported malaria in an ambulatory setting: prospective study. BMJ 2002;324:875–7.
59. Achan J, Tibenderana JK, Kyabayinze D, et al. Effectiveness of quinine versus artemether-lumefantrine for treating uncomplicated falciparum malaria in Ugandan children: randomised trial. BMJ 2009;339:b2763.
60. Nosten F, White NJ. Artemisinin-based combination treatment of falciparum malaria. Am J Trop Med Hyg 2007;77(Suppl 6):181–92.
61. Sinclair D, Donegan S, Lalloo D. Artesunate versus quinine for treating severe malaria [review]. Cochrane Database Syst Rev 2011;9:1–52.

62. Cramer JP, Lopez-Velez R, Burchard GD, et al. Treatment of imported severe malaria with artesunate instead of quinine - more evidence needed? Malar J 2011; 10(1):256.

63. Gasasira AF, Kamya MR, Achan J, et al. High risk of neutropenia in HIV-infected children following treatment with artesunate plus amodiaquine for uncomplicated malaria in Uganda. Clin Infect Dis 2008;46(7):985–91.

64. Bethell D, Se Y, Lon C, et al. Dose-dependent risk of neutropenia after 7-day courses of artesunate monotherapy in Cambodian patients with acute *Plasmodium falciparum* malaria. Clin Infect Dis 2010;51(12):e105–14.

65. Zoller T. Intravenous artesunate for severe malaria in travelers, Europe. Emerg Infect Dis 2011;17(5):771–7.

66. Dellinger RP, Levy MM, Carlet JM, et al. Surviving Sepsis Campaign: international guidelines for management of severe sepsis and septic shock: 2008. Crit Care Med 2008;36(1):296–327.

67. Maitland K, Kiguli S, Opoka RO, et al. Mortality after fluid bolus in African children with severe infection. N Engl J Med 2011;364(26):2483–95.

68. Maitland K, Nadel S, Pollard AJ, et al. Management of severe malaria in children: proposed guidelines for the United Kingdom. BMJ 2005;331(7512):337–43.

69. Hanson J, Lam SW, Mohanty S, et al. Central venous catheter use in severe malaria: time to reconsider the World Health Organization guidelines? Malar J 2011; 10(1):342.

70. Nguyen HP, Hanson J, Bethell D, et al. A retrospective analysis of the haemodynamic and metabolic effects of fluid resuscitation in Vietnamese adults with severe falciparum malaria. PLoS One 2011;6(10):e25523.

71. White NJ. Cardiotoxicity of antimalarial drugs. Lancet Infect Dis 2007;7(8): 549–58.

72. Chandy JC, Kutamba E, Mugarura K, et al. Adjunctive therapy for cerebral malaria and other severe forms of *Plasmodium falciparum* malaria. Expert Rev Anti Infect Ther 2010;8(9):997–1008.

73. Riddle MS, Jackson JL, Sanders JW, et al. Exchange transfusion as an adjunct therapy in severe *Plasmodium falciparum* malaria: a meta-analysis. Clin Infect Dis 2002;34(9):1192–8.

74. Behrens RH, Carroll B, Smith V, et al. Declining incidence of malaria imported into the UK from West Africa. Malar J 2008;7:235.

75. Behrens RH, Carroll B, Hellgren U, et al. The incidence of malaria in travellers to south-east Asia: is local malaria transmission a useful risk indicator? Malar J 2010;9:266.

76. Overbosch D, Schilthuis H, Bienzle U, et al. Atovaquone-proguanil versus mefloquine for malaria prophylaxis in nonimmune travelers: results from a randomized, double-blind study. Clin Infect Dis 2001;33(7):1015–21.

77. Schlagenhauf P, Adamcova M, Regep L, et al. The position of mefloquine as a 21st century malaria chemoprophylaxis. Malar J 2010;9(1):357.

78. Goodyer LI, Croft AM, Frances SP, et al. Expert review of the evidence base for arthropod bite avoidance. J Travel Med 2010;17(3):182–92.

79. Desai M, ter Kuile FO, Nosten F, et al. Epidemiology and burden of malaria in pregnancy. Lancet Infect Dis 2007;7(2):93–104.

Human African Trypanosomiasis

Reto Brun, PhD[a],*, Johannes Blum, MD[b]

KEYWORDS

- Human African trypanosomiasis • Sleeping sickness
- *Trypanosoma brucei gambiense* • *Trypanosoma brucei rhodesiense* • Epidemiology
- Diagnosis • Treatment

KEY POINTS

- Human African trypanosomiasis or sleeping sickness is caused by trypanosomes (protozoan parasites), transmitted by tsetse flies and restricted to countries in Subsaharan Africa.
- The disease is mainly found in rural populations in remote areas of Central Africa which are exposed to the tsetse flies, but rare among travellers with febrile disease.
- The disease shows two stages: A first stage with mainly fever, headache and adenopathy, and a second stage with mainly neuropsychiatric symptoms eventually leading to coma and death. However, most organs can be affected.
- Treatment is complicated and can be accompanied by severe adverse events. The disease is inevitably fatal if untreated.

BIOLOGY OF AFRICAN TRYPANOSOMES

Trypanosomes are unicellular organisms of 20 to 30 μm in length. The elongated cells are constantly moving in the insect vector or the human host with the help of a flagellum that is attached to the outside of the cell. In the human host, trypanosomes can initially be found in the lymph and blood system and after penetrating the blood-brain barrier also in the brain (second stage). African trypanosomes are always located extracellularly and their density is low, normally under the limit of detection.[1]

Trypanosomes are covered by a thick coat of variant surface glycoproteins that protect the parasite from the lytic factors in the blood. The patient's immune system is capable of developing an immune response (immunoglobulin [Ig]M and IgG) against these glycoproteins, which neutralizes the parasites. The trypanosomes have the

The authors have nothing to disclose.
[a] Department Medical Parasitology and Infection Biology, Swiss Tropical and Public Health Institute, Socinstrasse 57, CH-4002 Basel, Switzerland; [b] Outpatient Clinic, Department Medical Services and Diagnostics, Swiss Tropical and Public Health Institute, Socinstrasse 57, CH-4002 Basel, Switzerland
* Corresponding author.
E-mail address: Reto.brun@unibas.ch

Infect Dis Clin N Am 26 (2012) 261–273
doi:10.1016/j.idc.2012.03.003
0891-5520/12/$ – see front matter © 2012 Elsevier Inc. All rights reserved.

ability to change the glycoprotein to another type (antigenic variation), however, which is not recognized by the antibodies directed against the former type. One single trypanosome contains more than 1000 genes for these glycoproteins and thus can easily evade the immune response.[2] This is the reason why a host cannot overcome a trypanosome infection and eventually dies of the infection. Antigenic variation also prevents the development of a vaccine.

Trypanosomes are transmitted by more than 20 species of tsetse flies (*Glossina* spp.) while feeding on a mammalian host. Tsetse flies are viviparous insects (ie, a female deposits 1 larvae about every 10 days). The larvae pupates in the soil and after 30 days an adult fly hatches. This fly is not harboring trypanosomes and has first to get infected by feeding on an infected animal or human. The trypanosomes undergo a complex development during the following 3 to 5 weeks until they end in the salivary glands where they transform into infective forms. With the next feed on a human or animal, they transmit infective trypanosomes with their saliva. In the field, the proportion of flies with a mature infection is very low and in the range of 0.1%. Responsible for this low salivary gland infection rate is the long time it takes an infection to mature and the prerequisite that a fly can become infected only with its first blood meal.

Wild and domestic animals can harbor human pathogenic trypanosomes and thus act as a reservoir although not falling sick. For *Trypanosoma brucei rhodesiense,* the animal reservoir is important and comprises various antelopes, also warthogs and even carnivores, and cattle. Transmission is usually from animal to fly and later on to humans. *Trypanosoma brucei gambiense* is anthroponotic; infection spreads mainly from humans to fly to humans, only occasionally animal reservoirs are involved.

EPIDEMIOLOGY
Epidemiology in Endemic Countries

Human African trypanosomiasis (HAT) is a disease that is restricted to sub-Saharan Africa (**Fig. 1**). Its distribution overlaps with the distribution of tsetse flies, which are the vectors of the human and animal trypanosomiasis also known as Nagana. HAT is a disease of poor people in rural areas of more than 20 countries of tropical Africa.[1] There are 2 forms of human disease: the Central and West African form caused by *T brucei gambiense,* causing a chronic form of HAT leading on average to death in 3 to 4 years, and the East African form caused by *T brucei rhodesiense,* causing a more acute disease leading normally to death in 6 months.[1] The animal-pathogenic *Trypanosoma brucei brucei* is closely related to *T brucei gambiense* and identical with *T brucei rhodesiense* with the sole exception of the missing SRA (serum-resistance associated) gene.[3] The 2 disease forms are geographically separated with Uganda being the only country where both forms occur and the risk of an overlap exists.

In the past, major HAT epidemics ravaged Africa about the year 1900 and later on between 1920 and 1948 when hundreds of thousands of people were killed. The colonial powers put much emphasis in vector control and active surveillance of the populations, resulting in a decrease of the number of cases to the level where HAT was almost eliminated; however, after gaining independence, control activities were neglected in most countries, especially in those affected by civil conflicts. This led to a reemergence of cases almost to the level of 1945, mainly in the Democratic Republic of Congo, Angola, Uganda, and South Sudan.[4] A peak was reached in the late 1990s.[5] Since then, increased control activities and awareness of international organizations and not-for-profit organizations brought down the numbers of cases to the level of the lowest reported numbers. The World Health Organization published in 2009 fewer than 10,000 reported cases in fewer than 20 countries and estimated the

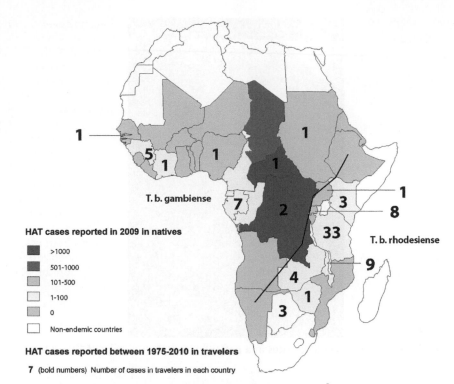

Fig. 1. HAT in endemic and nonendemic populations (travelers).[8] The black line divides the endemic regions of *T brucei gambiense* and *T brucei rhodesiense* HAT.

number of patients to 30,000.[6] Central Africa is not very well surveyed, however, and hidden pockets of HAT have to be suspected. A control program of Médecins sans Frontières in Chad and the Central African Republic revealed a prevalence of HAT of greater than 14% in some villages.[7]

Epidemiology in Travelers and Immigrants

HAT caused by *T brucei gambiense* is rare among travelers, but was sporadically reported in immigrants and long-term white residents living in rural settings in Central or West Africa (see **Fig. 1**). In contrast, *T brucei rhodesiense* HAT is mainly seen in short-term travelers. Travelers become infected mainly during safaris in *T brucei rhodesiense* endemic game parks in Eastern Africa and during hunting trips.[8]

CLINICAL PRESENTATION

The clinical presentation of HAT depends on the parasite species, the stage of the disease, and on the host.

Endemic Countries

T brucei gambiense HAT
T brucei gambiense HAT is characterized by a chronic progressive course leading to death if untreated. According to models based on survival analysis, the estimated duration of HAT is almost 3 years, evenly split between the first and second stage.[9] A trypanosome chancre (local reaction at the bite site of the tsetse fly) is only exceptionally observed. Fever, headache, pruritus (**Fig. 2**), lymphadenopathy (**Fig. 3**), and, to

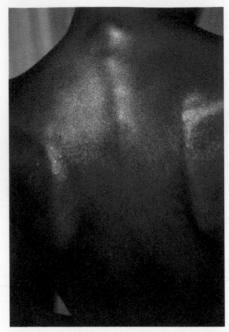

Fig. 2. Scratch marks owing to pruritus in a patient with HAT. (*Courtesy of* Blum J.)

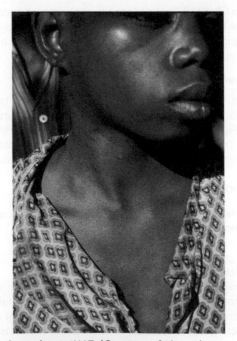

Fig. 3. Lymphadenopathy owing to HAT. (*Courtesy of* Blum J.)

a lesser extent, hepatosplenomegaly are the leading signs and symptoms of the first stage, but are also present to a lesser extent in the second stage. The fever is intermittent, with attacks lasting from a day to a week, separated by intervals of a few days to a month or longer, and is rarely seen in the second stage.[1]

In the second stage, sleep disturbances and neuropsychiatric disorders dominate the clinical presentation.[10]

Sleep disorder is the leading symptom, hence the name "sleeping sickness." It was already observed in the 19th century that patients with sleeping sickness have frequent sleep episodes of short duration, during the day and the night, and that the total time of sleep is equal to that of healthy persons. Lhermitte described sleeping episodes as follows: "Sleep overcomes the patient in a rapid and brutal way: the patient sleeps in during a conversation without finishing the sentence or during a meal with a full mouth, the head sinks to the breast and the sleep is complete. During the first crisis it is possible to awake the patient, but in repeated crisis attempts to awake the patient are fruitless." Somnographic studies have demonstrated that the disease causes dysregulation of the circadian rhythm of the sleep/wake cycle and a fragmentation of the sleeping pattern rather than the frequently reported "inversion of sleep."[11] The structure of sleep, and especially the sequence of the 2 types (rapid eye movement sleep and non–rapid eye movement sleep) is altered and is characterized by the occurrence of sleep-onset rapid-eye-movement episodes."[12,13] The circadian rhythm of secretion of prolactin, renin, growth hormone, and cortisol levels is disrupted in severe cases.[11]

The neurologic symptoms include tremor, fasciculations, general motor weakness, paralysis of an extremity, hemiparesis, akinesia, and abnormal movements, such as dyskinesia or choreoathetosis, parkinson-like movements, unspecific movement disorders, speech disorders, and abnormal archaic reflexes. Also, psychiatric symptoms, such as irritability, psychotic reactions, aggressive behavior, or inactivity with apathy may dominate the clinical picture. These neuropsychiatric disorders are rarely seen during the first stage and increase with the duration of the disease.[10,14]

Cardiac involvement documented by electrocardiogram (ECG) alterations is observed in more than 50% of patients in first-stage *T brucei gambiense* HAT and increases to 70% in the second stage; however, it rarely leads to relevant clinical heart failure.[15] The most frequent ECG changes are QTc prolongation, repolarization changes, and low voltage.[16] This QTc prolongation comprises a risk of fatal arrhythmias, but relevant arrhythmias are only rarely documented in endemic countries.[15] Endocrine disorders of the thyroid and adrenocortical function comprise hypofunction and hyperfunction, but rarely demand specific treatment.[17,18]

T brucei rhodesiense HAT

T brucei rhodesiense HAT is classically described as an acute disease progressing to second stage within a few weeks and death within 6 months. The clinical presentation is similar, but trypanosomal chancres are more frequently seen, the localization of enlarged lymph nodes is rather submandibular, axillary, and inguinal than nuchal, and edemas are more frequently observed. Recent descriptions of the clinical presentation show a high variability in different foci, however,[19,20] possibly because of different parasite strains. Whereas fever and headache were the leading symptom in the first stage in some foci, tremor and somnolence dominated in other foci.[19] In the second stage, fever is only moderate, rarely exceeding 38.4°C. Pruritus, sleeping disorders, reduced consciousness, or neurologic signs and symptoms, such as tremor, abnormal movements, or walking disabilities, may predominate in some foci. Compared with *T brucei gambiense* HAT, thyroid dysfunction, adrenal insufficiency, and hypogonadism are more frequently found and myopericarditis may be more severe. Liver involvement with hepatomegaly is usually moderate.[20]

Nonendemic Countries

The symptomatology of Europeans and North Americans is markedly different from the usual textbook descriptions of African patients with HAT. The onset of the disease is almost invariably acute and of the febrile type, regardless of the involved species.[8]

T brucei rhodesiense HAT has a short incubation period of a few days in travelers (<3 weeks). It is an acute, life-threatening disease with the cardinal symptoms of high fever, headache, and a trypanosomal chancre.[8] For *T brucei gambiense* HAT, the incubation period in travelers is often shorter than 1 month, but might be as long as 7 years in immigrants.

Fever is nearly always present in infections with either species and exceeds 38.5°C in more than 50% of cases.[8] If left untreated, the pyrexial episodes become irregular. Each attack may last from a day to a week and attacks may be separated by a few days to month-long intervals.[8,21] A trypanosomal chancre consists of a tender, purplish, indurated area that develops at the site of the tsetse fly bite. The lesion develops within 5 to 15 days, may ulcerate, and is often accompanied by a satellite lymphadenopathy. Within a few weeks, the chancre disappears without leaving a mark.[22] It is seen in more than 80% of patients with *T brucei rhodesiense* and 50% of patients with *T brucei gambiense*. A trypanosomal rash may appear in 25% to 35% of the cases at any time after the first febrile episode, consisting of nonitching blotchy irregular erythematous macules with a diameter of up to 10 cm. A large proportion of the macules develop a central area of normal-colored skin, giving the rash a circinate or serpiginous outline. The rash is evanescent, fading in one place and reappearing in another over a period of several weeks.[22]

The classical sleep disorders and neurologic findings of HAT are not a hallmark in travelers, irrespective of the species. Because most travelers are in the first stage and have a short duration of the disease, sleep disorders and neuropsychiatric findings may not be present at the time of the first clinical assessment.[8]

Headache, lymphadenopathy, splenomegaly, hepatomegaly, and even icterus are unspecific findings seen in about a quarter to half of the patients. Unspecific gastrointestinal symptoms, such as nausea, vomiting, and diarrhea may dominate the clinical presentation. ECG alterations owing to myopericarditis and conduction abnormalities, such as transient second-degree and third-degree atrioventricular block, supraventricular tachycardia, and ventricular premature captures, have been reported.[8] In a few travelers, HAT has been complicated by renal failure requiring hemodialysis, multiorgan failure, disseminated intravascular coagulopathy, and coma with even fatal outcome.[8]

The clinical presentation of HAT in immigrants is dominated by low-grade fever and neuropsychiatric disorders. Because of predominant psychiatric symptoms, some patients with HAT have even been admitted to psychiatric clinics.[8] Because of the long incubation period, HAT has to be considered even if the patient left the endemic country years earlier.

Radiological Findings

The knowledge on magnetic resonance imaging (MRI) alterations in patients with HAT is limited to a few case reports. The alterations are multifarious and include symmetric focal lesions,[23] diffuse hyperintensity,[24] brain edema with demyelination, brain atrophy, and multiple abnormal signals.[25–27] The alterations are localized in the brainstem, basal ganglia, white matter, and central gray matter. These lesions resolve after treatment.[26]

DIAGNOSIS

T brucei gambiense Suspects

Screening of patients in Africa has been extensively described and usually follows a screening cascade.[1,28,29] For suspects among travelers and immigrants in North America, a similar procedure can be chosen.[29] Patients who stayed in one of the *T brucei gambiense* endemic countries, traveled in the countryside, and report to have been bitten by biting flies should first be tested with the card agglutination test for trypanosomiasis/*T brucei gambiense* (CATT). This agglutination test requires a drop of blood, is fast and reliable with a high sensitivity and specificity, and can also be performed with blood on filter paper (**Fig. 4**).[30,31]

The next step is the parasitologic confirmation in blood or lymph node aspirate. An enlarged cervical lymph node is punctured and the aspirate examined under the microscope for moving trypanosomes (sensitivity of 40%–80%). Because the trypanosome density in the blood is very low and direct observation of a blood film is not sensitive enough, 2 concentration methods can be used. In the microhematocrit centrifugation technique, blood is centrifuged in capillary tubes and the buffy coat area examined for trypanosomes.[32] Even more sensitive is the miniature anion-exchange centrifugation technique, which separates the trypanosomes from the blood cells, which stick to the cellulose based on their charge.[33] Polymerase chain reaction (PCR) methods are also available to detect parasite DNA but kits are not yet available or validated.

Staging of positive patients is important for the selection of the appropriate drug for treatment. Cerebrospinal fluid (CSF) has to be collected, being careful not to have a contamination of blood. After centrifugation of the CSF, the pellet has to be examined for trypanosomes and for white blood cells. Trypanosomes or more than 5 white blood cells (WBC) per microliter are indicative for second-stage disease; some investigators tend to set the limit to 20 cells/μL. IgM in CSF is also considered an indication for second stage and can be determined by a latex agglutination test.[34]

T brucei rhodesiense Suspects

The diagnosis of patients with *T brucei rhodesiense* differs in many ways from the diagnosis for *T brucei gambiense*. The serologic CATT does not work for this

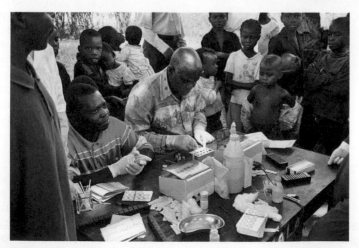

Fig. 4. CATT test performed in the field.

trypanosome species and can be skipped. The parasitologic tests have to be used in the first place and have a better chance to detect trypanosomes because patients with *T brucei rhodesiense* have a higher parasitemia as compared with patients with *T brucei gambiense* (**Fig. 5**). Research for better and less invasive diagnostic tests for detection as well as staging are being coordinated by the Foundation for Innovative Diagnostics, which was founded in 2006 (www.finddiagnostics.org). Projects are looking for methods to detect trypanosome antigens in blood and CSF, a new PCR technique called LAMP (loop-mediated isothermal amplification),[35] and new markers that are specific for the second stage of disease.

Diagnosis of Relapse

With increasing rates of drug resistance, the diagnosis of relapse becomes crucial. Control investigations of the CSF are recommended by the World Health Organization 3, 6, 12, 18, and 24 months after treatment.[36] However, different criteria defining a relapse according to WBC count in the CSF have been published and there is no consensus on the definition of a relapse.[37] An algorithm with CSF analysis at 6 and 12 months showed a sensitivity of 94% and a specificity of 98% for detection of relapses in patients with *T brucei gambiense* HAT: patients with a WBC of 5 cells/μL or fewer, without trypanosomes in CSF at 6 months had a low risk of treatment failure and did not need further tests. Patients with 50 cells/μL or more and/or trypanosomes in the CSF were considered as treatment failure. The group of 6 to 49 cells/μL and no trypanosomes in CSF needed further follow-up investigations.[38] Latex IgM trypanosome specific antibodies in the CSF were a less accurate indicator of relapse than WBC count.[38]

TREATMENT
Endemic Countries

The choice of the drug is directed by the species and the stage of the disease (**Table 1**). Recently, the recommended dose calculation for pentamidine has shifted from the base to the salt form, resulting in a significant reduction of the dosage of the active molecule while maintaining an excellent efficacy.

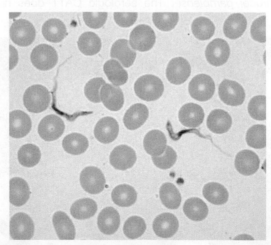

Fig. 5. *T brucei rhodesiense* trypomastigote forms in a Giemsa-stained blood smear. Morphologically, *T brucei rhodesiense* cannot be distinguished from *T brucei gambiense*. (*Courtesy of* Swiss TPH.)

Table 1
Treatment of HAT according to stage and species

	Trypanosoma brucei gambiense	*Trypanosoma brucei rhodesiense*
1st stage	Pentamidine 4 mg/kg at 24 hourly intervals Test dose of 4–5 mg kg^{-1} body weight at day 1, for 7 days IM (or as IV short infusion)	Suramin Test dose of 200 mg IV followed by 20 mg/kg on days 1, 3, 7, 14, and 21
2nd stage	Eflornithine intravenous eflornithine (100 mg/kg every 6 h) for 14 days Eflornithine/Nifurtimox combination IV eflornithine (200 mg/kg every 12 h) for 7 days and oral nifurtimox (15 mg/kg/d, every 8 h) for 10 days Melarsoprol 2.2 mg/kg IV 10 daily doses (and prednisone 1 mg/kg)	Melarsoprol 2.2 mg/kg IV 10 daily doses (and prednisone 1 mg/kg)

Abbreviations: IM, intramuscularly; IV, intravenous.

The main disadvantages of melarsoprol are the toxicity, including an encephalopathic syndrome (see later in this article), the long duration of treatment, and the increasing rate of treatment failures reaching up to 30%. A short-course melarsoprol treatment (daily injections of 2.2 mg/kg for 10 days) is established for *T brucei gambiense* HAT and recent results showed noninferiority to the previous treatment schedules for *T brucei rhodesiense* HAT.[39] In second-stage *T brucei rhodesiense* HAT, pretreatment with suramin is proposed in some national guidelines to reduce parasitemia before the initiation of melarsoprol, but the efficacy to avoid adverse events is not proven.

Eflornithine monotherapy clearly reduced the mortality (1.2%) in comparison with melarsoprol (4.2%–4.9%).[40] At present, the use of eflornithine against *T brucei rhodesiense* is not advised because of a lower susceptibility.[41] The main problems of eflornithine are the short half-life of the drug and the increasing rate of resistance to monotherapy. The total dosage of eflornithine can be reduced by half in the combination with nifurtimox (nifurtimox eflornithine combination treatment [NECT]), leading to increased cure rates (eflornithine monotreatment 92%; NECT 97%–98%). Although hematotoxic effects were reduced by half, nausea and vomiting increased to 50%.[42] Because cases of resistance against NECT were already observed, new drugs are desperately needed.

The most advanced new drug in the pipeline is fexinidazole, which belongs to the nitroimidazole class. The substance proved to be orally active against *T brucei gambiense* and *T brucei rhodesiense* in animal studies and had an excellent safety profile. Because it penetrates the blood-brain barrier, it should be effective in both stages of sleeping sickness.[43]

Non Endemic Countries

Because of the paucity of HAT outside Africa, treatment recommendations are based on studies conducted in endemic regions; however, the intravenous application of pentamidine is preferred in travelers because of the risk for rhabdomyolysis observed with intramuscular administration. Unfortunately, the limited availability of the drugs outside endemic regions and time pressure often determine the choice of drug.

Thus, in some patients with first-stage *T brucei rhodesiense* HAT, treatment was initiated with the more easily available pentamidine, switching to suramin as soon as it became available.[8] Because treatment of sleeping sickness is quite complex and might be associated with severe adverse events, it is advisable to consult a specialist in tropical medicine (**Table 2**).

Encephalopathic Syndrome

The encephalopathic syndrome is the most feared adverse event of treatment of sleeping sickness. It comprises convulsions, progressive coma, and psychotic reactions. It occurs in patients treated with melarsoprol with an average frequency of 4.7% for *T brucei gambiense* and 8.0% for *T brucei rhodesiense* HAT and has a fatality rate of about 50%. Dexamethasone 0.5 to 0.6 mg/kg/d divided in 4 to 6 doses against cerebral edema, anticonvulsive treatment in the presence of convulsions, correction of electrolyte dysbalance, and vasoactive substances to control arterial hypotension are recommended, but are not validated in a controlled trial. The prophylactic use of

Table 2
Adverse events of HAT treatment

Drug	Adverse Effect
Pentamidine	Aseptic abscess Diabetes, hypoglycemia Proteinuria Rhabdomyolysis Hypotension Subjective complaints of myalgia, nausea and gustative abnormalities, headache, pain at the injection side, abdominal pain
Suramin	Immediate reactions: nausea, vomiting, colic pain Anaphylactic shock (<1/2000), urticaria Late reactions (3–48 hours) Febrile reaction Photophobia, lacrimation Hyperesthesia Delayed reactions Common: Kidney damage, proteinuria (usually mild) Rare: Allergic dermatitis, polyneuropathia, agranulocytosis, hemolytic anemia
Melarsoprol	Encephalopathic reaction • Convulsions • Progressive coma Skin reactions Maculopapular or bullous eruptions, exfoliative dermatitis Polyneuropathy Diarrhea, hypotension Electrocardiogram alteration, arrhythmia
Eflornithine	Convulsions Anemia, leukopenia, thrombopenia Diarrhea, nausea, vomiting, abdominal pain
Eflornithine/Nifurtimox combination	Nausea, vomiting Convulsions Anemia, leukopenia, thrombopenia

prednisone (1 mg/kg) reduces incidence and mortality of the syndrome. A comparison of the encephalopathic syndrome between melarsoprol and eflornithine is difficult, because the definition of this syndrome has not been adopted in the eflornithine trials. Whereas alterations of the level of consciousness (ie, coma) appear more frequently with melarsoprol (4%–5%) than with eflornithine (1%–2%), convulsions are less frequently observed with melarsoprol (2%–5%) than with eflornithine/NECT (5%–13%).

PREVENTION/MANAGEMENT AFTER BITE OF A TSETSE FLY

A vaccine for sleeping sickness is not available and chemoprophylaxis is not recommended because of the toxicity of the available drugs and the low risk of infection. Travelers should take notice of the risk of sleeping sickness, and be informed on the transmission and clinical presentation of the disease and prevention. The only preventive measure is the protection from tsetse fly bites. The flies are attracted to bright or contrasting colors, particularly blue, as well as to the dust and motion of vehicles. They can bite through thin clothes and insect repellents provide only partial protection. As routine preventive measures, travelers should avoid known areas of tsetse flies, travel in endemic foci in cars with screened or closed windows, use insect repellent, and wear wrist-length and ankle-length clothes.

After a bite of a tsetse fly, the patient has to be observed. The risk of an infection is very low. In case of a chancre, fever, or other symptoms, trypanosomes have to be looked for in an aspirate of the chancre, in the blood, and eventually in a lymph node aspirate.

REFERENCES

1. Brun R, Blum J, Chappuis F, et al. Human African trypanosomiasis. Lancet 2010; 375(9709):148–59.
2. Horn D, McCulloch R. Molecular mechanisms underlying the control of antigenic variation in African trypanosomes. Curr Opin Microbiol 2010;13(6):700–5.
3. Vanhamme L. The human trypanolytic factor: a drug shaped naturally. Infect Disord Drug Targets 2010;10(4):266–82.
4. Simarro PP, Jannin J, Cattand P. Eliminating human African trypanosomiasis: where do we stand and what comes next? PLoS Med 2008;5(2):e55.
5. Steverding D. The history of African trypanosomiasis. Parasit Vectors 2008;1(1):3.
6. Simarro PP, Diarra A, Ruiz Postigo JA, et al. The Human African Trypanosomiasis Control and Surveillance Programme of the World Health Organization 2000-2009: the way forward. PLoS Negl Trop Dis 2011;5(2):e1007.
7. Chappuis F, Lima MA, Flevaud L, et al. Human African trypanosomiasis in areas without surveillance. Emerg Infect Dis 2010;16(2):354–6.
8. Urech K, Neumayr A, Blum J. Sleeping sickness in travelers: Do they really sleep? PLoS Negl Trop Dis 2011;5(11):e1358.
9. Checchi F, Filipe JA, Haydon DT, et al. Estimates of the duration of the early and late stage of gambiense sleeping sickness. BMC Infect Dis 2008;8:16.
10. Blum J, Schmid C, Burri C. Clinical aspects of 2541 patients with second stage human African trypanosomiasis. Acta Trop 2006;97(1):55–64.
11. Buguet A, Bisser S, Josenando T, et al. Sleep structure: a new diagnostic tool for stage determination in sleeping sickness. Acta Trop 2005;93(1):107–17.
12. Buguet A, Bourdon L, Bisser S, et al. [Sleeping sickness: major disorders of circadian rhythm]. Med Trop (Mars) 2001;61(4-5):328–39 [in French].
13. Lundkvist GB, Kristensson K, Bentivoglio M. Why trypanosomes cause sleeping sickness. Physiology (Bethesda) 2004;19:198–206.

14. Kennedy PG. Human African trypanosomiasis—neurological aspects. J Neurol 2006;253(4):411–6.
15. Blum JA, Burri C, Hatz C, et al. Sleeping hearts: the role of the heart in sleeping sickness (human African trypanosomiasis). Trop Med Int Health 2007;12(12): 1422–32.
16. Blum JA, Schmid C, Burri C, et al. Cardiac alterations in human African trypanosomiasis (T.b. gambiense) with respect to the disease stage and antiparasitic treatment. PLoS Negl Trop Dis 2009;3(2):e383.
17. Blum JA, Schmid C, Hatz C, et al. Sleeping glands? The role of endocrine disorders in sleeping sickness (T.b. gambiense human African trypanosomiasis). Acta Trop 2007;104(1):16–24.
18. Reincke M, Arlt W, Heppner C, et al. Neuroendocrine dysfunction in African trypanosomiasis. The role of cytokines. Ann N Y Acad Sci 1998;840:809–21.
19. MacLean LM, Odiit M, Chisi JE, et al. Focus-specific clinical profiles in human African trypanosomiasis caused by Trypanosoma brucei rhodesiense. PLoS Negl Trop Dis 2010;4(12):e906.
20. Kuepfer I, Hhary EP, Allan M, et al. Clinical presentation of T.b. rhodesiense sleeping sickness in second stage patients from Tanzania and Uganda. PLoS Negl Trop Dis 2011;5(3):e968.
21. Blum JA, Neumayr AL, Hatz C. Human African trypanosomiasis in endemic populations and travellers. Eur J Clin Microbiol Infect Dis 2011. [Epub ahead of print].
22. Duggan AJ, Hutchinson MP. Sleeping sickness in Europeans: a review of 109 cases. J Trop Med Hyg 1966;69(6):124–31.
23. Sabbah P, Brosset C, Imbert P, et al. Human African trypanosomiasis: MRI. Neuroradiology 1997;39(10):708–10.
24. Gill DS, Chatha DS, Carpio-O'Donovan R. MR imaging findings in African trypanosomiasis. AJNR Am J Neuroradiol 2003;24(7):1383–5.
25. Braakman HM, van de Molengraft FJ, Hubert WW, et al. Lethal African trypanosomiasis in a traveler: MRI and neuropathology. Neurology 2006;66(7):1094–6.
26. Serrano-Gonzalez C, Velilla I, Fortuno B, et al. [Neuroimaging and efficacy of treatment in advanced African trypanosomiasis]. Rev Neurol 1996;24(136): 1554–7 [in Spanish].
27. Bedat-Millet AL, Charpentier S, Monge-Strauss MF, et al. [Psychiatric presentation of human African trypanosomiasis: overview of diagnostic pitfalls, interest of difluoromethylornithine treatment and contribution of magnetic resonance imaging]. Rev Neurol (Paris) 2000;156(5):505–9 [in French].
28. Chappuis F, Loutan L, Simarro P, et al. Options for field diagnosis of human African trypanosomiasis. Clin Microbiol Rev 2005;18(1):133–46.
29. Lejon V, Boelaert M, Jannin J, et al. The challenge of Trypanosoma brucei gambiense sleeping sickness diagnosis outside Africa. Lancet Infect Dis 2003;3(12): 804–8.
30. Chappuis F, Pittet A, Bovier PA, et al. Field evaluation of the CATT/Trypanosoma brucei gambiense on blood-impregnated filter papers for diagnosis of human African trypanosomiasis in southern Sudan. Trop Med Int Health 2002;7(11): 942–8.
31. Magnus E, Lejon V, Bayon D, et al. Evaluation of an EDTA version of CATT/Trypanosoma brucei gambiense for serological screening of human blood samples. Acta Trop 2002;81(1):7–12.
32. Woo PT. The haematocrit centrifuge technique for the diagnosis of African trypanosomiasis. Acta Trop 1970;27(4):384–6.

33. Lumsden WHR, Kimber CD, Evans DA, et al. *Trypanosoma brucei*—miniature anion-exchange centrifugation technique for detection of low parasitemias—adaptation for field use. Trans R Soc Trop Med Hyg 1979;73(3):312–7.
34. Lejon V, Legros D, Richer M, et al. IgM quantification in the cerebrospinal fluid of sleeping sickness patients by a latex card agglutination test. Trop Med Int Health 2002;7(8):685–92.
35. Njiru ZK, Mikosza ASJ, Matovu E, et al. African trypanosomiasis: Sensitive and rapid detection of the sub-genus Trypanozoon by loop-mediated isothermal amplification (LAMP) of parasite DNA. Int J Parasitol 2008;38(5):589–99.
36. Control and surveillance of African trypanosomiasis. Geneva: WHO; 1998. Report No.881. WHO Technical rapport.
37. Mumba ND, Lejon V, N'Siesi FX, et al. Comparison of operational criteria for treatment outcome in gambiense human African trypanosomiasis. Trop Med Int Health 2009;14(4):438–44.
38. Mumba ND, Lejon V, Pyana P, et al. How to shorten patient follow-up after treatment for *Trypanosoma brucei gambiense* sleeping sickness. J Infect Dis 2010; 201(3):453–63.
39. Burri C, Nkunku S, Merolle A, et al. Efficacy of new, concise schedule for melarsoprol in treatment of sleeping sickness caused by *Trypanosoma brucei gambiense*: a randomised trial. Lancet 2000;355(9213):1419–25.
40. Chappuis F, Udayraj N, Stietenroth K, et al. Eflornithine is safer than melarsoprol for the treatment of second-stage *Trypanosoma brucei gambiense* human African trypanosomiasis. Clin Infect Dis 2005;41(5):748–51.
41. Iten M, Matovu E, Brun R, et al. Innate lack of susceptibility of Ugandan *Trypanosoma brucei rhodesiense* to Dl-alpha-difluoromethylornithine (Dfmo). Trop Med Parasitol 1995;46(3):190–4.
42. Priotto G, Kasparian S, Mutombo W, et al. Nifurtimox-eflornithine combination therapy for second-stage African *Trypanosoma brucei gambiense* trypanosomiasis: a multicentre, randomised, phase III, non-inferiority trial. Lancet 2009; 374(9683):56–64.
43. Burri C. Chemotherapy against human African trypanosomiasis: is there a road to success? Parasitology 2010;137(14):1987–94.

American Trypanosomiasis (Chagas Disease)

Anis Rassi Jr, MD, PhD[a],*, Anis Rassi, MD[a],
Joffre Marcondes de Rezende, MD[b]

KEYWORDS

- Chagas disease • Chagas heart disease • American trypanosomiasis
- *Trypanosoma cruzi* • Epidemiology • Treatment

KEY POINTS

- Chagas disease still represents a major public health challenge in Latin America, where 8 to 10 million people are infected. Because of growing population movements, the disease has also spread to other continents.

- The disease is caused by the protozoan parasite *T cruzi* and transmitted to humans usually by the faeces of triatomine bugs or occasionally by nonvectorial mechanisms, such as blood transfusion and mother to fetus.

- Chagas disease has 2 phases, acute and chronic. Acute-phase disease is often asymptomatic. Up to 40%-50% of chronically infected patients develop progressive cardiomyopathy and/or motility disturbances of the esophagus and colon.

- The disease, in both phases, is curable with the available antitrypanosomal drugs (benznidazole and nifurtimox). The sooner the treatment is initiated after infection, the greater the chance of cure.

- In patients with established chronic disease, several pharmacologic and nonpharmacologic interventions are available and may prevent or delay disease complications.

Chagas disease, or American trypanosomiasis, is caused by the parasite *Trypanosoma cruzi*, and was discovered in 1909 by the Brazilian physician Carlos Chagas (1879–1934).[1] While still at a young age he described the etiologic agent, vectors, principal reservoirs, and mechanism of infection, as well as the acute clinical manifestations of the first human case. However, Chagas disease is most likely an ancient disease: *T cruzi* DNA has been recorded in tissue specimens of mummies in pre-Colombian Andean countries from as early as 9000 years ago (~7050 BC).[2]

T cruzi is a protozoan of the *Sarcomastigophora* phylum, *Mastigophora* subphylum, *Kinetoplastida* order, and Trypanosomatidae family (**Fig. 1**). It has a flagellum and its

The authors have nothing to disclose.
[a] Division of Cardiology, Anis Rassi Hospital, Avenida José Alves 453, Setor Oeste, Goiânia, GO 74110-020, Brazil; [b] Instituto de Gastroenterologia de Goiânia, Avenida B, 435, Setor Oeste, Goiânia, GO 74435-010, Brazil
* Corresponding author.
E-mail address: arassijr@terra.com.br

Infect Dis Clin N Am 26 (2012) 275–291
doi:10.1016/j.idc.2012.03.002
0891-5520/12/$ – see front matter © 2012 Elsevier Inc. All rights reserved.

id.theclinics.com

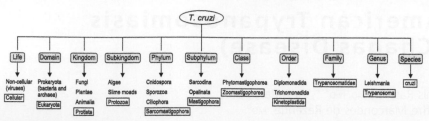

Fig. 1. Taxonomy of *Trypanosoma cruzi*. Eukaryota, cell organisms that have a cell nucleus and specialized organelles; Protista, a group of eukaryotic organisms (usually microorganisms), without the cardinal characteristics of plants and animals, also known as lower forms of plants and animals; Protozoa, the lowest form of animal life ("first animals"), typically unicellular; Sarcomastigophora, protozoa that locomote by flagellae, pseudopodia, or both; Mastigophora, use flagella for motility; Zoomastigophora, animal-like flagellates; Kinetoplastida, order of protozoa characterized by the possession of a kinetoplast (a region rich in DNA within the mitochondrion of the cell); *Trypanosoma*, name derived from the Greek *trypano* (auger, drill) and *soma* (body) because of their corkscrew-like motion; *cruzi*, species of *Trypanosoma* discovered by Carlos Chagas and named in honor of Dr Oswaldo Cruz, his mentor and a famous Brazilian bacteriologist.

single mitochondrion contains the kinetoplast, an extranuclear DNA network corresponding to the parasite's mitochondrial genome, which is localized near the flagellate's basal body.

This review discusses mechanisms of transmission and the life cycle of *T cruzi*, its epidemiology, pathogenesis, clinical manifestations, diagnosis, and treatment, with an emphasis on the effectiveness of antiparasitic treatment in the chronic phase of the disease.

MECHANISMS OF TRANSMISSION
Vector Transmission

Chagas disease is transmitted to human beings and to more than 150 species of domestic and wild mammals mainly by large, bloodsucking insects of the *Arthropoda* phylum, *Hexapoda* subphylum, *Hemiptera* order, Reduviidae family, and Triatominae subfamily. Although some 140 species of triatomines (kissing or cone-nosed bugs) have been identified, only a few are competent vectors for *T cruzi*. The main vectors are *Triatoma infestans, Triatoma brasiliensis*, and *Panstrongylus megistus* in the Southern Cone countries, *Rhodnius prolixus* and *Triatoma dimidiata* in the Andean Pact countries and parts of Central America, and *T dimidiata* and *Triatoma barberi* in Mexico.[3] Birds, reptiles, and amphibians are refractory to *T cruzi*; however, in some situations birds (mainly chickens) are important sources of blood meals for triatomines, which are strictly hematophagous.

Other Mechanisms of Transmission

Chagas disease can be transmitted to man by nonvector mechanisms: blood transfusion and congenital transmission are the main causes of infestation in urban zones and nonendemic countries. The risk of Chagas disease after transfusion of 1 unit of blood from an infected donor is as high as 10% to 20%.[4] Because trypomastigotes are predominantly separated into the platelet fraction during centrifugation, the transmission risk has been reported to be higher for transfusion of platelets than for other blood components. Congenital transmission occurs in at least 5% of pregnancies in chronically infected women in some regions of Bolivia, Chile, and Paraguay, and in 1% to 2% or less in most other endemic countries.[4]

Transmission can also occur from transplantation of a solid organ or bone marrow from a chronically infected donor, which has been well documented in Latin America. Furthermore, Chagas disease can be orally transmitted by ingestion of food or liquid contaminated with *T cruzi*. Such transmission is usually responsible for regional outbreaks of acute infection in areas devoid of domiciled insect vectors. More rarely, *T cruzi* can be transmitted through laboratory accidents to people who work with live parasites.

LIFE CYCLE OF *T CRUZI*

The life cycle of *T cruzi* is complex, with several developmental forms in insect vectors and mammalian hosts.[4] The insects become infected by sucking blood from animals or human beings who have circulating parasites (trypomastigote forms). In the digestive tract of triatomines, the trypomastigotes differentiate into epimastigotes (multiplicative form) and then to metacyclic trypomastigotes in the final portion of the intestine. Infection of mammals occurs when they come into contact with the infective metacyclic forms of the parasite that are eliminated with the feces of triatomines after feeding. This contact occurs through the mucosa or through injury, either preexistent or resulting from the bite of the bug.

Once in the vertebrate host, the metacyclic trypomastigotes invade the local reticuloendothelial and connective cells, and differentiate into amastigotes that begin replicating by binary fission. When the cell is swollen with amastigotes, they transform back into trypomastigotes by growing flagellae. The trypomastigotes lyse the cells, invade adjacent tissues, and spread via the lymphatics and bloodstream to distant sites, mainly muscle cells (cardiac, smooth, and skeletal) and ganglion cells, where they undergo further cycles of intracellular multiplication. The cycle of transmission is completed when circulating trypomastigotes are taken up in blood meals by vectors.[4]

EPIDEMIOLOGY AND GEOGRAPHIC DISTRIBUTION

T cruzi is restricted to South America, Central America, and parts of North America (Mexico and southern United States). The Caribbean islands are free of Chagas disease. In rural Latin America, poor housing conditions favor vector infestation and acute Chagas disease usually occurs in children younger than 12 years. Historically transmission and morbidity were concentrated in this region, but migration has brought chronic infected individuals to cities both in and outside of Latin America, making Chagas disease a public health problem of global concern. According to estimates by the Pan American Health Organization (PAHO)[5] and the World Health Organization (WHO),[6] 7.7 to 10 million people are chronically infected with *T cruzi*, and 10,000 to 14,000 deaths per year are caused by Chagas disease.

It is notable that as a result of successful programs involving vector control, blood bank screening, and education of at-risk populations, both of these estimates are substantially lower than a few decades ago. A major program, begun in 1991 in the Southern Cone nations of South America (Uruguay, Paraguay, Bolivia, Brazil, Chile, and Argentina), has provided the framework for much of this progress.[7] Uruguay and Chile were certified free of transmission by the main domiciliary vector species (*T infestans*) in the late 1990s, and Brazil was declared transmission-free in 2006. In addition, blood donor screening has steadily increased, with coverage now approaching 100% in most endemic countries.

The highest prevalences of Chagas disease have been reported from Bolivia (6.8%), Argentina (4.1%), El Salvador (3.4%), Honduras (3.1%), and Paraguay (2.5%).

However, 2 remaining countries with prevalences of about 1% (Brazil and Mexico), together with Argentina, are home to almost 60% of all people infected with *T cruzi* in Latin America.[4]

CHAGAS DISEASE IN THE UNITED STATES AND OTHER NONENDEMIC COUNTRIES

Acute Chagas disease is rare in the United States.[8] Six human cases of autochthonous transmission and 5 instances of transmission by blood transfusion have been reported. Furthermore, 3 infected donors transmitted *T cruzi* to 5 recipients of solid organs, 2 of whom received cardiac transplants. The rarity of autochthonous vector-borne transmission is presumably due to better housing conditions and less efficient vectors, but many infections probably go undetected. The 2 principal vectors in the United States (*Triatoma sanguisuga* and *Triatoma gerstaeckeri*) have relatively low infection rates (25% and 45%, respectively), display different feeding habits, and often defecate 30 minutes or more after feeding, making them likely to be somewhat inefficient at stercorarian transmission to hosts.[9]

By contrast, the prevalence of chronic *T cruzi* infections in the United States has increased substantially in the past 20 years. An estimated 23 million immigrants from endemic countries live in the United States, about 17 million of whom are Mexicans.[10] The United States ranks seventh worldwide for the total number of people infected with *T cruzi*: in 2009 an estimated 300,167 infected people lived in the United States.[11] Screening of United States blood donations for *T cruzi* infection began in January 2007, and now covers most of the blood supply. About 1 in 28,000 donors has *T cruzi* infection, and so far more than 1400 infected donors have been identified and deferred permanently from donation.[8]

The southern states of the United States have an active sylvatic transmission cycle involving many wild animal reservoirs. Recent serologic and parasitologic surveys suggest that raccoons, opossums, and woodrats are the main hosts, with prevalence of infections of 38.7%, 28.0%, and 33.2%, respectively.[9]

Many individuals with Chagas disease have emigrated from Latin America to countries other than the United States, such as Canada, Australia, Japan, France, Italy, Sweden, Switzerland, and England. But by far the largest population of these infected immigrants lives in Spain (47,000–67,000), with most originating from Ecuador, Argentina, Bolivia, and Peru.[12] Nonendemic countries with large immigrant populations have also begun to establish interventions to prevent transfusion-associated *T cruzi* infection. European legislation prevents people with a history of Chagas disease from donating blood. However, most infected people are asymptomatic and unaware of their status.

PATHOGENESIS

Chagas disease occurs in 2 phases: acute and chronic. Initial infection at the site of parasite entry is characterized by the presence of infective trypomastigotes in leukocytes and cells of subcutaneous tissues, and by the development of interstitial edema, lymphocytic infiltration, and reactive hyperplasia of adjacent lymph nodes. After dissemination through the lymphatic system and the bloodstream, parasites concentrate mainly in the muscles (including the myocardium) and ganglion cells. The characteristic pseudocysts that are present in some tissues are intracellular aggregates of multiplying forms (amastigotes).

Chagas disease is the most severe parasitic infection of the heart,[13] and the heart is the organ most often affected in individuals with chronic *T cruzi* infection.[14] Changes include thinning of the ventricular walls, biventricular enlargement, apical aneurysms, and mural thrombi. Widespread destruction of myocardial cells, diffuse fibrosis, edema, lymphocytic infiltration of the myocardium, and scarring of the conduction system are often apparent, but parasites are difficult to find in myocardial tissue by conventional histologic methods. In chronic Chagas disease of the gastrointestinal tract, the esophagus and colon can be dilated to varying degrees. On microscopic examination, focal inflammatory lesions with lymphocytic infiltration are seen, and the number of neurons in the myenteric plexus might be markedly reduced.

Evidence accumulated with highly powerful and sensitive methods, such as immunohistochemistry and polymerase chain reaction (PCR), indicates that myocardial damage in chronic *T cruzi* infection is due to the persistence of parasites and the accompanying chronic inflammation, rather than autoimmune mechanisms. Cardiac denervation (mainly parasympathetic), and abnormalities in the coronary microvasculature might also contribute to the pathogenesis of chronic lesions.[15]

CLINICAL MANIFESTATIONS
Acute Chagas Disease

In most individuals, irrespective of the mechanism of transmission, acute Chagas infection is asymptomatic, which is probably because the parasite load is fairly small.[4,10] Symptoms that develop at around 8 to 10 days after invasion by the parasites, or at 20 to 40 days after transfusion of *T cruzi*–infected blood, include prolonged fever, malaise enlargement of the liver, spleen, and lymph nodes, and subcutaneous edema (localized or generalized). In vector-borne transmission, there are signs of portal of entry of *T cruzi*: entry through the skin produces the chagoma, an indurated area of erythema and swelling, whereas entry via the ocular mucous membranes produces Romaña's sign, the classic finding in acute Chagas disease, which consists of unilateral painless edema of the palpebrae and periocular tissues. Severe myocarditis develops rarely; most deaths in acute Chagas disease are due to heart failure. Neurologic signs are not common, but meningoencephalitis occurs occasionally, especially in children younger than 2 years.[4,10]

An electrocardiogram (ECG) might show sinus tachycardia, first-degree atrioventricular block, low QRS voltage, or primary T-wave changes; and a chest radiograph might show variable degrees of cardiomegaly. Repetition of the ECG and chest radiograph is crucial for detection of these abnormalities.[16]

Echocardiography was recently introduced, which explains the lack of information about its performance during the acute phase because most of such cases were reported before this method was available. Nevertheless, variable degrees of pericardial effusion, mitral or tricuspid valve regurgitation, and concentric hypertrophy of the left ventricle have been described, with more than one abnormality often seen in the same patient.[17]

Chronic Chagas Disease

The chronic phase begins 2 to 3 months after initial infection, when the clinical manifestations (if present) of the acute disease will have resolved in virtually all infected individuals even if the infection has not been treated with trypanocidal drugs.[4] About 60% to 70% of these patients will have the indeterminate form of chronic Chagas disease, which has no clinical symptoms. This form is characterized by positivity for antibodies against *T cruzi* in serum, a normal 12-lead ECG, and normal radiologic examination of the chest, esophagus, and colon. The remaining patients (30%– 40%) will develop a determinate form—cardiac, digestive (mainly megaesophagus and megacolon), or cardiodigestive—usually 10 to 30 years after initial infection.[4]

Reactivation of Chagas disease can also occur in chronically infected patients who become immunologically compromised, for example, from coinfection with human immunodeficiency virus (HIV) or immunosuppressive drugs. Fever, myocarditis, panniculitis, and skin lesions are common in recipients of solid-organ or bone marrow transplants, whereas the most common manifestations of reactivation in patients with AIDS are meningoencephalitis and lesions of the central nervous system that resemble the lesions of cerebral toxoplasmosis.

Cardiac form

The cardiac form is the most serious and frequent manifestation of chronic disease.[14] This form develops in 20% to 30% of individuals and typically leads to abnormalities of the conduction system, bradyarrhythmias and tachyarrhythmias, apical aneurysms, cardiac failure, thromboembolism, and sudden death. The most common ECG abnormalities are right bundle branch block, left anterior fascicular block, ventricular premature beats, ST-T changes, abnormal Q waves, and low QRS voltage. The combination of right bundle branch block and left anterior fascicular block is very typical in Chagas heart disease.[4,13,14] Frequent, complex ventricular premature beats, including couplets and runs of nonsustained ventricular tachycardia, are a common finding on Holter monitoring or stress testing.[18]

Sustained ventricular tachycardia is another hallmark of the disease, and seems to result from an intramyocardial or subepicardial reentry circuit that is usually located at the inferior-posterior-lateral wall of the left ventricle.[4,14,18]

Heart failure is often a late manifestation of Chagas heart disease. Such failure is usually biventricular with a predominance of right-sided failure at advanced stages, with peripheral edema, hepatomegaly, and ascites more prominent than pulmonary congestion. Isolated left-sided failure can occur in the early stages of cardiac decompensation.[4,14] Heart failure of chagasic etiology is associated with higher mortality than is heart failure from other causes.[19] Systemic and pulmonary embolisms arising from mural thrombi in the cardiac chambers are frequent.

Sudden cardiac death accounts for nearly two-thirds of all deaths in Chagas heart disease, followed by refractory heart failure (25%–30%) and thromboembolism (10%–15%).[20] Sudden death can occur even in patients who were previously asymptomatic. It is usually associated with ventricular tachycardia and fibrillation or, more rarely, with complete atrioventricular block or sinus node dysfunction. **Fig. 2** summarizes the common findings associated with chronic Chagas heart disease.

Digestive form

The digestive form of Chagas disease is characterized by alterations in the motor, secretory, and absorptive functions of the esophagus and the gastrointestinal tract.[21] Lesions of the enteric nervous system are pivotal in the pathogenesis of Chagas digestive megasyndromes. The structure most often affected is the myoenteric plexus of Auerbach, which is located between the longitudinal and circular muscular layers of the digestive tract. Although most damage to the neurons of this plexus and the nervous fibers occurs during acute infection, further neuronal loss occurs slowly throughout the chronic phase. Denervation occurs to variable degrees, is irregular and noncontinuous, and probably depends on both parasitic and host factors. The esophagus and the distal colon, because of their physiology, are the most frequently compromised segments. Denervation leads to loss of motor coordination and achalasia of the sphincters, preventing these segments from emptying semisolid material, thereby causing dilatation; this is the pathophysiologic mechanism underlying chagasic megaesophagus and megacolon.

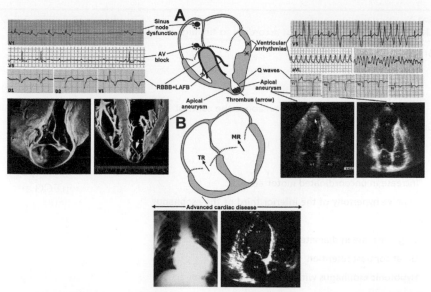

Fig. 2. Common findings in chronic Chagas heart disease. (*A*) Cardiac segmental form. (*B*) Cardiac global dilated form. AV, atrioventricular; LAFB, left anterior fascicular block; MR, mitral regurgitation; RBBB, right bundle branch block; TR, tricuspid regurgitation. (*Adapted from* Rassi A Jr, Rassi A, Marin-Neto JA. Chagas disease. Lancet 2010;375:1395; with permission.)

The digestive form is seen almost exclusively south of the Amazon basin (mainly in Brazil, Argentina, Chile, and Bolivia), and is rare in northern South America, Central America, and Mexico. This geographic distribution is probably due to differences in parasite strains. Gastrointestinal dysfunction (mainly megaesophagus, megacolon, or both) develops in about 10% to 15% of chronically infected patients.[4,21]

The megaesophagus causes dysphagia, regurgitation, and esophageal pain. Other less frequent symptoms are hiccups, pyrosis, and hypersalivation accompanied by parotid hypertrophy. Malnutrition occurs with progression of the disease. Radiologic examination, which is essential to confirm the diagnosis and stage of disease from the morphofunctional characteristics of the esophagus, identifies 4 groups and is very important for the selection of the most appropriate therapy (**Box 1**).[21]

Most cases of megacolon are associated with megaesophagus. The most common symptoms are constipation, meteorism, dyskinesia and, less often, abdominal colicky pain. Constipation can be absent in 25% to 30% of individuals who have radiologic dilatation of the colon. On physical examination, an increase in the abdominal volume is observed. Because the distal colon is the most affected segment, the distended sigmoid occupies a large part of the abdominal cavity and can be localized by palpation and percussion outside its normal topography. Prolonged retention of feces in the distal colon leads to formation of fecaloma, which can be diagnosed by simple abdominal palpation as an elastic tumor that can be molded by pressure. Rectal examination will detect a fecaloma at the rectal ampulla.[21]

Other segments and organs of the digestive system might be compromised in Chagas disease, causing functional and morphologic alterations that can be detected by different investigative methods, but with a much lower prevalence and impact than the lesions involving esophagus and colon.[21]

Nearly 20% of patients with megaesophagus have gastric involvement. The main changes are rapid gastric emptying for liquids and delayed emptying for solids,

---

Box 1
Classification of megaesophagus according to findings of radiologic examination

Group I

    Normal diameter

    Minimal contrast retention

    Presence of a residual air column above the contrast

Group II

    Moderate dilatation

    Some contrast retention

    Increase in uncoordinated motor activity

    Relative hypertony of the inferior third of the esophagus

Group III

    Large increase in diameter

    Great contrast retention

    Hypotonic esophagus with weak or absent motor activity

Group IV

    Large increase in volume

    Atonic, elongated esophagus, lying on the right diaphragmatic dome

---

reduced adaptive relaxation of the stomach in response to distension, altered gastric electric rhythm, chronic gastritis, and hypertrophy of pyloric muscle (pylorus achalasia). On radiologic examination the gastric volume is extremely variable, and patients with advanced megaesophagus typically do not have air in the stomach.[21]

Duodenum is, after the esophagus and colon, the segment that most often shows dilatation. Megaduodenum is nearly always associated with other visceromegaly. The dilatation can be localized only at the bulb (megabulb) or at the second and third segments, or can affect the entire duodenal arcade. Even when no dilatation is present, dyskinesia and hyperreactivity to cholinergic stimuli are common because of enteric denervation. Symptoms caused by megaduodenum can be confused with dyspepsia of gastric origin, of the dysmotility type.[21]

Findings of histopathologic studies have shown less denervation at the small intestine than at the esophagus and colon. Dilatation of jejunum or ileum, characterizing megajejunum or megaileum, is rare, with few published cases.[21]

An intrinsic denervation of the gallbladder might also be observed, leading to motor alterations in gallbladder filling and emptying. Manometric alterations have also been recorded at the Oddi sphincter. Nevertheless, cholecystomegaly and choledochodilatation are not frequent. An increased prevalence of cholelithiasis has been reported in chagasic patients with megaesophagus or megacolon, or both.[21]

Salivary glands, mainly parotids, are hypertrophic in patients with megaesophagus, a common finding in any obstructive esophageal disease because the esophageal-salivary reflex produces hypersalivation.[21] Patients with megaesophagus also have an increased prevalence of cancer of the esophagus. Conversely, an increased frequency of colorectal cancer has not been reported in patients with chagasic megacolon. The gastrointestinal manifestations of chronic Chagas disease are shown in **Fig. 3**.

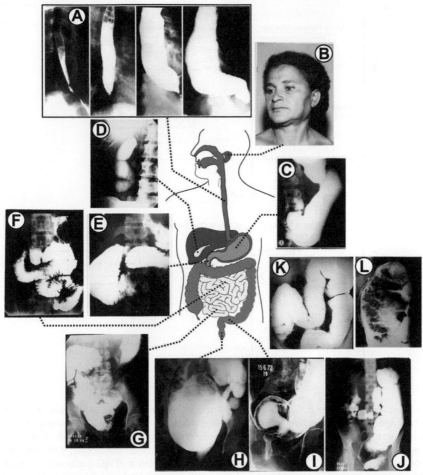

Fig. 3. Gastrointestinal manifestations of chronic Chagas disease. (*A*) Megaesophagus (groups, I, II, III, and IV). (*B*) Hypertrophic parotids in a patient with megaesophagus. (*C*) Megastomach associated with megaesophagus group IV. (*D*) Cholecystomegaly. (*E*) Megaduodenum. (*F*) Megajejunum. (*G*) Megaileum. (*H*) Megarectum. (*I*) Megasigmoid. (*J*) Megarectosigmoid. (*K*) Total megacolon. (*L*) Fecaloma. *C, D, E, F,* and *G* are rare manifestations.

Cardiodigestive form

The cardiodigestive form is a combination of heart disease with megaesophagus or megacolon, or both. In most countries, the development of megaesophagus usually precedes heart and colon disease, but the exact prevalence of the cardiodigestive form is not known because few appropriate studies have been done.

DIAGNOSIS

Diagnosis of acute infection is based on parasite detection (**Fig. 4**A). Microscopic examination of fresh anticoagulated blood or the buffy coat is the simplest way to see motile trypomastigotes. Parasites can also be seen in Giemsa-stained thin and thick blood smears.[4,10] Microhematocrit can be used for the same purpose, and is the method of choice to identify congenital infection because of its heightened

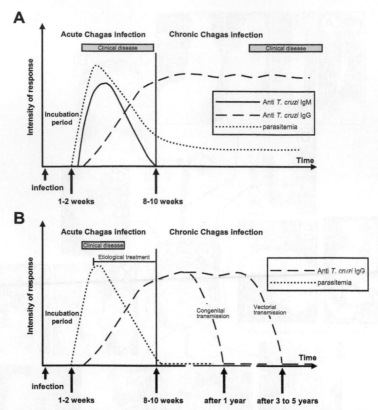

Fig. 4. Serologic and parasitologic evolution in acute Chagas infection. (*A*) Untreated patients. One to 2 weeks after infection with *T cruzi*, individuals undergo an acute phase that lasts approximately 2 months, and is characterized by intense parasitemia, high levels of anti *T cruzi* IgM antibodies, and increasing levels of immunoglobulin G (IgG) antibodies; with the resolution of the acute infection, parasitemia becomes extremely low and IgG antibodies reach their maximum level, persisting elevated and lifelong. (*B*) Treated and cured patients. Cure at the acute phase is accompanied by clearance of parasitemia, which occurs immediately after etiologic treatment, and by seronegative conversion, which occurs after about 1 year for congenital Chagas disease and after 3 to 5 years for vector-borne Chagas disease. Treated and uncured patients present a response that is similar to that of untreated patients.

sensitivity and the small amount of blood needed. Microscopic examination of cord blood or peripheral blood of the neonate by this technique is strongly recommended during the first month of life. Serologic testing is not helpful in diagnosing acute Chagas disease. Although the detection of anti–*T cruzi* immunoglobulin M (IgM) could be used (see **Fig. 4**A), IgM serology assays are not widely available and standardized.[4,10]

In the chronic phase, because of low and probably intermittent parasitemia, diagnosis relies on serologic detection of specific immunoglobulin G (IgG) antibodies that bind to *T cruzi* antigens (see **Fig. 4**A). Enzyme-linked immunosorbent assay, indirect immunofluorescence, and indirect hemagglutination are most common methods used. Two positive results from any of these 3 conventional techniques are recommended for a final diagnosis.

PCR is not helpful in routine diagnosis because of poor standardization, potential DNA cross-contamination, variable results across laboratories and countries, and the need for specific laboratory facilities. However, PCR has higher sensitivity than do other parasitologic methods, and therefore could be useful to confirm diagnosis in cases of inconclusive serology and as an auxiliary method to monitor treatment. PCR can identify treatment failure from positive detection of *T cruzi* DNA, but not treatment success, because even repeated negative PCR results do not necessarily indicate parasitologic cure. At best, such results indicate the absence of parasite DNA at the time of the test.[4,10]

Low parasitemia during the chronic phase means that hemoculture and xenodiagnosis have low sensitivity for parasite detection. However, these methods could be used to confirm diagnosis in rare cases of serologically doubtful results or to identify treatment failures at specialized centers when PCR is not available.[4,10]

Initial assessment of a patient newly diagnosed with chronic *T cruzi* infection includes a complete medical history and physical examination, and a resting 12-lead ECG.[4,22] Asymptomatic patients with a normal ECG have a favorable prognosis and should be followed up annually or biannually. Patients with ECG changes consistent with Chagas cardiomyopathy should undergo a routine cardiac assessment, including ambulatory 24-hour Holter monitoring (together with an exercise test whenever possible) to detect arrhythmias and assess functional capacity, chest radiography and 2-dimensional echocardiography to assess ventricular function, and other cardiologic tests as indicated. The results of these tests should be used to stratify individual patients by risk and implement appropriate therapy.[23–25] Barium swallow and enema are indicated for patients with symptoms of the digestive form.

TREATMENT

The aim of treatment is to cure infection in acute Chagas disease, to prevent organ damage in chronic asymptomatic infection, and to limit incapacity and prevent morbidity and mortality once the disease is already clinically manifested.[26] In patients with chronic long-standing *T cruzi* infection, research has not elucidated whether the parasite has to be eliminated from the body, or if only a reduction in the parasite burden is sufficient to prevent or delay disease progression.

Antitrypanosomal Treatment

Only 2 drugs, benznidazole and nifurtimox, are recommended for the treatment of Chagas disease. Benznidazole (a nitroimidazole derivative) has been more extensively investigated in clinical studies and has the better safety and efficacy profile, and therefore is usually used for first-line treatment. Children should be given 5 to 10 mg/kg benznidazole in 2 or 3 divided doses per day for 60 days, or 15 mg/kg nifurtimox in 3 divided doses per day for 60 to 90 days; both drugs should preferably be given after meals. For adults the recommended doses are 5 mg/kg benznidazole per day or 8 to 10 mg/kg nifurtimox per day, for the same duration as for children.[27]

The most common adverse effect of benznidazole is a generalized or, sometimes, localized allergic dermatitis, which affects about 20% to 30% of patients and consists of pruritic and nonbullous polymorphous erythematous rashes, often followed by desquamation. This dermatitis is autolimited, usually of mild to moderate intensity, and begins 8 to 10 days after treatment starts (occasionally later); the dose does not need to be reduced or interrupted in most patients. Another adverse effect, which occurs in about 5% to 10% of patients usually late in the treatment course, is a dose-dependent peripheral sensitive neuropathy, affecting mainly the distal parts of the lower limbs; in such cases, treatment should be stopped. Polyneuropathy is nearly always reversible but can take months to resolve. It is not relieved by the administration of B-complex vitamins, but might respond to systemic corticosteroids. Rare serious adverse events include leukopenia with granulocytopenia or agranulocytosis (sometimes followed by fever and tonsillitis), and thrombocytopenic purpura. Bone marrow suppression usually occurs by the third week of therapy, or eventually later, and should trigger immediate treatment interruption. Leukopenia usually resolves a few days after discontinuation of benznidazole, and tonsillitis should be treated with antibiotics. Additional reported side effects include nausea, vomiting, anorexia, weight loss, insomnia, loss of taste, and onycholysis.[26,28]

Nifurtimox is associated with various adverse effects that usually resolve when treatment is stopped. Gastrointestinal symptoms are the most common side effects reported in clinical studies, occurring in about 50% of patients, and include anorexia leading to weight loss, nausea, vomiting, abdominal discomfort, and occasionally diarrhea. Other common side effects include symptoms of central nervous system toxicity, such as insomnia, irritability, and disorientation. Polyneuropathy, paresthesias, and peripheral neuritis are more serious but less common adverse effects. Additional side effects include headache, myalgia, arthralgia, dizziness or vertigo, and mood changes.[26,28] In general, children treated with benznidazole or nifurtimox have fewer adverse effects than adults.

In acute Chagas disease, antitrypanosomal treatment clears the parasitemia, as shown by conversion to negative serologic and parasitologic tests, reduces the severity and duration of symptoms, and decreases mortality (**Fig. 4**B). Cure rates of up to 81% have been reported,[16] and treatment is mandatory for all patients with acute infection (vector borne, oral, or accidental), congenital infection, or reactivated infection from immunosuppressive treatment (eg, after organ transplantation) or coinfection with HIV.[29]

In children aged 6 to 12 years, findings of 2 randomized placebo-controlled trials showed that benznidazole cured about 60% of asymptomatic infections, as measured by conversion of IgG serologic tests to negative at 3 to 4 years after treatment completion.[30,31] Together with growing favorable anecdotal experiences of individual clinicians across Latin America, these studies prompted the WHO to recommend early diagnosis and antitrypanosomal treatment for all children with chronic *T cruzi* infection[32]; this recommendation was extended to children aged up to 18 years in the United States guidelines.[22]

Whether adults with the indeterminate or chronic symptomatic form of Chagas disease should be treated with benznidazole or nifurtimox has been debated for years. Some researchers argue that both drugs have frequent and unpleasant side effects, might be carcinogenic, need to be taken for a long period, and lack efficacy, as shown by low seroconversion rates.[33,34] However, none of these arguments is solid or compelling.[35] To improve benznidazole tolerability, the authors have adopted 3 strategies. First, the daily dose should not exceed 300 mg; in patients weighing more than 60 kg, a fixed daily dose of 300 mg should be given for a total number of days equal to the patient's weight in kilograms, resulting in a total dose that is equivalent to 5 mg/kg per day for 60 days.[26] Second, patients with mild to moderate allergic dermatitis should be treated immediately with low-dose systemic corticosteroids (eg, 20 mg/d prednisolone orally for 10 days, followed by 10 mg/d for 10 days), without the need for benznidazole interruption.[26,28] Third, in patients with severe dermatitis, the authors have achieved a tolerance rate of 72% by retreating 25 patients with benznidazole and prednisolone (20 mg/d during the first 14 days followed by 10 mg/d for the remaining days of treatment) at the same time (Rassi A, unpublished data, 2010).

Seroconversion might not be the most appropriate criterion to monitor drug efficacy after chemotherapy at a late stage of chronic infection. Contrary to parasitologic testing, serologic test results can take decades to convert from positive to negative in cured individuals (**Fig. 5**),[28] and drug-induced reduction (not necessarily eradication) of the parasite load could be sufficient to arrest evolution of the disease and avert the irreversible long-term consequences.[36] Moreover, even assuming that seroconversion is quite low after antitrypanosomal treatment in the late chronic phase (about 10%–20%), for every 10 patients treated, 1 or 2 will be cured. Therefore, thousands of infected individuals could derive some clinical benefit from treatment lasting 60 to 90 days,[35] which is a fairly short treatment period for a lifelong disease.

In several observational studies done in the past decades,[36–38] benznidazole treatment slowed the development and progression of cardiomyopathy in adults with long-standing chronic infection. In the largest study, 566 adults (aged 30–50 years) with chronic infection but without advanced heart disease were assigned, in alternating sequences, to receive benznidazole or no treatment.[36] After a median follow-up of 9.8 years, significantly fewer treated patients had a progression of disease or developed ECG abnormalities, despite seroconversion occurring in only 15% of patients.

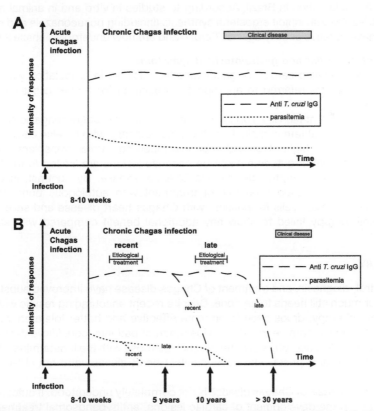

Fig. 5. Serologic and parasitologic evolution in chronic Chagas infection. (*A*) Untreated patients have low levels of circulating parasites and high levels of IgG antibodies directed against the antigens of *T cruzi*. (*B*) Treated and cured patients. Cure at the chronic phase is accompanied by clearance of parasitemia, which occurs immediately after etiologic treatment, and by seronegative conversion, which occurs after 5 to 10 years for those treated with less than 10 years after the initial infection (recent chronic infection), and after at least 20 years for those treated with more than 10 years after the initial infection (late chronic infection). Treated and uncured patients present a response that is similar to that of untreated patients.

Based on these results, in 2006 a panel of experts convened by the US Centers for Disease Control and Prevention[22] recommended that treatment be offered to adults younger than 50 years with presumably long-standing indeterminate T cruzi infections or even those with mild to moderate disease. In patients older than 50 years, treatment is optional because of the lack of data. By contrast, treatment is contraindicated during pregnancy and for patients with severe renal or hepatic insufficiency, and should generally not be offered to patients with advanced chagasic cardiomyopathy or megaesophagus with significantly impaired swallowing. A large, multicenter, randomized trial (BENEFIT)[39] has been designed to assess the parasitologic and clinical efficacy of benznidazole in adults (aged 18–75 years) with chronic Chagas heart disease (without advanced lesions), and is under way in Brazil, Argentina, Colombia, Bolivia, and El Salvador. The trial is expected to provide a more solid basis for treatment decisions in this group of patients.

Alternatives to benznidazole and nifurtimox, including allopurinol and itraconazole,[40,41] have had mostly unsuccessful results, with the exception of a small report from Chile[42] and anecdotal use of allopurinol to treat reactivation in patients after cardiac transplantation in Brazil. According to studies in vitro and in animal models, several triazoles that inhibit ergosterol synthesis (including posaconazole and ravuconazole) have curative activity against T cruzi, and are now undergoing phase 2 trials.[43]

Treatment of cardiac and gastrointestinal symptoms

Patients who develop cardiac or gastrointestinal disease in association with T cruzi infection should be referred to appropriate specialists for further assessment and treatment.

Cardiac transplantation is an option for patients with end-stage chagasic cardiomyopathy. The survival rate in patients with Chagas disease who receive cardiac transplants seems to be higher than that in people receiving cardiac transplants for other reasons.[44] This better outcome might be because lesions are limited to the heart in most patients with symptomatic chronic Chagas disease. By contrast, in the first placebo-controlled randomized trial of treatment with autologous bone marrow–derived mononuclear cells for patients with Chagas heart disease and severe heart failure, cell therapy failed to show any additional benefit compared with standard therapy.[45]

SUMMARY

The control, diagnosis, and treatment of Chagas disease have improved substantially lately, but much still needs to be done. Despite recent encouraging results with available chemotherapy, drugs need to be more effective and better tolerated. Although treatment is now recommended for a wide range of patients, conclusive data are still lacking for certain subgroups of patients, such as those with the indeterminate form or those in the chronic phase who have manifest heart disease and are older than 50 years.

The pathogenesis of Chagas disease is not completely understood. If autoimmunity participates in the development of cardiac lesions, antitrypanosomal treatment after the acute phase could be unsuccessful. However, if parasite persistence is the major pathogenic mechanism, the likelihood of curing a patient with treatment during the chronic phase would be greatly increased. In this regard, there is a great need to find better techniques to assess cure in chronically infected patients. Finally, whether a substantial reduction in parasite load from trypanocidal therapy, instead of parasitologic cure, is sufficient to prevent or delay progression of the disease needs to be rigorously evaluated.

ACKNOWLEDGMENTS

The authors thank Katrina Phillips for her comments, careful review, and editing of the text.

REFERENCES

1. Chagas C. Nova tripanozomiase humana. Estudos sobre a morfolojía e o ciclo evolutivo de Schizotrypanum cruzi n. gen., n. sp., ajente etiolójico de nova entidade morbida do homen. Mem Inst Oswaldo Cruz 1909;1:159–218 [in Portuguese].
2. Aufderheide AC, Salo W, Madden M, et al. A 9,000-year record of Chagas disease. Proc Natl Acad Sci U S A 2004;101:2034–9.
3. Gorla D, Noireau F. Geographic distribution of Triatominae vectors in America. In: Telleria J, Tibayrenc M, editors. American trypanosomiasis (Chagas disease). One hundred years of research. 1st edition. Burlington (VA): Elsevier Inc; 2010. p. 209–31.
4. Rassi A Jr, Rassi A, Marin-Neto JA. Chagas disease. Lancet 2010;375:1388–402.
5. Salvatella R. Organizacion panamericana de la salud. Estimacion cuantitativa de la enfermedad de chagas en las Americas. Report no. OPS/ HDM/CD/425–6. Montevideo (Uruguay): Organizacion Panamericana de la Salud; 2006 [in Spanish].
6. WHO. Chagas disease (American trypanosomiasis) fact sheet (revised in June 2010). Wkly Epidemiol Rec 2010;85:334–6.
7. Moncayo A. Chagas disease: current epidemiological trends after the interruption of vectorial and transfusional transmission in the Southern Cone countries. Mem Inst Oswaldo Cruz 2003;98:577–91.
8. Kirchhoff LV. Epidemiology of American trypanosomiasis (Chagas disease). Adv Parasitol 2011;75:1–18.
9. Kribs-Zaleta C. Estimating contact process saturation in sylvatic transmission of Trypanosoma cruzi in the United States. PLoS Negl Trop Dis 2010;4:e656.
10. Kirchhoff LV, Rassi A Jr. Chagas' disease and trypanosomiasis. In: Longo DL, Fauci AS, Kasper DL, et al, editors. Harrison's principles of internal medicine. 18th edition. New York: McGraw-Hill; 2011. p. 1716–21.
11. Bern C, Montgomery SP. An estimate of the burden of Chagas disease in the United States. Clin Infect Dis 2009;49:e52–4.
12. Gascon J, Bern C, Pinazo MJ. Chagas disease in Spain, the United States and other non-endemic countries. Acta Trop 2010;115:22–7.
13. Hidron A, Vogenthaler N, Santos-Preciado JI, et al. Cardiac involvement with parasitic infections. Clin Microbiol Rev 2010;23:324–49.
14. Rassi A Jr, Rassi A, Little WC. Chagas' heart disease. Clin Cardiol 2000;23:883–9.
15. Marin-Neto JA, Cunha-Neto E, Maciel BC, et al. Pathogenesis of chronic Chagas heart disease. Circulation 2007;115:1109–23.
16. Rassi A, Rassi A Jr, Rassi GG. Fase aguda da doença de Chagas. In: Brener Z, Andrade ZA, Barral-Netto M, editors. Trypanosoma cruzi e doença de Chagas. 2nd edition. Rio de Janeiro (Brazil): Guanabara Koogan; 2000. p. 231–45 [in Portuguese].
17. Pinto AY, Valente SA, Valente V da C, et al. Acute phase of Chagas disease in the Brazilian Amazon region: study of 233 cases from Pará, Amapá and Maranhão observed between 1988 and 2005. Rev Soc Bras Med Trop 2008;41:602–14 [in Portuguese].
18. Rassi A Jr, Gabriel Rassi A, Gabriel Rassi S, et al. Ventricular arrhythmia in Chagas disease. Diagnostic, prognostic, and therapeutic features. Arq Bras Cardiol 1995;65:377–87 [in Portuguese].

19. Freitas HF, Chizzola PR, Paes AT, et al. Risk stratification in a Brazilian hospital-based cohort of 1220 outpatients with heart failure: role of Chagas heart disease. Int J Cardiol 2005;102:239–47.

20. Rassi A Jr, Rassi SG, Rassi A. Sudden death in Chagas' disease. Arq Bras Cardiol 2001;76:75–96.

21. Rassi A, Rezende JM, Luquetti AO, et al. Clinical phases and forms of Chagas disease. In: Telleria J, Tibayrenc M, editors. American trypanosomiasis (Chagas disease). One hundred years of research. 1st edition. Burlington (MA): Elsevier Inc; 2010. p. 709–41.

22. Bern C, Montgomery SP, Herwaldt BL, et al. Evaluation and treatment of Chagas disease in the United States: a systematic review. JAMA 2007;298:2171–81.

23. Rassi A Jr, Rassi A, Little WC, et al. Development and validation of a risk score for predicting death in Chagas' heart disease. N Engl J Med 2006;355:799–808.

24. Rassi A Jr, Rassi A, Rassi SG. Predictors of mortality in chronic Chagas disease: a systematic review of observational studies. Circulation 2007;115:1101–8.

25. Rassi A Jr, Rassi A, Marin-Neto JA. Chagas heart disease: pathophysiologic mechanisms, prognostic factors and risk stratification. Mem Inst Oswaldo Cruz 2009;104(Suppl 1):152–8.

26. Rassi A Jr, Dias JC, Marin-Neto JA, et al. Challenges and opportunities for primary, secondary, and tertiary prevention of Chagas' disease. Heart 2009;95:524–34.

27. Ministério da Saúde Brasil. Brazilian Consensus on Chagas disease. Rev Soc Bras Med Trop 2005;38(Suppl 3):7–29 [in Portuguese].

28. Rassi A, Luquetti AO. Specific treatment for *Trypanosoma cruzi* infection (Chagas disease). In: Tyler KM, Miles MA, editors. American trypanosomiasis. Boston: Kluwer Academic; 2003. p. 117–25.

29. 811Control de La Enfermedad de Chagas. Série de Informes Técnicos de la OMS. Ginebra (Suiza): Comité de Expertos de la OMS; 1991 [in Spanish].

30. de Andrade AL, Zicker F, de Oliveira RM, et al. Randomised trial of efficacy of benznidazole in treatment of early *Trypanosoma cruzi* infection. Lancet 1996; 348:1407–13.

31. Sosa Estani S, Segura EL, Ruiz AM, et al. Efficacy of chemotherapy with benznidazole in children in the indeterminate phase of Chagas' disease. Am J Trop Med Hyg 1998;59:526–9.

32. Control of Chagas disease: report of a WHO expert committee. World Health Organ Tech Rep Ser 2002;905:1–109.

33. Mady C, Ianni BM, de Souza JL Jr. Benznidazole and Chagas disease: can an old drug be the answer to an old problem? Expert Opin Investig Drugs 2008;17: 1427–33.

34. Issa VS, Bocchi EA. Antitrypanosomal agents: treatment or threat? Lancet 2010; 376:768.

35. Rassi A Jr, Rassi A, Marin-Neto JA. Antitrypanosomal agents: treatment or threat? Lancet 2010;376:768–9 [authors' reply].

36. Viotti R, Vigliano C, Lococo B, et al. Long-term cardiac outcomes of treating chronic Chagas disease with benznidazole versus no treatment: a nonrandomized trial. Ann Intern Med 2006;144:724–34.

37. Gallerano RH, Sosa RR. Resultados de um estúdio a largo plazo com drogas antiparasitárias em infectados chagásicos crônicos. Rev Fed Arg Cardiol 2001; 30:289–96 [in Spanish].

38. Fabbro DL, Streiger ML, Arias ED, et al. Trypanocide treatment among adults with chronic Chagas disease living in Santa Fe city (Argentina), over a mean follow-up

of 21 years: parasitological, serological and clinical evolution. Rev Soc Bras Med Trop 2007;40:1–10.

39. Marin-Neto JA, Rassi A Jr, Morillo CA, et al. Rationale and design of a randomized placebo-controlled trial assessing the effects of etiologic treatment in Chagas' cardiomyopathy: the BENznidazole Evaluation For Interrupting Trypanosomiasis (BENEFIT). Am Heart J 2008;156:37–43.

40. Villar JC, Marin-Neto JA, Ebrahim S, et al. Trypanocidal drugs for chronic asymptomatic *Trypanosoma cruzi* infection. Cochrane Database Syst Rev 2002;1: CD003463.

41. Rassi A, Luquetti AO, Rassi A Jr, et al. Specific treatment for *Trypanosoma cruzi*: lack of efficacy of allopurinol in the human chronic phase of Chagas disease. Am J Trop Med Hyg 2007;76:58–61.

42. Apt W, Arribada A, Zulantay I, et al. Itraconazole or allopurinol in the treatment of chronic American trypanosomiasis: the results of clinical and parasitological examinations 11 years post-treatment. Ann Trop Med Parasitol 2005;99:733–41.

43. Leslie M. Infectious diseases. Drug developers finally take aim at a neglected disease. Science 2011;333:933–5.

44. Bocchi EA, Fiorelli A. First Guidelines Group for Heart Transplantation of the Brazilian Society of Cardiology. The paradox of survival results after heart transplantation for cardiomyopathy caused by *Trypanosoma cruzi*. Ann Thorac Surg 2001; 71:1833–8.

45. Feitosa G, dos Santos RR, Rassi S, et al. Cell therapy in dilated chagasic cardiomyopathy: the MiHeart study [abstract]. Eur Heart J 2010;31(Suppl):323–4.

Cutaneous and Mucocutaneous Leishmaniasis

Hiro Goto, MD, PhD[a,b],*, José Angelo Lauletta Lindoso, MD, PhD[b,c,d]

KEYWORDS

- Leishmaniasis • Cutaneous • Mucosal • Diagnosis • Antimonial • Amphotericin B

KEY POINTS

- Tegumentary leishmaniases are characterized by diversity of the species of *Leishmania*, of reservoirs and vectors occurring in sylvatic or peri-domestic environment and of clinical manifestations.
- Tegumentary leishmaniases prevail in tropical and subtropical areas but the human mobility makes them a medical problem also in non-endemic areas.
- Clinical manifestations may comprise cutaneous and mucocutaneous forms that may be localized, disseminated or diffuse in distribution and may differ in Old and New World.
- The process of diagnosis and treatment is intricate due to the diversity of *Leishmania* species involved, and to varied clinical manifestations.
- Leishmaniases in HIV-infected patients may present atypical clinical manifestations and augment the difficulty in the diagnosis and treatment.

Leishmaniases are diseases that are caused by protozoa of the genus *Leishmania*, which are prevalent in tropical and subtropical areas, and which consist of both visceral and tegumentary forms. The estimated incidence of tegumentary leishmaniasis is 1.5 million cases per year in 82 countries, with 90% of cases occurring in Afghanistan, Brazil, Iran, Peru, Saudi Arabia, and Syria.[1,2]

The authors have nothing to disclose.

Financial support: Laboratorio de Investigação Médica (LIM-38) do Hospital das Clínicas da Faculdade de Medicina, USP and Conselho Nacional de Pesquisa (fellowship to HG).

[a] Department of Preventive Medicine, Faculdade de Medicina, Universidade de São Paulo, São Paulo, SP, Brazil; [b] Laboratory of Soroepidemiology and Immunobiology, Instituto de Medicina Tropical de São Paulo, Universidade de São Paulo, Avenida Doutor Eneas de Carvalho Aguiar, 470, predio II, andar 4, São Paulo 05403-000, SP, Brazil; [c] Laboratório de Investigação Médica (LIM-38), Hospital das Clínicas da Faculdade de Medicina da Universidade de São Paulo, São Paulo, SP, Brazil; [d] Instituto de Infectologia Emílio Ribas, Secretaria do Estado da Saúde do Estado de São Paulo, São Paulo, SP, Brazil

* Laboratory of Soroepidemiology and Immunobiology, Instituto de Medicina Tropical de São Paulo, Universidade de São Paulo, Avenida Doutor Eneas de Carvalho Aguiar, 470, predio II, andar 4, São Paulo 05403-000, SP, Brazil.

E-mail address: hgoto@usp.br

Infect Dis Clin N Am 26 (2012) 293–307

doi:10.1016/j.idc.2012.03.001

id.theclinics.com

During its life cycle, *Leishmania* are present in the phlebotomine sandflies as pro-mastigotes (elongated forms of the protozoa with an external flagellum) and in the vertebrate host as amastigotes (round forms without any external flagellum).[3] In **Fig. 1**, both zoonotic (red arrows) and anthroponotic (black arrows) cycles of the *Leishmania* are shown. Infected female sandflies inject promastigotes into the skin of the vertebrate sylvatic or human hosts. Within vertebrate hosts, the parasites are phagocytized by macrophages in which they differentiate into amastigotes. The verte-brate hosts become reservoirs of the parasite that transmit it to the sandflies during blood feeding. The reservoirs may or may not present skin lesions.

Parasites causing tegumentary leishmaniases belong to the order Kinetoplastida, family Trypanosomatidae, genus *Leishmania*, subgenus *Leishmania* or *Viannia*. Approximately 15 different species are known: (1) *Leishmania (Leishmania) major*, *Leishmania (Leishmania) tropica*, *Leishmania (Leishmania) aethiopica*, and some strains of *Leishmania (Leishmania) infantum* in Asia, Africa, and Europe; (2) *Leishmania (Viannia) braziliensis*, *Leishmania (Leishmania) amazonensis*, *Leishmania (Viannia) guyanen-sis*, *Leishmania (Viannia) panamensis*, *Leishmania (Leishmania) mexicana*, *Leishmania (Leishmania) pifanoi*, *Leishmania (Leishmania) venezuelensis*, *Leishmania (Viannia) peruviana*, *Leishmania (Viannia) shawi*, and *Leishmania (Viannia) lainsoni* in the New World, mainly Latin America, with more diversity found in the Amazon region. *L (V) bra-ziliensis* is the more prevalent followed by *L (L) amazonensis* and *L (V) guyanensis*.[2,3]

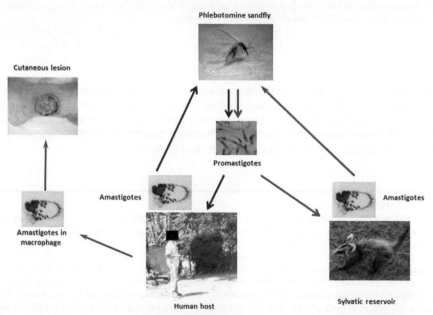

Fig. 1. Lifecycle of *Leishmania*. *Leishmania* is transmitted by phlebotomine sandfly (female *Lutzomyia whitmani* is shown), which inject promastigotes into the skin of the vertebrate sylvatic host or human host. Within vertebrate hosts, the parasites are phagocytized by macrophages in which they differentiate into amastigotes. Zoonotic cycle (*red arrow*). Anthroponotic cycle (*black arrow*). In humans, the infection can cause tegumentary lesions (*blue arrow*). (*Courtesy of* Eunice A.B. Galati from Faculdade de Sáude Pública-USP (sandfly photograph) and Roberto Hiramoto from Instituto Adolfo Lutz-São Paulo (sylvatic host photograph.)

Most leishmaniases are zoonotic diseases; the exceptions are those leishmaniases that are caused by L (L) tropica and Leishmania (Leishmania) donovani, which are considered to be anthroponotic.[2,3] The transmission of dermotropic species of Leishmania involves reservoirs and sandfly vectors of the order Diptera, family Psychodidae, subfamily Phlebotominae and genera Phlebotomus in the Old World or Lutzomyia in the New World.[4] The transmission cycles of each Leishmania species are diverse and involve different reservoirs and species of phlebotomine sandflies. The transmission can be predominantly peridomestic or sylvatic, as in the following examples. In the transmission of L (V) braziliensis in Brazil, peridomestic animals as equines and dogs (putative reservoirs), and sandflies Lutzomyia intermedia and Lutzomyia whitmani adapted to peridomestic habitat[5] are involved. In the transmission of L (V) guyanensis in the Amazon region of Brazil, sylvatic animals such as sloth Choloepus didactilus, and the sandfly Lutzomyia umbratilis, which are found in the forest canopy,[5] are involved.

Understanding the transmission cycles of Leishmania species in an area, the circadian and seasonal density of the vectors, feeding time of the vectors, the reservoirs, and the vector competence for transmission may aid in the prevention of the disease. Control and prevention measures are thus primarily directed at avoiding contact between man and phlebotomine sandflies.[4,6] Neither a vaccine nor prophylactic drugs are available for leishmaniasis. Contact with sandflies can be minimized by using garments to protect the body, including long-sleeved shirts and long trousers that are preferably white or light in color to facilitate the visualization of the insects. In addition, the use of repellents and a bed net that is impregnated with an insect repellent is advisable in high-risk areas.[4,6] It is also important to avoid the feeding period of the specific vectors; for most species, this period occurs at dusk and early night, although some vectors are active at dawn.[5]

LEISHMANIASES IN NONENDEMIC AREAS AND IN TRAVELERS

Leishmaniases are nowadays a concern in nonendemic areas, given the high global human mobility. Adventure tours and ecotourism place tourists in close contact with environments that can contain habitats that are reservoirs for vectors of leishmaniasis. In addition, Latin America and countries in the Old World are popular travel destinations.[7,8] Furthermore, cutaneous leishmaniasis caused by L (L) tropica is anthroponotic in Asia,[9] and there is an increase in vectors that are becoming more adapted to environments in periurban areas.[5] Among the dermatologic diseases that can occur in travelers, tegumentary leishmaniasis is frequent, and, in a survey of the GeoSentinel Surveillance Network covering a 10-year period (1997–2006), it represented 3.3% of 4594 patients.[7] Thus the prevention measures mentioned earlier have to be considered depending on the travel destination.

CLINICAL PRESENTATION

Tegumentary leishmaniases comprise various clinical forms that depend on the Leishmania species and strain that is involved as well as the host response. The initial lesion is in the site of the vector bite in the form of a macule, which from 2 weeks to 3 months onward may present as a small, pruritic, erythematous papule and/or nodule and may involve draining lymph nodes. The lesion may develop into a granuloma with a progressive increase in the nodule that may progress to a plaque.[10,11] This lesion may resolve spontaneously or may develop into a characteristic ulcer; some lesions may then develop into other chronic forms. Although some evidence suggests a correlation between the clinical features and the species and strains of Leishmania,[12,13] this relationship remains unclear, particularly in regions in which many different species coexist. Studies to address this question are needed but are difficult to perform, because these approaches are not easily available for processing the clinical specimens.

In general, dermotropic species from the Old World cause fewer clinical manifestations than New World species.[2,14–16] Viscerotropic *Leishmania* species can cause cutaneous lesion as well.[2,14,15] Post–kala-azar dermal leishmaniasis (PKDL) is caused by *L (L) donovani*,[17] and cutaneous leishmaniasis is caused by some zimodemes of *Leishmania (Leishmania) infantun* in Europe and Africa.[18] Based on their differing clinical presentations, tegumentary leishmaniases are classified as localized cutaneous leishmaniasis (LCL), diffuse cutaneous leishmaniasis (DCL), disseminated leishmaniasis, leishmaniasis recidiva cutis (LR), and mucosal leishmaniasis. This article briefly describes the main features (see Refs.[2,14–16] for detailed descriptions).

LCL is the most prevalent form and is caused by all of the dermotropic *Leishmania* species. The most common lesion type is characterized by an ulcer and can vary from 1 to 10 lesions that are localized in an exposed area of the body (**Fig. 2A**). Usually, the ulcer is painless, pink, and round, with well-delimited and raised edges, an indurated base, and a clean bottom where a central crust that may bleed can sometimes appear. A spontaneous resolution may occur, leaving a hypopigmented, smooth, thin scar. However, some cases evolve to other forms of the disease.

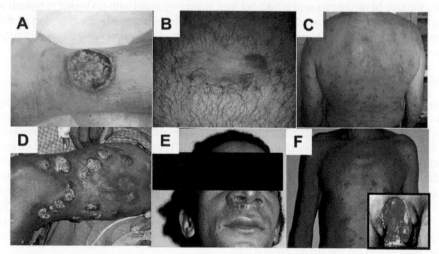

Fig. 2. Clinical forms of tegumentary leishmaniasis. (*A*) LCL presenting a single ulcer on the leg. (*B*) Leishmaniasis recidiva cutis presenting papules and vesicles around the healed lesion of cutaneous leishmaniasis on the leg. (*C*) Disseminated cutaneous leishmaniasis presenting numerous small ulcers on the back. (*D*) DCL presenting tumoral lesions and nodules associated with crusts and several scars from previous injuries on the left thigh. (*E*) Mucocutaneous leishmaniasis lesion in the nose and infiltration in nasal mucosa. (*F*) Atypical cutaneous leishmaniasis in a patient infected with human immunodeficiency virus presenting multiple macules on the chest and abdomen. (Insert in *F*) Extensive ulcer on the penis of a patient with acquired immune deficiency syndrome. ([*A*] *Courtesy of* Luiza K. Oyafuso, Instituto de Infectologia Emilio Ribas, São Paulo, Brazil; [*B*] *Courtesy of* Maria Edileuza Brito, Centro de Pesquisas Aggeu Magalhães, Fundação Oswaldo Cruz, Brazil; [*C*] *Courtesy of* Edgar M. Carvalho, Universidade Federal da Bahia, Brazil; [*D*] *Courtesy of* Jackson ML. Costa, Centro de Pesquisas Gonçalo Muniz, Fundação Oswaldo Cruz, Brazil.)

LR is more prevalent in the Old World (associated with *L (L) tropica* infection) but has also been observed in the New World. The lesion is characterized by an active lesion at (or near) the edge of the healed lesion or a scar (see **Fig. 2**B) that develops with or without treatment after a variable period of time. In the New World, LR is associated with *L (V) braziliensis* and *L (L) amazonensis* in Brazil[19] and *L (V) panamensis* in Ecuador.[20]

Disseminated leishmaniasis (DL) is characterized by the appearance of multiple (10–300) pleomorphic lesions in 2 or more noncontiguous areas of the body (see **Fig. 2**C), which are likely caused by hematogenous or lymphatic spread. The lesions are acneiform, ulcerated, and papular, and the mucosa is affected in 29% of cases. In Brazil, this presentation is attributed to *L (V) braziliensis*, although other species cannot be excluded.[21]

DCL is the anergic form of tegumentary leishmaniasis; thus, the lesions are full of parasites. DCL is a rare condition that is reported in South America, Central America, and Ethiopia. It evolves progressively from LCL; is characterized by multiple nodules, papules, or tubercles with diffuse cutaneous infiltration and no ulceration; and is localized primarily on exposed areas of the body (see **Fig. 2**D). The principal species involved include *L (L) mexicana* and *L (L) amazonensis* in the New World and *L (L) aethiopica* in the Old World.[2,22]

Mucosal leishmaniasis (ML) can occur simultaneously with a cutaneous manifestation (mucocutaneous leishmaniasis); however, ML usually occurs months or years after the cutaneous leishmaniasis. ML primarily affects the nasal mucosa (see **Fig. 2**E), but the oral mucosa can also be affected. The initial symptoms are nonspecific, making the diagnosis difficult. The symptoms can include itching in the nose that progresses to crust formation and bleeding. Initially, nasal inflammation and congestion are observed on a nostril examination; however, ulceration and perforation of the septum can slowly ensue. Parts of the face, soft palate, pharynx, and larynx may be affected. *L (V) braziliensis* is the primary species that is involved in New World mucosal leishmaniasis, although *L (V) panamensis*, *L (V) guyanensis*, and *L (L) amazonensis* can also be involved.[16] In the Old World, *L (L) major* and viscerotropic *L (L) infantum* are common.[23] The frequency of ML varies based on the geographic location. In Brazil, the incidence can range from 0.4% to 2.7%[16]; in Andean countries, the average incidence is 7.1%.[24]

Clinical manifestations of leishmaniasis in cases of human immunodeficiency virus (HIV)/*Leishmania* coinfection may present with different characteristics (see **Fig. 2**F). In the Old World, PKDL is reported in HIV-infected patients.[25] In the New World, the manifestations can vary from those that are similar to the symptoms that are found in non–HIV-infected patients to unusual manifestations. A wide variety of lesions, such as papules, nodules, plaques, and ulcerations, can occur, and some lesions can also affect the genital organs (see **Fig. 2**F, insert).[26] In the mucosa of the palate, a diffuse infiltration has been observed.[26] Tegumentary leishmaniasis may be the manifestation of an immune reconstitution inflammatory syndrome with newly disseminated lesions appearing or worsening while a recovery of the CD4+ T cell count and a decrease in viral load on antiretroviral treatment are detected.[27]

Some manifestations of infectious or noninfectious dermatologic diseases can be considered in the differential diagnosis and can include pyogenic skin infections, pyoderma gangrenosum, cutaneous mycobacterium infection, leprosy, syphilis, blastomycosis, chromoblastomycosis, sporotrichosis, sickle-cell anemia–related ulcers, idiopathic midline granuloma, sarcoidosis, Kaposi sarcoma, squamous cell carcinoma, basal cell carcinoma, B-cell cutaneous lymphoma, seborrheic keratosis, venous stasis, and traumatic ulcers.[16,28]

DIAGNOSIS OF LEISHMANIASIS
Laboratory Tests for Diagnosis

Parasite or parasite-related molecule detection

The presence of the parasite in the lesion is essential for diagnosis. Antigen-related or parasite-related molecules are occasionally detected, and these can serve as definitive markers in the diagnosis of leishmaniasis. The methods include a direct microscopic examination of a sample (**Fig. 3**A) that is taken from the lesion (by scraping, fine-needle puncture, or biopsy), an in vitro culture of a lesion sample to recover the parasite (see **Fig. 3**B), and immunohistochemistry to detect *Leishmania* antigens in the tissues (see **Fig. 3**C). The sensitivity of these methods is low and can be up to 58% using culture,[29] or 88% by immunohistochemistry.[30] The sensitivity can also depend on the clinical form; diffuse leishmaniasis lesions present with a high parasite density, whereas chronic lesions such as in ML and DL have few parasites. These methods can detect the parasite, but cannot identify the *Leishmania* species, which is possible only in reference laboratories that use recovered parasites from the lesion in culture and do tests for identification using *Leishmania* species–specific monoclonal antibodies[31] or by analyzing the isoenzyme profiles using electrophoresis.[32]

For etiologic diagnosis, alternatives include molecular approaches to detect *Leishmania* DNA using polymerase chain reaction (PCR) –based methods and can (1) detect the genus *Leishmania* to confirm leishmaniasis (as with other parasitologic methods) or (2) identify *Leishmania* species. The most commonly addressed targets are extrachromosomal DNA kinetoplast minicircle DNA (kDNA) and ribosomal RNA such as

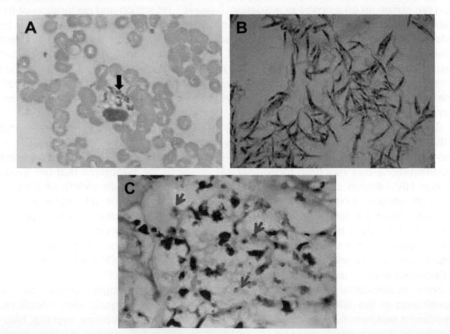

Fig. 3. Laboratory tests for the diagnosis of tegumentary leishmaniases. (*A*) Presence of *Leishmania* amastigotes within macrophages (*black arrow*) in smear from cutaneous lesion. (*B*) Presence of *Leishmania* promastigotes in culture. (*C*) Detection of *Leishmania* antigen (*red arrows*) by immunohistochemistry using polyclonal anti-*Leishmania* antibodies. 100×.

small subunit rRNA.[33] However, to be useful as a reference method, the protocols need to be standardized and optimized, and the sensitivity and specificity need to be evaluated in different centers to be considered comparable and reliable.

The identification of Leishmania species constitutes a challenge, and the available approaches are designed to analyze directly the genes for glucose-6-phosphate dehydrogenase,[34] mannose isomerase,[35] or restriction enzyme length polymorphism of kDNA, ribosomal internal transcribed spacer, heat shock protein 70,[36] or glycoprotein of molecular mass 63 (GP63)[37] gene products. Real-time PCR (qRT-PCR) has recently been evaluated as well for the diagnosis and identification of Leishmania species.[38]

Immunologic assays for diagnosis
Alternative or complementary approaches for diagnosis include the evaluation of indirect parameters using immunologic assays such as (1) anti-Leishmania delayed-type hypersensitivity (the Montenegro test or the leishmanin skin test) and (2) anti-Leishmania antibody assays.

Montenegro or leishmanin skin test At 48 or 72 hours after the injection of Leishmania antigen in the forearm, local induration is evaluated and considered positive when larger than 5 mm. This Leishmanin skin test is used in the diagnosis, but it can reveal both present and past infections,[39] even in infected asymptomatic individuals. Therefore, it is more appropriately used in epidemiologic studies to determine disease prevalence or for diagnosis in travelers who live in nonendemic areas and have no prior exposure to infection. In patients, only those who present with DCL test negative. One hundred percent of patients who present with ML or DL test positive, and 82% to 89% of patients with LCL test positive.[40]

Serologic diagnosis Indirect immunofluorescence assay (IIFA) and enzyme-linked immunosorbent assay (ELISA) are the methods that are commonly used in the diagnosis of leishmaniasis; however, in tegumentary leishmaniases, the sensitivity is considered to be low. In chronic lesions such as LR, MC, and DL, the sensitivity may be higher. In the case of ML (in which it is difficult to detect the parasite), positive serology may be the only criteria for diagnosis.[2] In addition, because the antibody level decreases after treatment,[41] a positive result may indicate a current infection.

In HIV/Leishmania coinfection, a diagnosis of leishmaniasis is difficult because of the varied clinical manifestations. A positive serologic test may help to provide an accurate diagnosis. In the Mediterranean region, serologic tests had low sensitivity in HIV/Leishmania-infected individuals,[42] but in Brazil, the sensitivity was higher, reaching 77%.[26] This finding might be explained by some patients having severe manifestations and/or a previous exposure to Leishmania in endemic areas and therefore likely having Leishmania-specific committed memory cells preserved, even in the face of immunosuppression from the HIV infection.

TREATMENT

For the definition of cases for treatment, see the flowcharts for cutaneous (**Fig. 4**A) and mucocutaneous leishmaniasis (see **Fig. 4**B), in which the contributions of each parameter are depicted.

Drug therapy for tegumentary leishmaniasis has not significantly changed since the beginning of the twentieth century, when it started. However, knowledge regarding the differences in the drug responses of the Leishmania species that are prevalent in different geographic areas and their clinical manifestation is slowly increasing. In

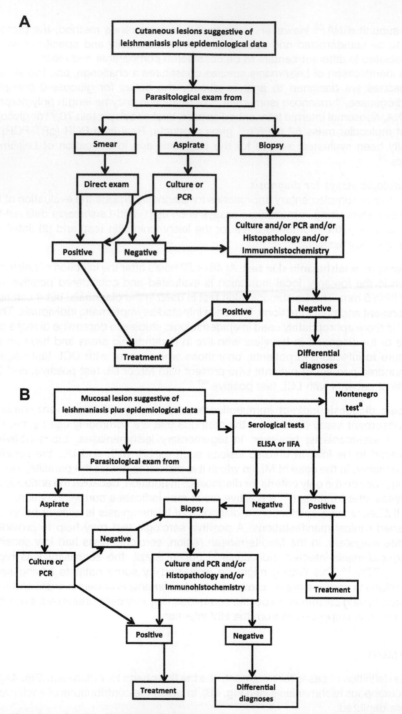

Fig. 4. Flowchart for the diagnosis of cutaneous (*A*) and mucocutaneous leishmaniasis (*B*). [a] Positive Montenegro test indicates present or past *Leishmania* infection; however, in a patient living outside an endemic area who presents a lesion that suggests leishmaniasis, it can be a criteria for definition of leishmaniasis.

addition, studies of resistance to drugs and the leishmaniases in immunosuppressed patients have been reported. However, in general terms, because the same drugs are used in both the Old World and New World, there is an urgent need to develop a more rational use of available treatments and to develop novel drugs.

On establishing a diagnosis, the treatment may be either local or systemic. There is growing evidence regarding the efficacy of local treatment in cutaneous leishmaniasis in the Old World, but less is known in the New World, which suggests the need for better designed studies there. Choosing systemic therapy instead of local therapy (which is more common in the New World) can minimize the potential risk for developing ML, which exists in the New World and has a more prolonged disease course[14,15] However, there is no conclusive study showing that systemic treatment is effective in preventing a severe outcome.[43] Therefore, in localities where the prevalence of this severe form is low (such as Venezuela and Colombia[24]), local treatment may be considered.

Recently, a report of the meeting of the World Health Organization (WHO) Expert Committee on the Control of Leishmaniases was published,[2] and the treatment recommendation was based on the grade of evidence, of geographic distribution, clinical manifestation, and Leishmania species. For the Old World L (L) major LCL, the following criteria to recommend local treatment were set: proven or strongly suggested L (L) major as the infecting agent; up to 4 lesions; the diameter of the lesions less than 5 cm; no potentially disfiguring or disabling lesion; no immunosuppression; and the possibility for follow-up. As summarized in **Table 1**, when indicated, the options for local therapy include the use of 15% paromomycin plus 12% methylbenzethonium chloride ointment or intralesional antimonials plus cryotherapy or thermotherapy. These procedures can cause discomfort, and many require local anesthesia.[2,44] For other conditions, systemic treatment should be chosen, with the use of fluconazole or pentavalent antimonials plus pentoxifylline for 10 to 20 days.[2,44]

To treat Old World LCL that is caused by L (L) tropica, L (L) aethiopica, or L (L) infantum, the local treatment mentioned earlier with intralesional antimonials alone, thermotherapy, or perhaps cryotherapy alone is recommended. In particular cases in which systemic treatment is indicated, the use of the pentavalent antimonials plus oral allopurinol is recommended when the disease involves L (L) tropica causing LR; pentavalent antimonials plus intramuscular paromomycin are indicated when the disease involves L (L) aethiopica causing DCL.[2,44]

In the New World, local treatment is considered in some situations, including the use of 15% paromomycin and 12% methylbenzethonium chloride ointment, thermotherapy (sometimes requiring 3 applications), or intralesional antimonials for all species.[2,45]

In the New World, systemic treatment is better established, and the efficacy depends on the Leishmania species that is involved. To treat LCL that is caused by L (L) mexicana, the use of ketoconazole or miltefosine is recommended. To treat LCL that is caused by other Leishmania species, pentavalent antimonials are commonly used. Alternate drugs for L (V) guyanensis and L (V) panamensis include pentamidine or miltefosine. For L (V) braziliensis, alternate drugs include amphotericin B deoxycholate or liposomal amphotericin B. To treat LCL that is caused by L (L) amazonensis, L (V) peruviana, or L (L) venezuelensis, the recommended initial treatment is exclusively based on pentavalent antimonials.[2,45]

Episodes of relapse are common in the New World, and this can be followed by amphotericin B deoxycholate, pentavalent antimonials plus topical imiquimod, or liposomal amphotericin B.

The only option for treating ML is systemic, sometimes using a higher dosage or prolonged treatment. The recommended drugs are (1) prolonged (30 days) pentavalent

Table 1
Local and systemic treatment regimens for tegumentary leishmaniasis

Local Treatment				
Therapy	Doses/Regimens	Period	Clinical Form	Leishmania Species
15% Paromomycin plus 12% Methylbenzetonyl chloride	Twice daily	20 d	CL	All species
Intralesional pentavalent antimonial	1–5 mL/session	Every 3–7 d, 1–5 sessions	CL	All species
Cryotherapy (liquid nitrogen: −195°C)[a]	Every 3–7 d	1–5 sessions	CL	Leishmania from Old World
Thermotherapy	50°C for 30 s	1–3 sessions	CL	All species
Imiquimod[b]	Every other day	20 d	CL	Leishmania from New World

Systemic Treatment				
Drug	Doses	Period	Clinical Form	Leishmania Species
Pentavalent antimonial	20 mg sb^{5+}/kg/d (IV or IM)	20 d	CL	All species
	20 mg sb^{5+}/kg/d (IV or IM)	30 d	ML	All species
Amphotericin B deoxycholate	0.7 mg/kg/d (IV infusion)	25–30 doses	CL	L (V) braziliensis
	0.7–1 mg/kg/d (IV infusion)	25–40 doses	ML	All species
Liposomal amphotericin B	2–3 mg/kg/d (IV infusion)	Total dose: 20–40 mg/kg	CL	L (L) aethiopica, L (V) braziliensis
	2–3 mg/kg/d (IV infusion)	Total dose: 40–60 mg/kg	ML	All species
Pentamidine isethionate	4 mg salt/kg/d, every other day (IM)	3 doses	CL	L (V) guyanensis, L (V) panamensis, L (L) mexicana
Miltefosine	2.5 mg/kg/d (oral) (maximum dose: 150 mg/d)	28 d	CL	L (V) guyanensis, L (L) mexicana L (V) panamensis
	2.5–3.3 mg/kg/d (oral) (maximum dose: 150 mg/d)	28 d	ML	L (V) braziliensis from Bolivia
Fluconazole	200 mg/d (oral)	6 wk	CL	L (L) major
Ketoconazole	600 mg/d (oral)	28 d	CL	L (L) mexicana
Pentoxifylline[b]	400 mg/every 8 h (oral)	10–20 d	CL	L (L) major
	400 mg/every 8 h (oral)	30 d	ML	All species
Allopurinol[b]	20 mg/kg/d	30 d	CL	L (L) tropica
Paromomycin[b]	15 mg (11 mg base)/kg/d (IM)	≥60 d	CL	L (L) aethiopica

Abbreviations: CL, cutaneous leishmaniasis; IM, intramuscular; IV, intravenous; ML, mucosal leishmaniasis.
[a] Could be used alone or in association with intralesional antimonial.
[b] Used only in association with other drugs.

antimonial treatment, (2) pentavalent antimonials plus oral pentoxifylline, (3) amphotericin B deoxycholate, or (4) liposomal amphotericin B.[2,45] In Bolivia, miltefosine can be used to treat ML that is caused by L (V) braziliensis.[2,46]

In HIV-infected patients, relapses of tegumentary leishmaniasis are more frequent; thus, only systemic drug treatment is indicated. Because of more frequent side effects that are associated with pentavalent antimonial use in HIV-infected patients, amphotericin B is the drug of choice (at the same dose and duration as in non–HIV-infected patients). No secondary prophylaxis is indicated for patients with tegumentary leishmaniasis who also have acquired immune deficiency syndrome.[47]

A detailed description of the drug actions and the efficacy of other drugs are provided in a recently published review by Goto and Lindoso[16] and in the report of the meeting of the WHO Expert Committee on the Control of Leishmaniases.[2] Briefly, among the antileishmanial drugs, pentavalent antimonials (including sodium stibogluconate and meglumine antimoniate) are most commonly prescribed. Varied efficacy among the different species, but also within the same species, has been observed. For example, in ML, the cure rates range from 30% to 90%, depending on the geographic area and the dose of the drug.[48,49] Another example is the failure rate for treating Leishmania (V) braziliensis versus Leishmania (V) guyanensis, which is higher for the former in Peru[50] and lower for the former in Brazil.[51] Various dosages have been studied, and doses other than the recommended dose are occasionally used; however, such a decision must be based on structured studies within the same area and with the same Leishmania species.[52,53] Contraindications for the use of pentavalent antimonials include pregnancy and renal, heart, or hepatic failure.

Amphotericin B is found in 4 different formulations: amphotericin B deoxycholate, liposomal amphotericin, cholesterol dispersion amphotericin, and lipid complex amphotericin. They all present similar efficacy but differ in side effects. Renal injury is more frequent with amphotericin B deoxycolate.[54]

Pentamidine presents the same efficacy as antimonials[55] in cutaneous leishmaniasis caused by L (V) panamensis or L (V) guyanensis in Brazil, Colombia, French Guiana, and Suriname, but less with L (V) braziliensis. Hypoglycemia and hyperglycemia are its main adverse effects.[54]

Using miltefosine, cure rates of 75% and 88%, respectively, were reported in Bolivia and Brazil, in LCL caused by L (V) braziliensis,[56,57] and 71.4% was reported in LCL caused by L (V) guyanensi.[58] Its use is contraindicated during pregnancy.

Azoles such as fluconazole, ketoconazole, and itraconazole have shown cure rates between 55% and 79% in the Old World.[59] In the New World, ketoconazole has shown efficacy against L (L) mexicana and L (V) panamensis and is recommended to treat LCL in Guatemala and Panama.[45]

As shown earlier, pentoxifylline, an immunomodulatory drug inhibitor of TNF-α, has been used in conjunction with antimonials to treat mucosal and cutaneous leishmaniasis and led to a reduction in healing time.[60,61] Conversely, immunotherapy using Leishmania antigen alone or in combination with bacille Calmette-Guérin has been used with partial success in Brazil and Venezuela, although it is not in routine use.[62,63] Regarding the use of immunomodulatory drugs or immunotherapy, it is important to better understand the immunopathogenesis of cutaneous leishmaniasis and ML, because immunotherapy can increase the immune inflammatory process that may interfere with the manifestations of cutaneous and mucosal leishmaniasis that are caused by hypersensitivity rather than immunosuppression,[64] with the exception of DCL.

On treatment, it should be emphasized that the criteria of cure are only clinical because neither parasitologic nor laboratory parameters meet this purpose. In cutaneous leishmaniasis, the criteria of cure are total epithelialization of the lesion and the disappearance of the induration at the base of the ulcer that should occur up to 3 months after treatment. In ML, cure is total regression of clinical signs that should ensue within 6 months after treatment. If clinical cure according to these criteria is not achieved, it is considered as relapse and new treatment should be provided with the same or an alternative regimen.[47]

SUMMARY

Tegumentary leishmaniasis is a disease characterized by an extreme diversity of the various species of the causal agent, their different geographic distribution, diverse reservoirs, and diverse vectors occurring in sylvatic or peridomestic environments and varied clinical manifestations. Global human mobility, climate changes, civil wars, and HIV infection have increased the complexity of an already multifaceted disease in recent years. These characteristics complicate the process of diagnosis and treatment. This article provides an overall guide to assist patients with tegumentary leishmaniasis.

ACKNOWLEDGMENTS

We would like to acknowledge Edite H. Kanashiro-Yamashiro, Fredy G. Ovallos, and Luiza C. Reis for technical assistance. We would like to thank Edgar M. Carvalho, Eunice A. B. Galati, Luiza K. Oyafuso, Maria Edileuza Brito, and Roberto M. Hiramoto for kindly providing and authorizing the publication of pictures.

REFERENCES

1. Desjeux P. Leishmaniasis: current situation and new perspectives. Comp Immunol Microbiol Infect Dis 2004;27:305–18.
2. Control of leishmaniases. Report of a meeting of the WHO Expert Committee. Geneve: WHO; 2010. WHO Technical Report Series 949. p. 1–186.
3. Banuls AL, Hide M, Prugnolle F. *Leishmania* and the leishmaniases: a parasite genetic update and advances in taxonomy, epidemiology and pathogenicity in humans. Adv Parasitol 2007;64:1–109.
4. Sharma U, Singh S. Insect vectors of *Leishmania*: distribution, physiology and their control. J Vector Borne Dis 2008;45:255–72.
5. Rangel EF, Lainson R. Proven and putative vectors of American cutaneous leishmaniasis in Brazil: aspects of their biology and vectorial competence. Mem Inst Oswaldo Cruz 2009;104:937–54.
6. Magill AJ. Cutaneous leishmaniasis in the returning traveler. Infect Dis Clin North Am 2005;19:241–66, x-xi.
7. Faulde M, Schrader J, Heyl G, et al. Differences in transmission seasons as an epidemiological tool for characterization of anthroponotic and zoonotic cutaneous leishmaniasis in northern Afghanistan. Acta Trop 2008;105:131–8.
8. Lederman ER, Weld LH, Elyazar IR, et al. Dermatologic conditions of the ill returned traveler: an analysis from the GeoSentinel Surveillance Network. Int J Infect Dis 2008;12:593–602.
9. El Hajj L, Thellier M, Carriere J, et al. Localized cutaneous leishmaniasis imported into Paris: a review of 39 cases. Int J Dermatol 2004;43:120–5.
10. Machado P, Araujo C, Da Silva AT, et al. Failure of early treatment of cutaneous leishmaniasis in preventing the development of an ulcer. Clin Infect Dis 2002; 34:E69–73.

11. Walton BC. American cutaneous and mucocutaneous leishmaniasis. In: Peters W, Killick-Kendrick R, editors. The leishmaniases in biology and medicine, vol. 2. London: Academic Press; 1987. p. 637–64.

12. Vendrame CM, Souza LD, Carvalho MD, et al. Insulin-like growth factor-I induced and constitutive arginase activity differs among isolates of Leishmania derived from patients with diverse clinical forms of Leishmania braziliensis infection. Trans R Soc Trop Med Hyg 2010;104:566–8.

13. Schriefer A, Wilson ME, Carvalho EM. Recent developments leading toward a paradigm switch in the diagnostic and therapeutic approach to human leishmaniasis. Curr Opin Infect Dis 2008;21:483–8.

14. Weigle K, Saravia NG. Natural history, clinical evolution, and the host-parasite interaction in New World cutaneous leishmaniasis. Clin Dermatol 1996;14:433–50.

15. Akilov OE, Khachemoune A, Hasan T. Clinical manifestations and classification of Old World cutaneous leishmaniasis. Int J Dermatol 2007;46:132–42.

16. Goto H, Lindoso JA. Current diagnosis and treatment of cutaneous and mucocutaneous leishmaniasis. Expert Rev Anti Infect Ther 2010;8:419–33.

17. Zijlstra EE, Musa AM, Khalil EA, et al. Post-kala-azar dermal leishmaniasis. Lancet Infect Dis 2003;3:87–98.

18. Pratlong F, Rioux JA, Marty P, et al. Isoenzymatic analysis of 712 strains of Leishmania infantum in the south of France and relationship of enzymatic polymorphism to clinical and epidemiological features. J Clin Microbiol 2004;42:4077–82.

19. Bittencourt AL, Costa JM, Carvalho EM, et al. Leishmaniasis recidiva cutis in American cutaneous leishmaniasis. Int J Dermatol 1993;32:802–5.

20. Calvopina M, Uezato H, Gomez EA, et al. Leishmaniasis recidiva cutis due to Leishmania (Viannia) panamensis in subtropical Ecuador: isoenzymatic characterization. Int J Dermatol 2006;45:116–20.

21. Turetz ML, Machado PR, Ko AI, et al. Disseminated leishmaniasis: a new and emerging form of leishmaniasis observed in northeastern Brazil. J Infect Dis 2002;186:1829–34.

22. Barral A, Costa JM, Bittencourt AL, et al. Polar and subpolar diffuse cutaneous leishmaniasis in Brazil: clinical and immunopathologic aspects. Int J Dermatol 1995;34:474–9.

23. Faucher B, Pomares C, Fourcade S, et al. Mucosal Leishmania infantum leishmaniasis: specific pattern in a multicentre survey and historical cases. J Infect 2011;63:76–82.

24. Davies CR, Reithinger R, Campbell-Lendrum D, et al. The epidemiology and control of leishmaniasis in Andean countries. Cad Saude Publica 2000;16:925–50.

25. Puig L, Pradinaud R. Leishmania and HIV co-infection: dermatological manifestations. Ann Trop Med Parasitol 2003;97(Suppl 1):107–14.

26. Lindoso JA, Barbosa RN, Posada-Vergara MP, et al. Unusual manifestations of tegumentary leishmaniasis in AIDS patients from the New World. Br J Dermatol 2009;160:311–8.

27. Posada-Vergara MP, Lindoso JA, Tolezano JE, et al. Tegumentary leishmaniasis as a manifestation of immune reconstitution inflammatory syndrome in 2 patients with AIDS. J Infect Dis 2005;192:1819–22.

28. Reithinger R, Dujardin JC, Louzir H, et al. Cutaneous leishmaniasis. Lancet Infect Dis 2007;7:581–96.

29. Weigle KA, de Davalos M, Heredia P, et al. Diagnosis of cutaneous and mucocutaneous leishmaniasis in Colombia: a comparison of seven methods. Am J Trop Med Hyg 1987;36:489–96.

30. Sotto MN, Yamashiro-Kanashiro EH, da Matta VL, et al. Cutaneous leishmaniasis of the New World: diagnostic immunopathology and antigen pathways in skin and mucosa. Acta Trop 1989;46:121–30.
31. Grimaldi G, McMahon-Pratt D. Monoclonal antibodies for the identification of New World *Leishmania* species. Mem Inst Oswaldo Cruz 1996;91:37–42.
32. Cupolillo E, Grimaldi G Jr, Momen H. Discrimination of *Leishmania* isolates using a limited set of enzymatic loci. Ann Trop Med Parasitol 1995;89:17–23.
33. Reithinger R, Dujardin JC. Molecular diagnosis of leishmaniasis: current status and future applications. J Clin Microbiol 2007;45:21–5.
34. Castilho TM, Shaw JJ, Floeter-Winter LM. New PCR assay using glucose-6-phosphate dehydrogenase for identification of *Leishmania* species. J Clin Microbiol 2003;41:540–6.
35. Zhang WW, Miranda-Verastegui C, Arevalo J, et al. Development of a genetic assay to distinguish between *Leishmania viannia* species on the basis of isoenzyme differences. Clin Infect Dis 2006;42:801–9.
36. Garcia L, Kindt A, Bermudez H, et al. Culture-independent species typing of neotropical *Leishmania* for clinical validation of a PCR-based assay targeting heat shock protein 70 genes. J Clin Microbiol 2004;42:2294–7.
37. Marfurt J, Niederwieser I, Makia ND, et al. Diagnostic genotyping of Old and New World *Leishmania* species by PCR-RFLP. Diagn Microbiol Infect Dis 2003;46: 115–24.
38. Antinori S, Calattini S, Piolini R, et al. Is real-time polymerase chain reaction (PCR) more useful than a conventional PCR for the clinical management of leishmaniasis? Am J Trop Med Hyg 2009;81:46–51.
39. Sassi A, Louzir H, Ben Salah A, et al. Leishmanin skin test lymphoproliferative responses and cytokine production after symptomatic or asymptomatic *Leishmania major* infection in Tunisia. Clin Exp Immunol 1999;116:127–32.
40. Shaw JJ, Lainson R. Leishmaniasis in Brazil: X. Some observations of intradermal reactions to different trypanosomatid antigens of patients suffering from cutaneous and mucocutaneous leishmaniasis. Trans R Soc Trop Med Hyg 1975;69: 323–35.
41. Romero GA, de la Gloria Orge Orge M, de Farias Guerra MV, et al. Antibody response in patients with cutaneous leishmaniasis infected by *Leishmania* (*Viannia*) *braziliensis* or *Leishmania* (*Viannia*) *guyanensis* in Brazil. Acta Trop 2005;93: 49–56.
42. Alvar J, Aparicio P, Aseffa A, et al. The relationship between leishmaniasis and AIDS: the second 10 years. Clin Microbiol Rev 2008;21:334–59, table of contents.
43. Schubach A, Haddad F, Oliveira-Neto MP, et al. Detection of *Leishmania* DNA by polymerase chain reaction in scars of treated human patients. J Infect Dis 1998; 178:911–4.
44. Gonzalez U, Pinart M, Reveiz L, et al. Interventions for Old World cutaneous leishmaniasis. Cochrane Database Syst Rev 2008;4:CD005067.
45. Gonzalez U, Pinart M, Rengifo-Pardo M, et al. Interventions for American cutaneous and mucocutaneous leishmaniasis. Cochrane Database Syst Rev 2009; 2:CD004834.
46. Soto J, Toledo J, Valda L, et al. Treatment of Bolivian mucosal leishmaniasis with miltefosine. Clin Infect Dis 2007;44:350–6.
47. Saude MD. Manual de recomendações para diagnóstico, tratamento e acompanhamento de pacientes com coinfecção *Leishmania*/HIV. Ministerio da Saúde do Brasil, 2011 [in Portuguese].

48. Franke ED, Wignall FS, Cruz ME, et al. Efficacy and toxicity of sodium stibogluconate for mucosal leishmaniasis. Ann Intern Med 1990;113:934–40.
49. Amato VS, Tuon FF, Imamura R, et al. Mucosal leishmaniasis: description of case management approaches and analysis of risk factors for treatment failure in a cohort of 140 patients in Brazil. J Eur Acad Dermatol Venereol 2009;23: 1026–34.
50. Arevalo J, Ramirez L, Adaui V, et al. Influence of Leishmania (Viannia) species on the response to antimonial treatment in patients with American tegumentary leishmaniasis. J Infect Dis 2007;195:1846–51.
51. Romero GA, Guerra MV, Paes MG, et al. Comparison of cutaneous leishmaniasis due to Leishmania (Viannia) braziliensis and L. (V.) guyanensis in Brazil: therapeutic response to meglumine antimoniate. Am J Trop Med Hyg 2001;65:456–65.
52. Oliveira-Neto MP, Mattos M, Pirmez C, et al. Mucosal leishmaniasis ("espundia") responsive to low dose of N-methyl glucamine (Glucantime) in Rio de Janeiro, Brazil. Rev Inst Med Trop Sao Paulo 2000;42:321–5.
53. de Oliveira-Neto MP, Mattos Mda S. Successful therapeutic response of resistant cases of mucocutaneous leishmaniasis to a very low dose of antimony. Rev Soc Bras Med Trop 2006;39:376–8.
54. Seifert K. Structures, targets and recent approaches in anti-leishmanial drug discovery and development. Open Med Chem J 2011;5:31–9.
55. Tuon FF, Amato VS, Graf ME, et al. Treatment of New World cutaneous leishmaniasis–a systematic review with a meta-analysis. Int J Dermatol 2008;47:109–24.
56. Soto J, Rea J, Balderrama M, et al. Efficacy of miltefosine for Bolivian cutaneous leishmaniasis. Am J Trop Med Hyg 2008;78:210–1.
57. Machado PR, Ampuero J, Guimaraes LH, et al. Miltefosine in the treatment of cutaneous leishmaniasis caused by Leishmania braziliensis in Brazil: a randomized and controlled trial. PLoS Negl Trop Dis 2011;4:e912.
58. Chrusciak-Talhari A, Dietze R, Chrusciak Talhari C, et al. Randomized controlled clinical trial to access efficacy and safety of miltefosine in the treatment of cutaneous leishmaniasis Caused by Leishmania (Viannia) guyanensis in Manaus, Brazil. Am J Trop Med Hyg 2011;84:255–60.
59. Khatami A, Firooz A, Gorouhi F, et al. Treatment of acute Old World cutaneous leishmaniasis: a systematic review of the randomized controlled trials. J Am Acad Dermatol 2007;57:335.e331–9.
60. Machado PR, Lessa H, Lessa M, et al. Oral pentoxifylline combined with pentavalent antimony: a randomized trial for mucosal leishmaniasis. Clin Infect Dis 2007;44:788–93.
61. Sadeghian G, Nilforoushzadeh MA. Effect of combination therapy with systemic glucantime and pentoxifylline in the treatment of cutaneous leishmaniasis. Int J Dermatol 2006;45:819–21.
62. Convit J, Ulrich M, Zerpa O, et al. Immunotherapy of American cutaneous leishmaniasis in Venezuela during the period 1990-99. Trans R Soc Trop Med Hyg 2003;97:469–72.
63. Mayrink W, Botelho AC, Magalhaes PA, et al. Immunotherapy, immunochemotherapy and chemotherapy for American cutaneous leishmaniasis treatment. Rev Soc Bras Med Trop 2006;39:14–21.
64. Carvalho LP, Passos S, Bacellar O, et al. Differential immune regulation of activated T cells between cutaneous and mucosal leishmaniasis as a model for pathogenesis. Parasite Immunol 2007;29:251–8.

Visceral Leishmaniasis

Johan van Griensven, MD, PhD, MSc[a],*, Ermias Diro, MD[a,b]

KEYWORDS

- Visceral leishmaniasis • Neglected disease • Chronic fever
- Human immunodeficiency virus

KEY POINTS

- Visceral leishmaniasis is a neglected but typically fatal vector-borne protozoan disease reported from all continents except Antarctica and Australia.
- The parasite targets the reticuloendothelial system, with infiltration of the spleen, liver, bone marrow and lymph nodes causing organomegaly and pancytopenia.
- Parasitologic diagnosis relies on invasive procedures like spleen or bone marrow aspirate, but most cases can be detected using molecular or serological testing.
- The commonly used drugs for the treatment of visceral leishmaniasis include antimonials, conventional and liposomal amphotericin B and miltefosine.
- Besides the emergence of drug resistance, the increase in VL-HIV coinfection in disease-endemic countries poses an important challenge.

Visceral leishmaniasis (VL), also known as kala-azar, is a disseminated protozoan infection caused by *Leishmania donovani* complex.[1,2] VL is essentially caused by *L donovani* and *Leishmania infantum* (synonym *Leishmania chagasi* in South-America). Exceptionally, visceralization of species typically associated with cutaneous leishmaniasis has been observed. Most commonly, this has been reported with *Leishmania tropicalis* in the Middle East and *Leishmania amazonensis* in South-America. In individuals infected with human immunodeficiency virus (HIV), visceralization of a number of dermatotropic species has been documented as well (see section on VL-HIV coinfection).[3]

EPIDEMIOLOGY AND TRANSMISSION

VL is transmitted through the bite of female hematophageous sand flies from the genus *phlebotomus* in the old world and *Lutzomiya* in the new world. At the global

Conflict of interest: the authors have nothing to disclose.
[a] Department of Clinical Sciences, Institute of Tropical Medicine, Nationalestraat 155, Antwerp, Belgium; [b] Department of Internal Medicine, University of Gondar, Post Office Box 196, Gondar, Ethiopia
* Corresponding author.
E-mail address: jvangriensven@itg.be

Infect Dis Clin N Am 26 (2012) 309–322
doi:10.1016/j.idc.2012.03.005
0891-5520/12/$ – see front matter © 2012 Elsevier Inc. All rights reserved.

id.theclinics.com

level, there are over 10 species of sand flies playing a role in the transmission of VL, with at least 1 species involved per geographic region.[1,2] The adult fly, about 2 to 4 mm long, is most active during dusk and night time. Resting sites are dark, moist places including soil cracks, termite hills, and other shady places. Whereas transmission is predominantly peri-domestic in the Indian subcontinent, it mostly occurs outside villages in East Africa. Rare modes of transmission for VL include intravenous drug use, blood transfusion, organ transplantation, congenital transmission, and laboratory accidents.[4]

Depending on the transmission characteristics, 2 types of VL exist (**Fig. 1**). The zoonotic form, with dogs as main reservoir, occurs in the Mediterranean basin, China, the Middle East, and South America. This form is caused by *L infantum*. At the global level, the antroponotic form, with human-to-human transmission without animal reservoir, is clearly more common. This form is caused by *L donovani* and is prevalent in East Africa, Bangladesh, India, and Nepal.[1,4] Whereas *L infantum* predominantly affects children and immunocompromised individuals, *L donovani* tends to affect all age groups.

VL is reported in over 70 countries from 5 continents, with the exception of Australia and Antarctica, with 200 million people at risk. Overall, it is estimated that around 500,000 new cases occur annually, with and estimated 50,000 deaths, although the real number is probably much higher.[1,5] Ninety percent of all cases occur in 5 countries: India, Bangladesh, Nepal, Sudan, and Brazil (see **Fig. 1**). With an estimated 300,000 cases per year, India carries the largest VL burden.

VL typically affects poor communities in remote, rural areas, although periurbanization has been reported in some countries like Brazil.[1,5] Outbreaks occur during massive migration or resettlement of susceptible hosts into endemic areas, or disturbance to the habitat of the sand fly like deforestation for expansion of agricultural sites. The increase in immunosuppressed individuals, related to the HIV epidemic, has additionally contributed to increased case loads in certain areas, predominantly East Africa.

PATHOGENESIS

The parasite exists in 2 distinct forms: a promastigote form found in the vector, and an amastigote form, which develops intracellularly in the susceptible mammalian host.

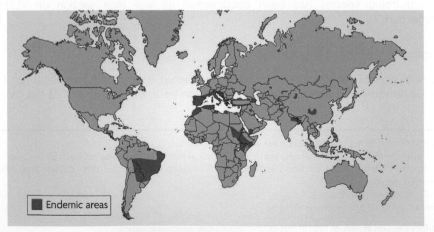

Fig. 1. Geographic distribution of visceral leishmaniasis. (*Reprinted from* Desjeux P. Leishmaniasis. Nat Rev Microbiol 2004;2:692; with permission.)

Infection occurs after inoculation of promastigotes into the skin following the bite of an infected sand fly. Promastigotes are taken up by macrophages, where they develop into amastigotes and multiply within phagolysosomes (**Fig. 2**). Subsequently, the parasites can disseminate and infect cells of the reticuloendothelial system in various tissues, predominantly infiltrating the spleen, bone marrow, liver, and lymph nodes.[1,2,5]

However, infection does not progress to overt disease in the majority of individuals, and in some highly endemic areas, up to 30% of habitants demonstrate evidence of asymptomatic infection. Asymptomatic infection can be detected early on by serologic tests. The subsequent development of cell-mediated immunity can be revealed by leishmanin skin testing (similar as the purified protein derivative [PPD] skin test for tuberculosis).[1,2,5] Oligosymptomatic, self-limiting forms have been described in South America. Most likely, viable parasites persist after primary infection, leading to reactivation and disease in case of immunosuppression like HIV infection and malnutrition.[3]

Although the determinants of progression to disease after primary infection are only partly understood, parasitic virulence, nutritional status, age, and host genetic factors are thought to contribute. Control of infection relies on activated, leishmanicidal macrophages and an intact T-helper cell type 1 (Th1) response. Overt disease is associated with a mixed Th1/Th2 response. High levels of regulatory T cells are thought to contribute to the pronounced immunosuppression seen during VL.[1,2] Upon successful treatment, increased production of Th1 cytokines and decreased interleukin (IL)-10

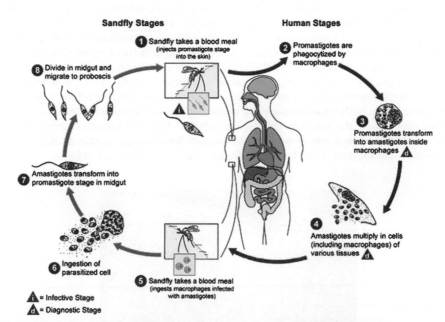

Fig. 2. Life cycle of the leishmania parasite. *Leishmania donovani/infantum* exists in 2 forms: promastigotes in the sandfly, amastigotes localized in macrophages in the mammalian host. After inoculation in the skin following a bite of an infected sandfly, a systemic infection can occur mainly targeting the reticulo-endothelial system in bone marrow, spleen, liver, and lymph nodes. (*From* Centers for Disease Control and Prevention DPDx. Leishmaniasis. Available at: http://www.dpd.cdc.gov/dpdx/HTML/Leishmaniasis.htm.)

levels are seen. Current evidence suggests that after cure of VL, apparent immunity is established.

CLINICAL PRESENTATION

The incubation period for VL typically ranges from 2 to 6 months, but can vary from weeks to several years. Patients present with insidious onset fever, weight loss, and organomegaly that persists for months. Splenomegaly is prominent (**Fig. 3**). It is often soft on palpation and can complicate with infarction or spontaneous subcapsular bleeding. Hepatomegaly is less marked.[2,4] Lymphadenopathy is usually observed in Sudan but is rare in other endemic regions. Darkening of the skin is mainly described in South Asia, where it got the name kala-azar (meaning black fever in Hindi). Anemia, thrombocytopenia, and neutropenia are usually seen, reflecting bone marrow suppression and splenic sequestration. Hyperglobulinemia is common. Mild-to-moderate increases in liver enzymes can be documented as well. The patients may become cachexic and edematous from hypoalbuminemia or congestive heart failure due to anemia. Epistaxis, gum bleeding, petechial, and bleeding from other sites can occur. Hepatic dysfunction, jaundice, and ascites can occur in advanced disease.[2,4] Patients are at high risk for additional infections like otitis media, gastrointestinal (GI) infections, and pneumonia and complicate easily with sepsis. A raised white blood cell count in the peripheral blood should trigger investigations for concomitant infections. Atypical localizations, like the GI and respiratory tract, have been documented, but seem to be especially more common in VL-HIV coinfection.[3] Without treatment, VL is almost universally fatal.

Post-kala-azar dermal leishmaniasis (PKDL) is a chronic skin rash that appears after effective treatment of VL due to *L donovani* (**Fig. 4**).[6] It is considered a sign of immune reconstitution against the parasite, with recovery of the cell-mediated immunity. PKDL is very common (50%–60%) in Sudan occurring during or within 6 months of VL treatment, while it is less frequent (5%–10%) in India and usually occurs years after treatment. Exceptionally, it can occur in patients without history of VL. It starts with erythematous macules and papules around the perinasal areas and often progresses to plaques and nodules, subsequently spreading to the shoulders, the trunk, and extremities. Since the parasite can be detected in the skin lesions, such patients can potentially have a role in the transmission of the disease, acting as reservoirs. Whereas most forms are self-healing in Sudan, this is not the case in India.[6]

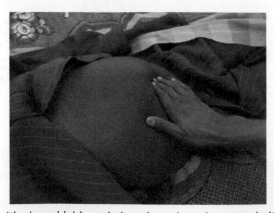

Fig. 3. A patient with visceral leishmaniasis and massive splenomegaly (Gondar, Ethiopia).

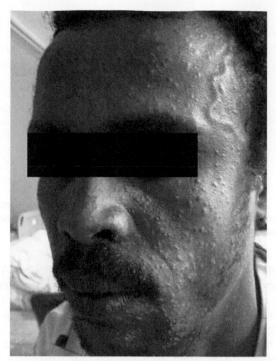

Fig. 4. A patient with post-kala-azar dermal leishmaniasis (PKDL) (Gondar, Ethiopia). PKDL typically starts with erythematous macules and papules around the perinasal areas, which often progresses to plaques and nodules and spreads to the shoulders, the trunk, and extremities.

DIAGNOSIS
Parasitologic Diagnosis

The current gold standard for diagnosis relies on the visualization of the amastigote form of the parasite within macrophages by microscopic examination of tissue aspirates (spleen, bone marrow, or lymph nodes) after Giemsa staining (**Fig. 5**).[1,7] Whereas in Europe bone marrow aspiration is most commonly done, spleen aspiration is predominantly used in Africa and Asia, although the later is associated with a risk of life-threatening bleeding of around 0.1%. Specificity of microscopy is high, but its sensitivity varies between spleen (93%–99%), bone marrow (52%–85%), and lymph node (52%–58%) aspirates. Culture can additionally improve sensitivity, but requires special media (Novy-MacNeal-Nicolle [NNN] media) and is not widely available in most disease-endemic regions. Growth can take up to several weeks. Promising findings have been reported with a microculture method using peripheral blood samples, with high sensitivities and shorter growth duration obtained.[7] Species identification is usually not needed for patient management.

Serologic Diagnosis

Several serologic tests have been developed. High diagnostic accuracy has been reported with indirect fluorescence antibody (IFA) tests, enzyme-linked immunosorbent assays (ELISA), and immunoblotting. Although test performance varies across different studies, more recent studies have reported high sensitivities (96%–100%)

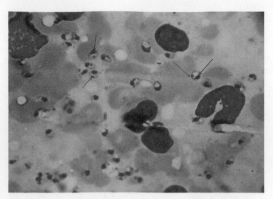

Fig. 5. Leishmania amastigotes (small purple bodies) in spleen tissue from a patient with visceral leishmaniasis (Gondar, Ethiopia). *Red arrows* show the kinetoplast, and the *black arrows* show the marginalized nucleus.

and specificities (96%–98%).[7] However, all suffer from 2 limitations. The fact that antibody response tends to persist (albeit at lower levels) after cure hampers the use of serologic tests to diagnose relapse. Moreover, asymptomatic infections—with positive serologic tests—are common in disease-endemic regions. Since they are technologically demanding, these tests are not routinely available in most disease-endemic areas. Two tests have been specifically developed for field use and have undergone substantial validation.[1,7] The direct agglutination test (DAT) is a semiquantitative test. Agglutination is observed after overnight incubation of dilutions of patient's serum and killed parasites in microtiter plates. Sensitivity has been estimated at 95%, with specificity of 86%. An rK39-based immunochromatographic (ICT) strip test has been developed as well, with sensitivity and specificity estimated at 94% and 95%, respectively, although sensitivity was lower in East Africa.[1] This test currently has an increasing role in VL control programs, since it is easy to perform, cheap (approximately 1$/test), and rapid (10–20 minutes), making it ideal for the remote settings where most VL cases occur.

Antigen Detection Tests

Antigen tests have been explored as well, given their theoretical potential to differentiate active from previous infections and their potential use as noninvasive markers of treatment response (test of cure).[1] The most studied test is the kala-azar latex agglutination test (KAtex), detecting a heat-stable leishmania antigen in the urine of VL patients. Whereas specificity was excellent, sensitivity was low (48%–87%) and variable.[1,7] Although the test correlated well with treatment response,[8] it is currently not sufficiently accurate to serve as a test of cure. Attempts to improve the sensitivity and the format of the test are ongoing.

Molecular Diagnosis

Polymerase chain reaction (PCR)-based assays to detect parasite DNA are being increasingly used in high-income countries, particularly in Europe.[9] High sensitivity and specificity have been reported both on peripheral blood and bone marrow aspirates. PCR on peripheral blood has been recommended as a noninvasive first-line screening test, for both immunocompetent and immunocompromised patients.[10] The different techniques have only poorly been standardized. A point-of-care test adapted to field conditions is still lacking. The frequent demonstration of PCR-positive tests in asymptomatic infected individuals in disease-endemic regions obviously hampers their clinical use in these settings. Real-time PCR now also allows quantification of parasite burden, which could help in determining active disease and enhance its use as a noninvasive prognostic marker.[11] This has been especially explored in the long-term monitoring of HIV-infected patients, as a way to reduce the need of invasive investigations.[12]

Diagnosis of PKDL relies on microscopic demonstration of parasites in skin specimens (biopsy or slit skin samples).[6] However, sensitivity is low in mild clinical cases. The highest yield can be expected from nodular lesions. Molecular testing of blood and skin samples has been explored in some areas to increase sensitivity.

TREATMENT

Traditionally, treatment of VL has relied on the use of pentavalent antimonials (Sb^{5+}), introduced in the 1940s.[2,13] From the 1980s on, conventional amphotericin B deoxycholate has been increasingly used in high-income countries. Subsequently, different lipid formulations of amphotericin B, most notably liposomal amphotericin B, have been developed, which combine a high efficacy with low toxicity.[14] Liposomal amphotericin B is the only treatment approved by the US Food and Drug Administration (FDA). Several studies have been conducted in low- and middle-income countries with paromomycin, a cheap and effective parenteral drug with an acceptable toxicity profile that can easily be administered in an ambulatory way by intramuscular injection.[15] The development of miltefosine, the first oral drug for VL, has been a major breakthrough.[16,17] This drug is the pillar of the recently launched VL elimination plan in the Indian subcontinent. Both paromomycin and miltefosine are rarely available or used in the United States and Europe. Although other compounds are in the pipeline, these previously mentioned drugs, all belonging to chemically unrelated classes, will probably constitute the main therapeutic options for VL for the next years to come.[13,18] Although the mechanism of action remains poorly defined for some of these, all are thought to have distinct targets. All of these drugs face a number of important disadvantages (**Table 1**).

Clear differences in clinical efficacy of antileishmanials have been observed between different geographic areas, which have to be taken into consideration in treatment decisions.[13,19] In line with this, current World Health Organization (WHO) treatment recommendations differ according to the geographic region (**Box 1**).[20] These differences are thought to be at least partially explained by differences in parasite susceptibility.[13,19]

Individual Drugs

The pentavalent antimonials (sodium stibogluconate and meglumine antimoniate) have been the cornerstone for first-line treatment of VL over the last 70 years. This is now slowly changing due to the availability of alternative treatment options and the emergence of resistance in India over the last 20 years, with treatment failure now observed in up to 60% of cases in certain areas of India.[13,21] Antimonials can be given via intravenous or intramuscular – injections. A major concern is cumulative toxicity, particularly pancreatitis and cardiotoxicity.[22] Pancreatic enzyme elevations are seen frequently, but clinical pancreatitis is uncommon. Whereas mild electrocardiogram (ECG) changes (T-wave flattening or inversion) are seen in around 50% of the patients, serious, but potentially life-threatening, cardiotoxicity is uncommon, occurring in less than 9% of cases.[23] Features of dangerous cardiotoxicity include

Table 1
The main drugs currently used for treatment of visceral leishmaniasis

Drugs	Regimen	Marketing[a]	Clinical Efficacy	Resistance	Toxicity	Cost/Course	Issues
Pentavalent antimonials	20 mg/kg iv or im daily for 28–30 days	Albert David (SSG); GSK (Pentostam) Sanofi Aventis (Glucantime)	35%–95% (depending on geographic area)	As high as 60% (Bihar, India)	Frequent, potentially severe; Cardiac toxicity, Pancreatitis, Nephro + hepatotoxicity	Generic ~ $53 Branded ~ $70	Quality control Length of treatment Painful injection Toxicity Resistance in India
Amphotericin B	0.75–1 mg/kg iv for 15–20 doses (daily or alternate days)	Bristol Meyers Squibb (Fungizone) Generic companies	>97% all regions	Not documented	Frequent Infusion-related reactions, Nephrotoxicity (in-patient care needed)	Generic price: ~ $21	Need for slow iv infusion Dose-limiting nephrotoxicity Heat stability
Liposomal Amphotericin B	10–30 mg/kg Total dose iv; usually 3–5 mg/kg/dose Single dose (10 mg/kg) in India	Gilead (AmBisome)	Europe and Asia: >95%; Africa: not fully established (higher dose required?)	Not documented	Uncommon and mild; Nephrotoxicity (limited)	Preferential price: $280 (20 mg/kg total dose) Commercial price: ~ 10x	Price Need for slow iv infusion Heat stability (stored <25° C)
Miltefosine	2–2.5 mg/kg/d orally daily over 28 days	Paladin (Impavido)	Asia: 94% (India) Africa: single field study (93% in HIV(-)	Readily obtained in laboratory isolates	Common, usually mild and transient; gastro-intestinal (20%–55%), Nephro + hepatotoxicity Possibly teratogenic	Preferential price: ~ $74 Commercial price: ~ $150	Price Possibly teratogenic Potential for resistance (half-life) Patient compliance
Paromomycin sulfate	15 mg/kg im daily for 21 days (India only)	IOWH/Gland Pharma	Asia: 95% (India) Africa: 15 mg/kg: 64% (Sudan <50%) 20 mg/kg: 80% (Sudan)	Readily obtained in laboratory isolates	Uncommon, Nephrotoxicity Ototoxicity Hepatotoxicity	~ $15	Efficacy variable between and within regions Potential for resistance (?)

Abbreviations: im, intramuscular; iv, intravenous; SSG, sodium stibugluconate.
[a] Marketing authorization holder.
Data from Drugs for Neglected Diseases initiative (DNDi), from data provided during presentation of DNDi during Fourth World Congress on Leishmaniasis (3–7 February, 2009).

Box 1
Treatment recommendations for visceral leishmaniasis per geographic region, as recommended by the World Health Organization (in order of preference)

L donovani—Indian subcontinent

1. Liposomal amphotericin B: 3–5 mg/kg/d intravenously over 3 to 5 days for a total dose of 15 mg/kg or 10 mg/kg intravenously single dose

2. Combination regimens (sequential coadministration)

   a. Liposomal amphotericin B (5 mg/kg intravenously single dose) plus miltefosine (dosage as below) for 7 days

   b. Liposomal amphotericin B (5 mg/kg intravenously single dose) plus paromomycin (dosage as below) for 10 days

   c. Paromomycin plus miltefosine (dosages as below) for 10 days

3. Amphotericin B deoxycholate 0.75–1 mg/kg/d intravenously, daily or on alternate days, for 15 to 20 doses

4. Miltefosine: children 2 to 11 years: 2.5 mg/kg/d; 12 years and older and less than 25 kg body weight: 50 mg/day; 25 to 50 kg: 100 mg/d; over 50 kg: 150 mg/d, orally for 28 days

5. Paromomycin 15 mg (11 mg base)/kg/d intramuscularly for 21 days

6. Pentavalent antimonials: 20 mg Sb^{5+}/kg/d intramuscularly or intravenously for 30 days in areas where they remain effective (including Nepal, Bangladesh, and certain areas in India)

7. Rescue treatment in case of nonresponse: conventional amphotericin B deoxycholate or liposomal amphotericin B at higher doses

L donovani—East Africa

1. Combination therapy: pentavalent antimonials plus paromomycin for 17 days (dosages as above)

2. Pentavalent antimonials monotherapy as above

3. Liposomal amphotericin B 3–5 mg/kg/d intravenously over 6 to 10 days for a total dose of 30 mg/kg

4. Amphotericin B deoxycholate as above

5. Miltefosine as above

L infantum

1. Liposomal amphotericin B 3–5 mg/kg/d intravenously in 3 to 6 doses for a total dose of 18–21 mg/kg

2. Pentavalent antimonials 20 mg/kg Sb5+/kg/d intramuscularly or intravenously for 28 days

3. Amphotericin B deoxycholate 0.75–1 mg/kg/d intravenously, daily or on alternate days for 20 to 30 doses, total dose of 2 to 3 g

---

a concave ST segment and prolongation of the corrected QT interval. ECG monitoring is warranted while on treatment, and particular attention should be given to those with pre-existing cardiac conditions.[23,24] Cardiac effects are usually reversible within days to weeks after treatment discontinuation. Within the United States, the drug is not licensed, but requests can be addressed to the Centers for Disease Control and Prevention (CDC).

Conventional amphotericin B is an effective treatment option, with toxicity and need of prolonged hospitalization as major disadvantages. Traditionally it has been most often used as second-line or rescue treatment.[13] Liposomal amphotericin B has enhanced tissue distribution and longer tissue half-life, resulting in less toxicity and less demanding treatment regimens.[14] Whereas liposomal amphotericin B is currently the preferential treatment regimen in high-income countries, it is increasingly being explored in low-income countries as well. Recommended treatment regimens vary between geographic regions, and the optimal treatment schedule remains to be determined. Traditionally, a total dose of 18 to 21 mg/kg of liposomal amphotericin B has been recommended, with varying treatment schedules being used.[14] FDA recommendations, based on studies with confirmed or presumed *L infantum,* propose a total dose of 21 mg/kg (3 mg/kg at days 1–5, 14 and 21).[25] Two consecutive doses of 10 mg/kg have been used for treatment of children in Europe. More recent evidence suggests that lower total doses could suffice in the Indian subcontinent, where even a single dose of 10 mg/kg of liposomal amphotericin B has been proved effective.[26] Probably, higher doses might be needed in East Africa, at least in some areas.[27]

Paromomycin is a novel option for treatment of antroponotic VL, which can entirely be given in an ambulatory way.[28] It is now an option for first-line treatment in the Indian subcontinent, and in combination with antimonials in East Africa. Whereas high efficacy of paromomycin has been consistently documented in India, treatment response has been lower in East Africa, and higher doses have been required. Of interest, within this region, clear differences in efficacy have been seen in between and within different countries.[29] Paromomycin is hardly used or available outside Africa and the Indian subcontinent. No clinical trials have been conducted with *L infantum*. Similarly, most data on miltefosine come from areas with antroponotic VL. The long terminal half-life (~150 hours) combined with the observed poor treatment compliance when given as self-administered outpatient therapy has raised concerns of rapid emergence of drug resistance in disease-endemic countries.[30] Miltefosine is potentially teratogenic, requiring effective contraception until several months after its use. Miltesosine is licensed in a limited number of countries, including Germany, Colombia, and India. Special FDA regulations exist for miltefosine use in the United States.

Combination Therapy

Combination therapy has increasingly been explored, particularly in highly endemic regions, aiming to identify a short, cheap, well-tolerated combination regimen that can preferably be given in an ambulatory way and requiring minimal clinical monitoring. Combination therapy could also help to delay the emergence of resistance and increase the therapeutic lifespan of the respective drugs, as has been used for diseases like malaria, tuberculosis, and HIV.[30] A 17-day combination of antimonials with paromomycin was found effective in East Africa (93% efficacy). Combination regimens including liposomal amphotericin B (5 mg/kg single dose), paromomycin and/or miltefosine were also found highly effective (98%–99%) and safe, and are now included in WHO recommendations for the Indian subcontinent (see **Box 1**).[20]

Treatment Monitoring

In routine clinical practice, treatment response is usually assessed clinically (resolution of fever, weight gain and splenomegaly, and improvement in hematological abnormalities), with parasitologic evaluation performed on clinical indication. Clinical improvement is typically seen within 7 to 10 days after treatment initiation. Splenomegaly might need several months to disappear completely. In some centers, tissue aspiration or PCR on peripheral blood is performed routinely at the end of treatment besides clinical evaluation, particularly in coinfected patients. Close follow-up for relapse for at least 6 months is recommended. In general, over 90% to 95% of immunocompetent patients demonstrate a good clinical response to treatment, with treatment unresponsiveness, death, or severe toxicity seen in less than 5% to 10% of patients.[2,13]

However, treatment outcomes vary widely between different geographic regions and depending on severity of disease and the presence of coinfections. Up to 5% to 10% of immunocompetent individuals with apparent cure develop relapse, most commonly within 6 months after treatment. Ideally, patients should also be monitored for the occurrence of PKDL.

Special Situations: PKDL

With most cases resolving without treatment in East Africa, treatment is only indicated for severe, complicated, or persisting cases.[6] On the other hand, treatment is generally recommended for all in the Indian subcontinent, except perhaps for those with very mild disease. Limited data are available to guide treatment of PKDL. In East Africa, prolonged administration of antimonials (20 mg Sb^{5+}/kg/d for 30–60 days) or liposomal amphotericin B (2.5 mg/kg/d for 20 days) has been recommended. For the Indian subcontinent, conventional amphotericin B (1 mg/kg/d for 20 days, to be repeated up to 3–4 times with 20-day intervals) or miltefosine for 12 weeks is currently recommended by WHO.[20] Promising findings have been reported with therapeutic vaccination in Sudan.[31]

PREVENTIVE MEASURES FOR TRAVELERS

No vaccine or chemoprophylaxis to prevent infection currently exists. Preventive measures are particularly important for individuals traveling in rural areas and in more primitive conditions, although the parasite has now also spread to peri-urban areas in some regions. Other people at risk include soldiers. Preventive measures aiming at reducing contact with sand flies include the use of (ideally insecticide-treated) bed nets and the use of insecticide sprays in the sleeping room. It is advised to avoid outdoor activities, especially from dusk to dawn, when activity of sand flies is highest. Chances of bites can be reduced by wearing protective clothing and applying insect repellent. Spraying of clothing with permethrin-containing insecticides can additionally be considered. The CDC Web site can be consulted for more information (http://www.dpd.cdc.gov/dpdx/HTLM/Leishmaniasis.htm).

VL-HIV COINFECTION

VL has emerged as an important opportunistic infection in VL-endemic areas in the era of HIV. The HIV epidemic has significantly influenced the epidemiology, the clinical manifestations, and course of VL. In return, VL also accelerates HIV disease progression by increasing the viral replication, leading to further immunosuppression. HIV contributed to the re-emergence of VL in Europe in the 1990s, with 50% to 60% of all VL cases coinfected at some point.[3] Subsequently, VL-HIV coinfection was reported from 35 countries. The highest prevalence of HIV among VL patients is reported from northwest Ethiopia, ranging from 20% to 30%.

In the presence of HIV coinfection, VL tends to be more severe and manifest atypically, particularly with advanced HIV disease.[3] Patients tend to have less organomegaly, while nonreticulo-endothelial organs are commonly involved. The disease may present with concomitant cutaneous, GI, or other tissue involvement.[32] Patients can even present without fever or without splenomegaly. Resemblance of VL clinical features with several other HIV-associated opportunistic conditions leads to additional diagnostic difficulties.

In general, serologic tests have lower performance among HIV patients. The sensitivity of rK39 ELISA was found to be as low as 22% in Spain.[33] However, detailed studies on the performance of the different methods and how sensitivity varies across regions and populations are lacking. On the other hand, parasite load in peripheral blood seems to be higher in coinfected individuals. Consequently, sensitivity of PCR-based methods, microscopy of peripheral blood, and antigen-based tests seems to be higher in this population. In some centers in Europe, the first diagnostic step consists of PCR or microscopy on peripheral blood.[3]

Treatment of VL in coinfected patients is also challenging. HIV coinfection is associated with poor treatment responses, higher initial failure and relapse rates, more drug toxicity, and higher treatment-associated mortality.[3,34] Current WHO guidelines recommend liposomal amphotericin B at a high dose (40 mg/kg), although lower doses might suffice in some regions.[35] Toxicity of antimonials is enhanced in HIV coinfection. In an Ethiopian study, miltefosine was found safer but less effective than antimonials.[36] The role of combination therapy in VL-HIV coinfection is currently being explored.

Antiretroviral treatment should be initiated as soon as antileishmanial drugs are tolerated, usually within the second week after VL treatment initiation. Although widespread use of antiretroviral treatment has resulted in dramatic reductions in the incidence of VL-HIV coinfection in southern Europe, it appears to have only a partially protective effect against relapses. Repeated relapses tend be become progressively less acute, more atypical, and less responsive to treatment. Even while on highly active antiretroviral therapy (HAART), 1-year relapse rates of 30% to 60% have been reported.[3] Consequently, secondary prophylaxis is currently given in Europe, after achieving parasitologic cure. Administration of liposomal amphotericin B, antimonials, or pentamidine every 3 to 4 weeks has been most commonly used. Experience with miltefosine for secondary prophylaxis is limited. In the Mediterranean, transmission is essentially zoonotic, although transmission through needles among intravenous drug users has probably occurred as well. It is currently unclear whether and how prophylaxis can be safely implemented in areas with antroponotic transmission, where the risk of rapid spread of drug-resistant strains is a concern. Additional information can be found at http://www.cdc.gov/mmwr/pdf/rr/rr5804.pdf.

SUMMARY

VL is one of the major neglected infectious diseases. Whereas the development of rapid diagnostic tests has been a significant progress, non-invasive cheap tests to assess treatment response and diagnose relapse are currently lacking. Molecular testing is increasingly used in high-income countries. Significant progress has been made in terms of treatment, including the development of combination therapy. The emergence of drug resistance in disease-endemic countries is concerning and should be closely monitored. VL-HIV coinfection is increasing worldwide and brings additional challenges in terms of diagnosis and treatment. Concerted efforts from scientists, implementers and funding agents will be required to ensure access to VL diagnosis and treatment at the global level and achieve improved VL control. This should go hand in hand with VL prevention efforts.

REFERENCES

1. Chappuis F, Sundar S, Hailu A. Visceral leishmaniasis: what are the needs for diagnosis, treatment and control? Nat Rev Microbiol 2007;5:873–82.
2. Murray HW, Berman JD, Davies CR, et al. Advances in leishmaniasis. Lancet 2005;366:1561–77.

3. Alvar J, Aparicio P, Aseffa A, et al. The relationship between leishmaniasis and AIDS: the second 10 years. Clin Microbiol Rev 2008;21:334–59.
4. Herwaldt BL. Leishmaniasis. Lancet 1999;354:1191–9.
5. Guerin PJ, Olliaro P, Sundar S, et al. Visceral leishmaniasis: current status of control, diagnosis, and treatment, and a proposed research and development agenda. Lancet Infect Dis 2002;2:494–501.
6. Zijlstra EE, Musa AM, Khalil EA, et al. Post-kala-azar dermal leishmaniasis. Lancet Infect Dis 2003;3:87–98.
7. Srivastava P, Dayama A, Mehrotra S, et al. Diagnosis of visceral leishmaniasis. Trans R Soc Trop Med Hyg 2011;105:1–6.
8. Sundar S, Agrawal S, Pai K, et al. Detection of leishmanial antigen in the urine of patients with visceral leishmaniasis by a latex agglutination test. Am J Trop Med Hyg 2005;73:269–71.
9. Reithinger R, Dujardin JC. Molecular diagnosis of leishmaniasis: current status and future applications. J Clin Microbiol 2007;45:21–5.
10. Antinori S, Calattini S, Longhi E, et al. Clinical use of polymerase chain reaction performed on peripheral blood and bone marrow samples for the diagnosis and monitoring of visceral leishmaniasis in HIV-infected and HIV-uninfected patients: a single-center, 8-year experience in Italy and review of the literature. Clin Infect Dis 2007;44:1602–10.
11. Mary C, Faraut F, Drogoul MP, et al. Reference values for *Leishmania infantum* parasitemia in different clinical presentations: quantitative polymerase chain reaction for therapeutic monitoring and patient follow-up. Am J Trop Med Hyg 2006;75:858–63.
12. Riera C, Fisa R, Ribera E, et al. Value of culture and nested polymerase chain reaction of blood in the prediction of relapses in patients co-infected with leishmania and human immunodeficiency virus. Am J Trop Med Hyg 2005;73:1012–5.
13. Alvar J, Croft S, Olliaro P. Chemotherapy in the treatment and control of leishmaniasis. Adv Parasitol 2006;61:223–74.
14. Bern C, Adler-Moore J, Berenguer J, et al. Liposomal amphotericin B for the treatment of visceral leishmaniasis. Clin Infect Dis 2006;43:917–24.
15. Sundar S, Chakravarty J. Paromomycin in the treatment of leishmaniasis. Expert Opin Investig Drugs 2008;17:787–94.
16. Berman JD. Development of miltefosine for the leishmaniases. Mini Rev Med Chem 2006;6:145–51.
17. Croft SL, Engel J. Miltefosine–discovery of the antileishmanial activity of phospholipid derivatives. Trans R Soc Trop Med Hyg 2006;100(Suppl 1):S4–8.
18. Maltezou HC. Visceral leishmaniasis: advances in treatment. Recent Pat Antiinfect Drug Discov 2008;3:192–8.
19. Croft SL, Sundar S, Fairlamb AH. Drug resistance in leishmaniasis. Clin Microbiol Rev 2006;19:111–26.
20. World Health Organization. Control of the leishmaniasis. Report of a meeting of the WHO Expert Committee on the Control of Leishmaniases. Geneva (Switzerland): World Health Organization; 2010. Available at: http://whqlibdoc.who.int/trs/WHO_TRS_949_eng.pdf. Accessed March 7, 2012.
21. Sundar S. Drug resistance in Indian visceral leishmaniasis. Trop Med Int Health 2001;6:849–54.
22. Sundar S, Chakravarty J. Antimony toxicity. Int J Environ Res Public Health 2010; 7:4267–77.
23. Chulay JD, Spencer HC, Mugambi M. Electrocardiographic changes during treatment of leishmaniasis with pentavalent antimony (sodium stibogluconate). Am J Trop Med Hyg 1985;34:702–9.

24. Herwaldt BL, Berman JD. Recommendations for treating leishmaniasis with sodium stibogluconate (Pentostam) and review of pertinent clinical studies. Am J Trop Med Hyg 1992;46:296–306.
25. Meyerhoff A. U.S. Food and Drug Administration approval of AmBisome (liposomal amphotericin B) for treatment of visceral leishmaniasis. Clin Infect Dis 1999;28:42–8.
26. Sundar S, Jha TK, Thakur CP, et al. Single-dose liposomal amphotericin B in the treatment of visceral leishmaniasis in India: a multicenter study. Clin Infect Dis 2003;37:800–4.
27. Mueller M, Ritmeijer K, Balasegaram M, et al. Unresponsiveness to AmBisome in some Sudanese patients with kala-azar. Trans R Soc Trop Med Hyg 2007;101: 19–24.
28. Davidson RN, Den BM, Ritmeijer K. Paromomycin. Trans R Soc Trop Med Hyg 2009;103:653–60.
29. Hailu A, Musa A, Wasunna M, et al. Geographical variation in the response of visceral leishmaniasis to paromomycin in East Africa: a multicentre, open-label, randomized trial. PLoS Negl Trop Dis 2010;4:e709.
30. van Griensven J, Balasegaram M, Meheus F, et al. Combination therapy for visceral leishmaniasis. Lancet Infect Dis 2010;10:184–94.
31. Musa AM, Khalil EA, Mahgoub FA, et al. Immunochemotherapy of persistent post-kala-azar dermal leishmaniasis: a novel approach to treatment. Trans R Soc Trop Med Hyg 2008;102:58–63.
32. Rosenthal E, Marty P, Del GP, et al. HIV and leishmania coinfection: a review of 91 cases with focus on atypical locations of leishmania. Clin Infect Dis 2000;31: 1093–5.
33. Medrano FJ, Canavate C, Leal M, et al. The role of serology in the diagnosis and prognosis of visceral leishmaniasis in patients coinfected with human immunodeficiency virus type-1. Am J Trop Med Hyg 1998;59:155–62.
34. Pintado V, Martin-Rabadan P, Rivera ML, et al. Visceral leishmaniasis in human immunodeficiency virus (HIV)-infected and non-HIV-infected patients. A comparative study. Medicine (Baltimore) 2001;80:54–73.
35. Sinha PK, van Griensven J, Pandey K, et al. Liposomal amphotericin B for visceral leishmaniasis in human immunodeficiency virus-coinfected patients: 2-year treatment outcomes in bihar, India. Clin Infect Dis 2011;53:e91–8.
36. Ritmeijer K, Dejenie A, Assefa Y, et al. A comparison of miltefosine and sodium stibogluconate for treatment of visceral leishmaniasis in an Ethiopian population with high prevalence of HIV infection. Clin Infect Dis 2006;43:357–64.

Protozoan Infections of the Gastrointestinal Tract

Stephen G. Wright, FRCP

KEYWORDS

- Protozoan • Infection • Gastrointestinal tract • Parasites

KEY POINTS

- Studies of parasite epidemiology and molecular typing of organisms have contributed to increased recognition of the zoonotic transmission of several species of gut protozoa.
- Diarrheal disease lasting for longer than 14 days in the tropics is likely to be caused by protozoan parasite infection.
- Fecal microscopy is the most readily available means of diagnosis though PCR based testing gives higher yields of parasite diagnosis.
- Treatment with metronidazole and related compounds is effective against giardia and amebiasis but not against cryptosporidium and cyclospora infections.

GIARDIA LAMBLIA
Life Cycle

Infection occurs by ingestion of giardia cysts (**Fig. 1**). The infecting dose is as low as 10 cysts, whereas 100 cysts consistently caused infection.[1] In vitro exposure to pH 2.2 and then pH 8.0 is necessary[2] for excystation. Protein kinase A is important for excystation and motility.[3,4] Trophozoites (**Fig. 2**) divide asexually every 8 hours,[5] with peak populations at 14 days in mouse infections.[6] Encystation involves selective gene activation[7,8] induced by altered concentrations of bile, cholesterol, and lactic acid.

Distribution

Giardiasis occurs worldwide as determined by opportunities for fecal-oral transmission of cysts in food and water. The malfunction of water treatment and the ineffective disposal of feces provide opportunities for giardia transmission.

Transmission
Infection is caused by the ingestion of cysts in contaminated food and water, through licking fingers or hands contaminated with cysts from the earth, and in the course of sexual activity when cysts adherent to perianal skin are ingested via fingers or tongue. Levels of chlorination in swimming pools do not inactivate cysts.[9]

Private Consulting Rooms, Emmanuel Kaye House, 37a Devonshire Street, London, W1G 6QA
E-mail address: stephenwright1@doctors.net.uk

Infect Dis Clin N Am 26 (2012) 323–339
doi:10.1016/j.idc.2012.03.009
0891-5520/12/$ – see front matter © 2012 Elsevier Inc. All rights reserved.

id.theclinics.com

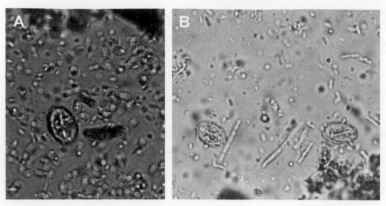

Fig. 1. Cyst of *Giardia lamblia* ([A] unstained, [B] iodine, original magnification ×400). (Copyright Monika Manser; with permission.)

Epidemiology

Giardiasis is most common among the pediatric age group in the tropics, with peak infection rates at age 6 years of age, with subsequent decline caused by acquired immunity or reduced exposure. Infection occurs at any age among those from nonendemic areas. Outbreaks have occurred in preschool nurseries.

Giardiasis is a zoonotic disease. Beavers trapped around a surface water source implicated in the Camas, Washington outbreak[10] excreted cysts. Hikers were infected from spring water they drank above human dwellings.[11] Giardia infection in dogs, cats, and birds had molecular typing identical with human infections. Eight assemblages (genotypes), A to H, are recognized, only A & B cause disease in humans.[12] Nucleotide sequence data differences meriting separate species status were found in 2 human isolates from different assemblages.[13]

Clinical

Giardia causes a range of severity of upset: from severe diarrhea with malabsorption to mild diarrhea with normal absorption. The incubation period is 8 days[14] (median). Acute infections cause the sudden onset of watery diarrhea with yellow foul-smelling stools and foul-smelling flatus, abdominal distension, and occasionally

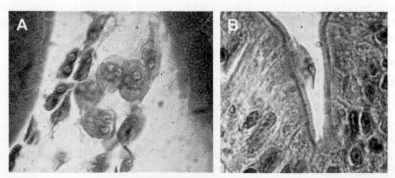

Fig. 2. (*A*) Giardia trophozoites in the intervillous space in jejunum, (*B*) a giardia trophozoite on the microvillous border of the jejunum (hematoxylin-eosin, original magnification ×400).

feverish symptoms with no parasites in stools. Appetite declines and anorexia is exacerbated by nausea, energy is markedly depleted, and weight loss is prominent. Symptoms may be present for some days before positive stool microscopy.[14] Asymptomatic cyst excreters can infect others.

Malabsorption of fat, xylose, and vitamin B12 with high stool weights are found in those who are most markedly symptomatic.[15] Impaired digestion and absorption involve altered events in the gut lumen to impair fat absorption.[16] A mannose-binding lectin[17] mediates parasite adhesion to the enterocyte brush border. Upregulation of apoptosis, loosening adhesion of enterocytes at tight junctions and damage to the luminal enterocyte membrane all contribute to impairing digestion and absorption.[6,18–20] Ileal mucosa is normal in giardiasis.[21] Vitamin B12 absorption improves rapidly after treatment (Wright SG, unpublished observations, 1978), suggesting that luminal rather than mucosal events underlie this finding. Folate deficiency is rare.

Mucosal changes comprise reduced villous height, increased crypt depth, lamina propria infiltrate with lymphocytes and plasma cells, and increased interepithelial lymphocytes with trophozoites in intervillous spaces (see **Fig. 2**). The changes are not as severe as in celiac disease. Patients with pan-hypogammaglobulinemia have a persisting infection until immunoglobulin therapy is started.

The diagnosis is made by microscopy, and fecal antigen detection testing supplements fecal microscopy. Real-time polymerase chain reaction (PCR) is the most sensitive diagnostic test[22] and will become the standard method in the future.

Complications

Infected children were more likely to be stunted (51.7% vs 33.1%; odds ratio of 2.16; confidence interval 1.13–4.15).[23] Two or more giardia infections by 2 years of age was associated with a 4.1 points lower Wechsler Intelligence Scale for Children score on testing at 9 years of age.[24]

Management

Metronidazole is an effective treatment: 250 mg 3 times daily for 10 days or single daily doses of 2 g on 3 successive days. Tinidazole (2 g), with a longer half-life than metronidazole, is an effective single-dose treatment, which cures 93% of cases with a better side-effect profile.[25] Secnidazole and ornidazole have similar pharmacokinetics to tinidazole. Treatment is usually effective, with the resolution of symptoms and intestinal changes. Occasionally, the initial improvement is followed by a subsequent relapse of symptoms, which requires repeat treatment. Infection among home contacts should be excluded. Some relapsing patients needed combination therapy in a large Norwegian outbreak[26]; metronidazole with albendazole was effective in 30 out of 38 patients, paromomycin in 3 of 6, and quinacrine with metronidazole in 3. Screening home contacts may be needed. Persisting intestinal symptoms after eradication of the parasite can relate to lactose intolerance and to post-infective intestinal irritability. These are managed in the usual ways but in those patients who fail to gain weight after treatment it is essential to exclude underlying intestinal disease, particularly celiac disease.

Prevention

Clean water provision and the effective disposal of fecal wastes would prevent giardiasis, but this is expensive and will not be achieved in the near future for many populations in the tropics. In temperate parts of the world, continued vigilance of the performance of the water treatment plant is essential.

CRYPTOSPORIDIUM
Life Cycle

The cryptosporidium life cycle involves asexual and sexual phases (**Fig. 3**).

Human infections are mainly caused by *Cryptosporidium hominis* and *C parvum*. Sixteen species are recognized, and there are several that can infect man. Cryptosporidiosis is a zoonosis. *C parvum* infects calves, lambs, and kids; *C meleagridis* infects birds; and *C cuniculus* infects rabbits.

Distribution

This infection occurs worldwide in temperate and tropical regions, with prevalent infection in calves, kids, and lambs, giving the opportunity for infection in children by close contact on farms or in family groups herding animals. Animals kept in houses expose humans to oocysts. Many animal species infect humans via fecal contamination of surface water and earth.

Cause

Cryptosporidium is found intracellularly but extracytoplasmically effacing the brush border at the apex of the enterocyte (**Fig. 4**). Cryptosporidiosis in calves caused increased intestinal permeability, reduced d-xylose absorption and reduced weight gain. Functional recovery occurred by 20 days after infection though calves were still underweight.[27] Mucosal levels of substance P (SP), a gut hormone that causes glucose malabsorption and chloride ion secretion, were high in cryptosporidium-infected mucosa from macaque monkeys that were simian immunodeficiency virus positive, volunteers who were human immunodeficiency virus (HIV) negative with cryptosporidium infections, and patients who were HIV positive with chronic diarrhea

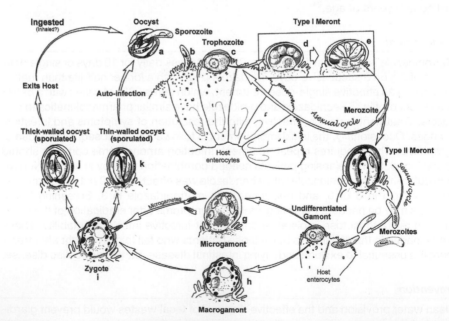

Fig. 3. Life cycle of cryptosporidium. (*From* Hunter GW, Swartzwelder JC, Clyde DF. Hunter's tropical medicine. 5th edition. Philadelphia: WB Saunders; 1976. p. 595, Fig. 88-1; with permission.)

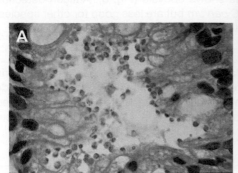
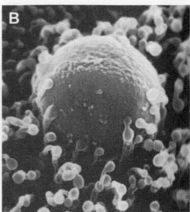

Fig. 4. (*A*) Cryptosporidia at apical sites in enterocytes from small intestine, (hematoxylin & eosin stain, original magnification ×1000). (*B*) Scanning electron micrograph of a parasite effacing the microvillous brush border (original magnification ×40,000). ([*A*] Copyright SB Lucas, with permission; and [*B*] *From* Hunter GW, Swartzwelder JC, Clyde DF. Tropical medicine, 5e. WB Saunders; 1976. p. 595, Fig. 88–5, with permission.)

associated with the organism. In the macaque model, the SP antagonist, aprepitant, reversed the changes.[28,29] Parasite-induced apoptotic responses destroy organisms but cryptosporidium voids this by inducing antiapoptotic effects.[30]

Transmission

The lowest infecting dose was 10 oocysts.[31] Mild short-lived symptoms occurred in 16 subjects and no symptoms in 8 subjects. Contamination of surface water sources has been repeatedly shown as the source of infection in communities stressing clean water provision. Water chlorination in swimming pools does not kill oocysts. Heating water to 64°C for 2 minutes kills oocysts, and municipal water authorities have issued such directives in waterborne outbreaks.[32] Cooking and freezing kill oocysts. Person-to-person spread is recognized through sexual activity among men who have sex with men (MSM).[33]

Epidemiology

Human cryptosporidiosis was first reported in patients who were immunodeficient and later as the cause of self-limiting diarrhea in immunocompetent people, particularly children in rural communities. Large waterborne outbreaks have occurred in the United States, for example, in Milwaukee, involving 400,000 people.[34]

Prospective studies in the tropics found that cryptosporidium caused 6% of 1216 diarrheal episodes.[35] Among 100 children followed for a year in Zambia cryptosporidiosis was more common than giardiasis and was significantly associated with diarrhea (RR 1.23, 95% CI 1.03-147).[36]

Clinical

Cryptosporidiosis in immunocompetent patients causes a small bowel infection with mild, short-lived, watery diarrhea lasting 5.5 days (median; range 1–40), with a longer duration in *C hominis* infections.[37] Pain is not prominent and systemic upset is absent. There is no fecal cellular exudate. AIDS is associated with prolonged cryptosporidial diarrhea that is fulminant when CD4 counts are less than 50 with stool outputs of

2L/d and median survival of 5 weeks.[33] Malnutrition in the tropics causes immune deficiency, with cryptosporidiosis as a recognized consequence.

Ziehl-Neelsen staining of fecal smears shows oocysts (**Fig. 5**). Antigen detection tests are satisfactory for *C hominis* and *C parvum* but are less good for other species. Real-time PCR performs better than both methods and detects any species.[38]

Management

Nitazoxanide, 500 mg twice a day for 3 days in adults with lower doses of the pediatric suspension for children, is effective in treatment of cryptosporidiosis.[39] Nitazoxanide given to HIV-negative Zambian children with diarrhea eradicated infection, stopped diarrhea, and reduced mortality, whereas no benefit was seen in children who were HIV positive.[40]

Prevention

The provision of a safe water supply and sanitation will prevent cryptosporidiosis. Surface water sources for villages in the tropics are likely to be contaminated with oocysts.

ENTAMOEBA HISTOLYTICA
Life Cycle

Entamoeba histolytica (*Eh*) parasitizes the human colon. Cysts are ingested and the cyst wall broken down to release trophozoites though where this process occurs in the gut lumen and how the trophozoites localize to the colon are uncertain. The cecum and the rectum are areas of predilection, but any length of colonic mucosa can be affected. In some human hosts, amebae live on the surface epithelium generating cysts passed in feces.

Cause

In 1925, Emile Brumpt suggested there were 2 separate species: (1) *E histolytica* associated with invasive disease and (2) *E dispar*, a noninvasive commensal with identical cyst morphology. This notion was rejected. Sargeaunt and colleagues[41] identified 2 isoenzyme patterns: one associated with amebae from invasive cases and the other with asymptomatic cyst excretion. Tannich and colleagues[42] defined molecular distinctions between pathogenic and nonpathogenic amebae, and Clarke and

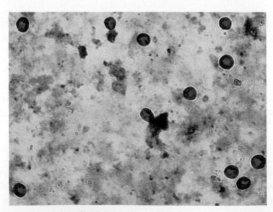

Fig. 5. Cryptosporidium oocysts. (Ziehl-Neelsen, original magnification ×400.) (Copyright Monika Manser; with permission.)

Diamond[43] provided definitive evidence supporting separate species status for invasive and noninvasive organisms. A technique based on the enzyme-linked immunosorbent assay identified *Eh* adhesin to make the distinction though this will progressively be replaced by PCR testing. Amebae cause disease by a direct contact-mediated cytotoxicity on host cells producing necrosis. The perforinlike molecule, amoebapore,[44] mediates cytotoxicity, although its actions in the colon are less certain.

Transmission

Cysts (**Fig. 6**) are ingested in food or water or taken in via the contamination of hands and fingers. Cysts adherent to the perianal skin may be transmitted from one person to another in sexual activity. High-risk sexual activity was associated more frequently with positive amebic serology among MSM than those with low-risk sexual activity.[45] The infecting dose for *E histolytica* cysts is unknown. Effective defense mechanisms may explain the commensal colonic carriage of *Eh*.

Epidemiology

Invasive disease affects adults rather than children, although amebiasis caused diarrhea among children in Bangladesh,[46] and amebae were commonly detected in stools by PCR from patients of all age groups during a 1-year follow-up.

Prospective studies in Vietnam showed a high, initial prevalence of *E histolytica* cyst excretion, 11%, among a group of people who then had repeated fecal examinations over a year. Twelve months later 28 out of 43 were still infected with the same strain. Reinfection after eradication occurred in 11.4% over the next 12 months, whereas 4.1% of the uninfected individuals acquired infection. One case of liver abscess occurred in the infected group.[47]

Amebiasis among adults with learning disabilities in Japan showed the importance of personal and environmental sanitation.[48]

Clinical

Intestinal amebiasis presents with large bowel–type diarrhea. Stools vary in consistency and contain blood (**Fig. 7**). Disease severity varies from mild to severe to life threatening. The rectum and cecum are areas of predilection for disease, but the

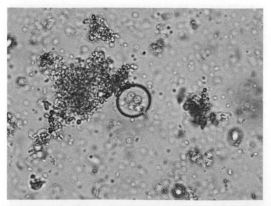

Fig. 6. Quadrinucleate cyst of *Entamoeba histolytica* or *Entamoeba dispar* (the two are indistinguishable morphologically) (iodine, original magnification ×400). (Copyright Monika Manser; with permission.)

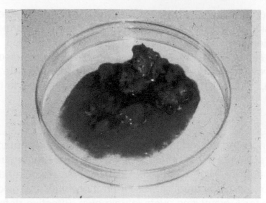

Fig. 7. Amebic dysentery: fragments of formed stool with bloodstained mucus. (Copyright Wright SG; with permission.)

greater extent of disease is associated with more severe diarrhea, more obvious bloodstaining of stools, and increasing abdominal pain. Fevers occur in more severe cases. All forms of invasive disease are more common in men than women, ratio M:F 3.2:1, despite equal carrier rates.[49] *Eh* is relatively infrequent among travelers. Using PCR, Herbinger and colleagues[49] found *Eh* in 9.5% of travelers with diarrhea after returning to Germany.

The physical signs relate to the severity of the disease, with anemia, dehydration, and abdominal tenderness determined by the extent and duration of the disease. Scattered ulcers (**Fig. 8**) with basal slough on normal mucosa are a common appearance, although diffuse inflammation with overlying exudate is seen. Amebae are seen on the microscopy of saline preparations of material from ulcerated mucosa or in bloodstained mucus (**Fig. 9**) or in fixed and stained sections of affected mucosa (**Fig. 10**). Serology is positive in 66% of patients with colonic amebiasis.

Complications

Toxic dilatation, perforation, and hemorrhage can complicate amebic dysentery. Among 55 cases of Fulminant amebic colitis, there was an excess of men with

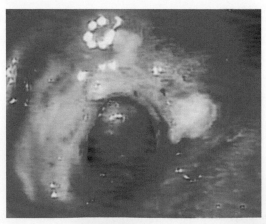

Fig. 8. Ulcerated mucosa in the cecum caused by amebiasis. (Copyright Bloom SR; with permission.)

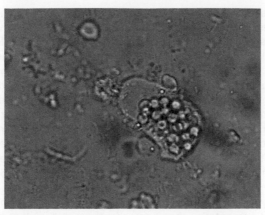

Fig. 9. Amebic trophozoite with ingested red cells. An unstained preparation in saline showing a trophozoite with numerous ingested red cells (original magnification ×400). (Copyright Monika Manser; with permission.)

diabetes mellitus and alcoholism as co-morbidities. Nineteen out of 25 having surgery died.[50] Colonic perforation occurred in a patient taking loperamide for diarrhea caused by unrecognized amebiasis.[51] Rarely, amebae undermine the mucosa and a tube of surface mucosa is sloughed off leaving a denuded area of colon that bleeds and exudes protein-rich fluid.

Ameboma, a constricting colonic lesion comprising granulation tissue with few amebae, occurs most often in the cecum or rectum though any location in the colon is possible with multiple amebomata rarely recorded. Local extension of amebiasis onto the perianal, penile, and labial skin is recognized but not common.

There are reports suggesting that amebiasis in men infected with HIV is increasingly common, with the usual clinical features.[52] One hundred and seventy patients with invasive amebiasis were identified retrospectively over a 13 year period with 102 having dysentery, 63 ALA and 5 perianal abscess. Recurrent amebiasis occurred in 16 patients with dysentery and 9 with amebic liver abscess (ALA).

Hematogenous spread via the portal vein takes trophozoites to the liver to cause ALA. Fever, pain, and signs related to the site and size of the abscess are usual, although small abscesses only cause fever. Most abscesses are in the right lobe,

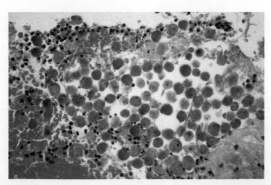

Fig. 10. Numerous amebae seen in the slough overlying the ulcerated mucosa shown in **Fig. 8** above. Amebic trophozoites are much larger than human macrophages (hematoxylin-eosin, original magnification ×400). (Copyright Wright SG; with permission.)

fewer in both lobes, and least commonly in the left lobe. Abscess in the lower part of the right lobe cause palpable liver enlargement and tenderness with occasionally localized tenderness on the liver surface and occasionally a palpable swelling. Laterally sited lesion will cause chest wall pain that may be pleuritic. There may be intercostal tenderness and a rub. When the liver beneath the right hemidiaphragm is involved, pain is usually referred to the right shoulder region and there are signs at the base of the right lung with consolidation, collapse, or effusion. Neutrophil leukocytosis, elevated markers of inflammation, positive amebic serology, and negative blood cultures are usual. These clinical and laboratory features are similar to those of pyogenic liver abscess (PLA) in which amebic serology would be negative and blood cultures often positive. Lodhi and colleagues[53] showed more frequent ALA (ALA/PLA 4:1) and a lower mean age in ALA (40 vs 51 years), with a preponderance of men in both groups.

Amebic serology is virtually always positive in ALA, but occasionally patients with small abscesses at presentation may have negative serology that becomes positive when repeated 5 days later. Computed tomography (CT) or ultrasound scanning localizes the abscess within the liver (**Fig. 11**). The latter has widespread availability, ease of repetition without concerns about x-rays, and usefulness in guiding aspiration.

Management

Metronidazole is the most commonly used medication for invasive amebiasis, giving doses of 400 mg 3 times daily for 5 to 10 days. The efficacy of available treatments was assessed by the Cochrane Collaboration.[54] Tinidazole, in doses of 2 g daily for 2 or 3 days, was better than metronidazole at reducing clinical failure and was better tolerated. Supportive care is also needed for those more severely affected. The management of ALA comprises (1) drug therapy with metronidazole 800 mg 3 times daily for 7 days or tinidazole 2 g daily for 5 days and (2) consideration of the need for aspiration, which is indicated with the failure to respond to drug treatment, imminent rupture, or doubt regarding the diagnosis. A prospective study showed no difference in outcome among patients with uncomplicated ALA treated with oral treatment with or without aspiration.[55] The Cochrane review of the management of ALA did not find adequate evidence to allow a conclusion on the role of aspiration as a *routine* part of management.[56] Treatment with a tissue amebicide for colitis or ALA should be followed by the eradication of luminal amebae. A small prospective treatment study showed that paromomycin was significantly better than diloxanide furoate.[57]

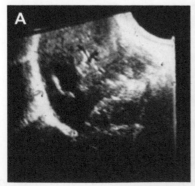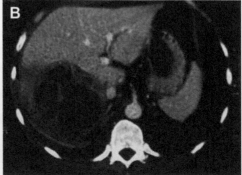

Fig. 11. Imaging in ALA: (*A*) ultrasound scanning, (*B*) CT scan. In both images, the irregular cavity is clearly seen in the right lobe of the liver. (Copyright Wright SG; with permission.)

Prevention

Clean domestic water supplies for use in food preparation and hand washing prevent infection. Heating water to 60°C for 2 minutes kills cysts and sand filtration removes them from water supplies. Attention to personal and public sanitation is a major factor in controlling amebiasis.[48]

CYCLOSPORA CAYETANENSIS

Cyclospora are a genus of coccidian parasites. *C cayetanensis* causes acute diarrheal disease in humans.

Life Cycle

The life cycle is complex, with asexual and sexual phases in the intestine similar to that of cryptosporidium except that cysts take 7 to 14 days to sporulate, forming an oocyst with 2 sporocysts, each with 2 sporozoites. Infection occurs by ingesting oocysts. Sporozoites infect enterocytes, divide asexually, and produce type I meronts, which invade other cells, and type II meronts differentiate into gametocytes for the sexual phase of reproduction to generate oocysts. *C cayetanensis* is solely a parasite of humans.

Distribution

Since the description of this parasite as a human pathogen in Peru and Nepal, it has been recognized as a cause of endemic gut infection, epidemic gut infection, and imported gut infection from more locations in temperate and tropical regions.

Cause

The pathophysiological mechanisms causing this diarrheal illness are likely to be similar to those in cryptosporidiosis. The presence of organisms in enterocytes produces interactions activating apoptosis, promoting secretion, and loosening adhesion mechanisms of columnar enterocytes.

The host response is effective because this infection is self-limiting, although when diarrhea persists co-trimoxazole treatment shortens its duration.

Transmission

Oocysts (**Fig. 12**) in water and food transmit infection.[58] Infected foods are those eaten uncooked, such as basil and raspberries. Snow peas have also been a source of

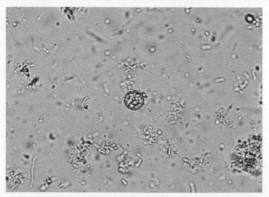

Fig. 12. Cyclospora oocyst: unstained preparation from fecal concentrate (original magnification ×400). (Copyright Monika Manser; with permission.)

infection. The stickiness of oocysts and the hairiness of raspberries may account for the efficiency of this route of transmission.[58]

Epidemiology

The infection has been misdiagnosed as cryptosporidiosis because of similar staining using the modified Ziehl-Neelsen technique. The time required for sporulation prevents person-to-person spread. Surface contamination allows sporulation, and food contaminated on those surfaces provides a route of transmission.

Clinical

Cyclosporiasis causes acute watery diarrhea with an incubation period of about 12 days (range 7–14). Mild systemic upset is reported. The infection causes small bowel diarrhea with griping abdominal pains. Flatulence is reported and patients are fatigued. Children are more commonly, more frequently, and more markedly affected than adults in endemic areas. Stools are watery or soft and nondysenteric. Symptoms resolve spontaneously, diarrhea lasting up to 8 weeks at presentation. Asymptomatic oocyst excretion is well recognized. Cyclosporiasis is an opportunist pathogen, although it is not common in HIV/AIDS. Duodenal mucosal biopsies show blunting of villi, increased crypt depth, and increased inflammatory infiltrate in the lamina propria. Changes resolve after treatment. Cyclospora is recognized as a cause of persisting diarrhea in patients who are HIV positive.

Management

The treatment of choice is co-trimoxazole in a dose of 160/800mg taken twice daily for 7 days.

Prevention

There is a need for the provision of clean water and safe disposal of fecal wastes. Filtration removes oocysts from water because the organism is resistant to disinfecting agents. Heating to 70°C or freezing to -70°C inactivates oocysts.

MICROSPORIDIOSIS
Life Cycle

Encephalitozoon intestinalis and Enterocytozoon bieneusi are the common microsporidian fungal parasites that cause disease in immunosuppressed patients, most often HIV/AIDS, but also immunosuppression related to transplantation and chemotherapy. There are at least 1200 species, with new opportunist species continuously being reported. It is an intracellular pathogen that undergoes initial asexual reproduction and later sporogony producing thick-walled spores. After ingestion, the organism is expelled from the spore and the polar tube penetrates the host cell wall. The cytoplasm and nucleus are injected through the polar tube to initiate infection.

Distribution

Microsporidia have a worldwide distribution. A study of microsporidiosis in travelers showed a range of countries visited that included India, Thailand, Indonesia, Zaire, and Nigeria.

Cause

Microsporidia are intracellular parasites and so control of the infection depends on cell mediated immune responses with CD8+ lymphocytes particularly important.[59] Median spore counts in the stool of patients with AIDS were 4.5×10^7/mL of stool.

Duodenal morphology was normal in most patients, with rare instances of villous atrophy. There was some increase in lamina propria inflammatory infiltrate.[60]

Transmission

Microsporidiosis is transmitted via food and water and perhaps from person to person. Water from drinking water treatment plants, wastewater treatment plants, and recreational water bodies were examined, with 2, 5, and 1 samples positive, respectively.[61] Animal microsporidia species are infectious for humans; cattle, pigs, and birds of all types, including swans, ducks, and geese, contaminate surface water sources.[62] Pet guinea pigs bring the organism into the home.[63]

Epidemiology

Prospective testing in men who are HIV positive with diarrhea the United States showed that the prevalence of this infection was low: 1.5% in 737 samples from men who are HIV positive and 0.16% in a larger national database. When found, microsporidiosis was associated with low CD4+ counts.[64] Fourteen species of microsporidia are presently recognized as causes of diarrhea in humans.

Clinical

Acute diarrheal disease has been recognized in children and adults whose immune responses are normal. The major interest in these organisms has been as causes of diarrhea and impaired absorption in immunodeficiency, most often HIV/AIDS but also in the context of organ transplantation and chemotherapy.

The laboratory diagnosis of this condition is difficult. Trichrome (**Fig. 13**A) and more recently Calcofluor (see **Fig. 13**B) staining have been used, but PCR has greater sensitivity: 10^2 to 10^4 detectable by PCR versus 10^6/mL of feces by staining.[65]

Complications

Microsporidia have been identified in material from sites, such as bile ducts in patients with HIV/AIDS with cholangiopathy, but the certainty with which the cause can be ascribed to this microbe is questionable because of the way in which multiple infectious agents are the rule rather than the exception in this setting. Keratitis caused by microsporidia is caused by other species that are not primarily gut pathogens.

Management

For infections other than *E bieneusi*, albendazole is effective in doses of 400 or 800 mg twice daily in adults, 15 mg/kg twice daily in children, for 7 days. A randomized trial in

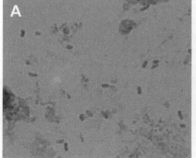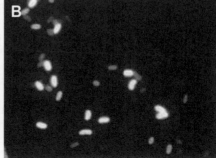

Fig. 13. Microsporidium trophozoites ([A] Trichrome, [B] Calcofluor, ×). (Copyright Monika Manser; with permission.)

children showed improvement within 48 hours of starting treatment in 95% of the treated children and 30% of the untreated group.[66] *Encephalitozoon bieneusi* does not respond to albendazole but does respond to fumagillin which is more toxic. For all patients with HIV/AIDS anti-retroviral treatment to raise the CD4 count is a major element in management. Where immunosuppression relates to organ transplantation careful monitoring of immunosuppressant drugs and drug-induced toxicity.

Prevention

It is probably difficult to prevent this infection because exposure and infection take place early in life, with latency of infection to cause disease in the setting of immune deficiency.

SUMMARY

A range of protozoan parasites is accepted as intestinal pathogens in individuals with normal and impaired immune responses and these are discussed previously. Although these parasites are more common in the tropics and subtropics where sanitation is lacking, their transmission in temperate regions is well recognized. In patients with clinical features suggesting malabsorption, giardiasis should come to mind. Dysenteric diarrhea caused by amebiasis should be considered in the differential diagnosis of someone with a colitic illness if they have previously spent time in the tropics. Latency of amebic infection is recognized, and treatment of patients with amebic dysentery for nonspecific ulcerative colitis with immunosuppressant medications can have disastrous consequences. It seems likely that molecular techniques for parasite diagnosis will become increasingly used in the near future, although clinical awareness will always be needed to prompt their use. The range of medications available for treatment is limited, and there remains a need to identify new compounds for use in treatment.

REFERENCES

1. Rendtorff CE. The experimental transmission of human intestinal protozoan parasites II *Giardia lamblia* cysts given in capsules. Am J Hyg 1954;59:209–20.
2. Rice EW. Schaefer III Improved *in vitro* excystation procedure for *Giardia lamblia* cysts. J Clin Microbiol 1981;14:709–10.
3. Abel ES, Davids BJ, Robles LD, et al. Possible roles of protein kinase A in cell motility and excystation of the early diverging eukaryote *Giardia lamblia*. J Biol Chem 2001;276:10320–9.
4. Birkeland SR, Preheim SP, Davids BJ, et al. Transcriptome analysis of the *Giardia lamblia* life cycle. Mol Biochem Parasitol 2010;174:62–5.
5. Binz N, Thompson RC, Lymbery AJ, et al. Comparative studies on the growth dynamics of two genetically distinct isolates of *Giardia duodenalis in vitro*. Int J Parasitol 1992;22:195–202.
6. Ferguson A, Gillon J, al Thamery D. Intestinal abnormalities in murine giardiasis. Trans R Soc Trop Med Hyg 1980;74:445–8.
7. Yu-Jiao P, Chao-Cheng C, Yu-Yun K, et al. A novel WRKY-like protein involved in transcriptional activation of cyst wall protein genes in *Giardia lamblia*. J Biol Chem 2009;284:17975–88.
8. Morf LM, Spycher C, Rehrauer H, et al. The transcription response to encystation stimuli by *Giardia lamblia* is restricted to a small set of genes. Eukaryot Cell 2010; 9:1566–76.

9. Porter JD, Ragazzoni HP, Buchanon JD, et al. Giardia transmission in a swimming pool. Am J Public Health 1988;78(6):659–62.

10. Dykes AC, Juranek DD, Lorenz RA, et al. Municipal waterborne giardiasis: an epidemiologic investigation. Beavers implicated as a possible reservoir. Ann Intern Med 1980;92(2 Pt 1):165–70.

11. Barbour AG, Nichols CR, Fukushima T. An outbreak of giardiasis in a group of campers. Am J Trop Med Hyg 1980;25:384–9.

12. Caccio SM, Ryan U. Molecular epidemiology of giardiasis. Mol Biochem Parasitol 2008;160:75–80.

13. Jerlström-Hutqvits J, Anarklev J, Staffan SG. Is human giardiasis caused by two different Giardia species? Gut Microbes 2010;1:379–82.

14. Jokipii AM, Jokipii L. Prepatency of giardiasis. Lancet 1977;1:1095–7.

15. Wright SG, Tomkins AM, Ridley DS. Giardiasis: clinical and therapeutic aspects. Gut 1977;18:343–50.

16. Katelaris P, Seow F, Ngu M. The effect of Giardia lamblia trophozoites on lipolysis in vitro. Parasitology 1991;103:35–9.

17. Farthing MJ, Pereira ME, Keusch GT. Description and characterization of a surface lectin from *Giardia lamblia*. Infect Immun 1986;51:661–77.

18. Chin AC, Teoh DA, Scott KG, et al. Strain-dependent induction of enterocyte apoptosis by *Giardia lamblia* disrupts epithelial barrier function in a caspase – 3 dependent manner. Infect Immun 2007;70:3673–80.

19. Panaro MA, Cianciulli A, Mitolo V, et al. Caspase dependent apoptosis of the HCT-8 epithelial cell line induced by the parasite *Giardia intestinalis*. FEMS Immunol Med Microbiol 2007;51:302–9.

20. Troeger H, Epple HJ, Schneider T, et al. Effect of chronic *Giardia lamblia* infection on epithelial transport and barrier function in human duodenum. Gut 2007;56: 328–35.

21. Oberhuber G, Stolte M. Histologic detection of trophozoites of *Giardia lamblia* in the terminal ileum. Scand J Gastroenterol 1995;30:905–8.

22. Calderaro A, Gorrini C, Montecchini S, et al. Evaluation of a real-time polymerase chain reaction assay for the laboratory diagnosis of giardiasis. Diagn Microbiol Infect Dis 2010;66:261–7.

23. Sackey ME, Weigel MM, Armijos RX. Predictors and nutritional consequences of intestinal parasitic infections in rural Ecuadorian children. J Trop Pediatr 2003;49: 17–23.

24. Berkman DS, Lescano AG, Gilman RH, et al. Effects of stunting, diarrhoeal disease and parasitic infection during infancy on cognition in late childhood: a follow up study. Lancet 2002;359:564–71.

25. Jokipii L, Jokipii AM. Single-dose metronidazole and tinidazole as therapy for giardiasis: success rates, side effects, and drug absorption and elimination. J Infect Dis 1979;140(6):984–8.

26. Mørch K, Hanevik K, Robertson LJ, et al. Treatment-ladder and genetic characterization of parasites in refractory giardiasis after an outbreak in Norway. J Infect 2008;56(4):268–73.

27. Klein P, Kleinová T, Volek Z, et al. Effect of Cryptosporidium parvum infection on the absorptive capacity and paracellular permeability of the small intestine in neonatal calves. Vet Parasitol 2008;152:53–9.

28. Garza A, Lackner A, Aye P, et al. Substance P receptor antagonist reverses intestinal pathophysiological alterations occurring in a novel ex-vivo model of Cryptosporidium parvum infection of intestinal tissues derived from SIV-infected macaques. J Med Primatol 2008;37:109–15.

29. Robinson P, Okhuysen PC, Cappell CL, et al. Substance P expression correlates with severity of diarrhea in cryptosporidiosis. J Infect Dis 2003;188:290–6.

30. Castellano-Gonzalez A, Yancey LS, Wang HC, et al. *Cryptosporidium* infection of human intestinal epithelial; cells increases expression of osteoprotegerin: a novel mechanism for evasion of host defense. J Infect Dis 2008;197:916–23.

31. DuPont HL, Chappell CL, Sterling CR, et al. The infectivity of Cryptosporidium parvum tin healthy volunteers. N Engl J Med 1995;332:855–9.

32. Sattar SA, Chauret C, Springthorpe VS, et al. Giardia cyst and Cryptosporidium oocyst survival in watersheds and factors affecting inactivation. Denver (CO): American Water Works Association Research Foundation; 1999. p. 1–10.

33. Blanshard C, Jackson AM, Shanson DC, et al. Cryptosporidiosis in HIV-seropositive patients. Q J Med 1992;85:813–23.

34. MacKenzie WR, Hoxie NJ, Proctor ME, et al. A massive outbreak in Milwaukee of cryptosporidium infection transmitted through the public water supply. N Engl J Med 1994;331:161–7.

35. Molbak K, Hojlyng N, Ingholt L, et al. An epidemic of cryptosporidiosis: a prospective community study from Guinea Bissau. Pediatr Infect Dis J 1990; 9:566–70.

36. Siwila J, Ohiri IG, Enemark HL, et al. Seasonal prevalence and incidence of *Cryptosporidium spp* and *Giardia duodenalis* and associated diarrhoea in children attending pre-school in Kafue, Zambia. Trans R Soc Trop Med Hyg 2011;105:102–8.

37. Cama VA, Bern C, Roberts J, et al. *Cryptosporidium* species and subtypes and clinical manifestations in children, Peru. Emerg Infect Dis 2008;14:1567–74.

38. Hadfield SJ, Robinson G, Elwin C, et al. Detection and differentiation of *Cryptosporidium* spp. In clinical samples by use of real time PCR. J Clin Microbiol 2011;49:918–24.

39. Rossignol JF, Ayoub A, Ayer MS. Treatment of diarrhea caused by *Cryptosporidium parvum*: a prospective randomized double-blind placebo-controlled study of nitazoxanide. J Infect Dis 2001;184:103–6.

40. Amadi B, Mwiya M, Musuku J, et al. Effect of nitazoxanide on morbidity and mortality in Zambian children with cryptosporidiosis: a randomized controlled trial. Lancet 2002;360:1375–80.

41. Sargeaunt P, Williams P, Greene JD. The differentiation of invasive and non-invasive *Entamoeba histolytica* by isoenzyme electrophoresis. Trans R Soc Trop Med Hyg 1978;72:519–21.

42. Tannich E, Horstmann RD, Knobloch J, et al. Genomic differences between pathogenic and nonpathogenic *Entamoeba histolytica*. Proc Natl Acad Sci U S A 1989;86:5118–22.

43. Diamond LS, Clarke CG. A redescription of *Entamoeba histolytica* Schaudin 1903 (Emended Walker 1911) to separate *Entamoeba histolytica* it from *Entamoeba dispar* (Brumpt 1925). J Eukaryot Microbiol 1993;40:340–4.

44. Zhang X, Zhang Z, Alexander D, et al. Expression of amoebapore is required for full expression of *Entamoeba histolytica* virulence in amebic liver abscess but is not necessary for the induction of inflammation or tissue damage in amebic colitis. Infect Immun 2004;72:678–83.

45. James R, Barratt J, Marriott D, et al. Seroprevalence of *Entamoeba histolytica* among men who have sex with men in Sydney Australia. Am J Trop Med Hyg 2010;83:914–6.

46. Haque R, Mondal D, Karim A, et al. Prospective case control study of the association between common enteric protozoal parasites and diarrhea in Bangladesh. Clin Infect Dis 2009;48:1191–7.

47. Blessmann J, Ibne K, Phuong A, et al. Longitudinal study of intestinal *Entamoeba histolytica* infections in asymptomatic adult carriers. J Clin Microbiol 2003;41: 4745–50.
48. Nishise S, Fiujishima T, Kobayashi S, et al. Mass infection with *Entamoeba histolytica* in a Japanese institution for individuals with mental retardation: epidemiology and control measures. Ann Trop Med Parasitol 2010;104:383–90.
49. Herbinger KH, Fleischmann E, Weber C, et al. Epidemiological, clinical and diagnostic data on intestinal infections with *Entamoeba histolytica* and *Entamoeba dispar* among returning travelers. Infection 2011;39(6):527–35.
50. Takahashi T, Gambon-Dominguez A, Gomez-Mendez TJ, et al. Fulminant amebic colitis: an analysis of 55 cases. Dis Colon Rectum 1997;40:1362–7.
51. McGregor A, Brown M, Thway K, et al. Fulminant amoebic colitis following loperamide use. J Travel Med 2007;14:61–2.
52. Watanabe K, Gatanag H, Escueta de Cadiz A, et al. Amebiasis in HIV-1 infected Japanese men: clinical features and response to therapy. PLoS Negl Trop Dis 2011;5:e13418.
53. Lodhi S, Sarwar AR, Muzammil M, et al. Features distinguishing amoebic liver abscess from pyogenic liver abscess: a review of 577 cases. Trop Med Int Health 2004;9:718–23.
54. Gonzalez ML, Dans LF, Martinez EG. Antiamoebic drugs for treating amoebic colitis. Cochrane Database Syst Rev 2009;15:CD006085.
55. Blessmann J, Binh HD, Hung DM, et al. Treatment of amoebic liver abscess with metronidazole alone or in combination with ultrasound-guided needle aspiration: a comparative, prospective and randomized study. Trop Med Int Health 2003;8: 1030–4.
56. Chavez-Tapia NC, Hernandez-Callerros J, Tellez-Avila FI, et al. Image-guided procedure plus Metronidazole versus Metronidazole alone for uncomplicated amebic liver abscess. Cochrane Database Syst Rev 2009;1:CD00488.
57. Blessmann J, Tannich E. Treatment of asymptomatic intestinal *Entamoeba histolytica* infection. N Engl J Med 2002;347:1384.
58. Ortega YR, Sanchez R. Update on cyclosporiasis: a food-borne and waterborne parasite. Clin Microbiol Rev 2010;23:218–34.
59. Moretto M, Weiss LM, Combe CL, et al. IFN-Y producing dendritic cells are important for priming of gut intraepithelial lymphocyte response against intracellular parasitic infection. J Immunol 2007;179:2485–92.
60. Goodgame R, Stager C, Marcantel B, et al. Intensity of infection in AIDS-related intestinal microsporidiosis. J Infect Dis 1999;180:929–32.
61. Izquierdo F, Catillo Hermida JA, Fenoy S, et al. Detection of microsporidia in drinking water, waste water and recreational rivers. Water Res 2011;45:4837–43.
62. Slodkowicz-Kowalska A. Animal reservoirs of human virulent microsporidian species. Wiad Parazytol 2009;55:63–5.
63. Cama V, Pearson J, Cabrera L, et al. Transmission on Enterocytozoon bieneusi between a child and guinea pigs. J Clin Microbiol 2007;45:2708–10.
64. Dworkin MS, Buskin SE, Davidson AJ, et al. Prevalence of intestinal microsporidiosis in human immunodeficiency virus infected patients with diarrhea in major United States cities. Rev Inst Med Trop Sao Paulo 2007;49:339–42.
65. Wolk DM, Schneider SK, Wengwenack NL, et al. Real time PCR for detection of Encephalitozoon intestinalis from stool samples. J Clin Microbiol 2002;40:3922–8.
66. Tremoulet AH, Avila-Aguero ML, Paris MM, et al. Albendazole therapy for Microsporidium diarrhea in immunocompetent children. Pediatr Infect Dis J 2004;23: 915–8.

Nematode Infections
Soil-Transmitted Helminths and *Trichinella*

Stefanie Knopp, PhD[a,b,*], Peter Steinmann, PhD[a,b],
Jennifer Keiser, PhD[a,c], Jürg Utzinger, PhD[a,b]

KEYWORDS

- Soil-transmitted helminths • *Enterobius vermicularis* • *Strongyloides stercoralis*
- *Toxocara* • *Trichinella* • Burden • Diagnosis • Control

KEY POINTS

- Soil-transmitted helminth and *Trichinella* infections belong to the "neglected tropical diseases" and the "neglected infections of poverty".
- Intestinal nematode infections considerably impact on people's health in the tropics and subtropics, and also occur in temperate and arctic regions of the United States and Europe.
- Early diagnosis and adequate treatment of infections at an early stage can help to avoid chronic morbid sequelae as infection progresses.
- Access to clean water, improved sanitation, personal hygiene, and food protection measures are key factors to avoid infection and transmission of intestinal nematodes.
- Diagnosis, prevention, and treatment of intestinal nematode infections gain importance in western travel clinics due to growing tourism, travel, migration, and food imports.

Intestinal nematode infections caused by soil-transmitted helminths (ie, *Ascaris lumbricoides*, *Strongyloides stercoralis*, *Trichuris trichiura*, and the 2 hookworm species *Ancylostoma duodenale* and *Necator americanus*), *Enterobius vermicularis*, *Toxocara* spp, and *Trichinella* spp belong to both the "neglected tropical diseases" and the "neglected infections of poverty."[1–3] Given the sheer number of the at-risk population

---

Funding Statement: While preparing the current review, Stefanie Knopp was financially supported by the "Forschungsfonds" of the University of Basel. At present, Stefanie Knopp is financially supported by the University of Georgia Research Foundation Inc., which is funded by the Bill & Melinda Gates Foundation (SCORE project).
Conflict of Interests: The authors have nothing to disclose.
[a] University of Basel, Petersplatz 1, CH-4003 Basel, Switzerland; [b] Department of Epidemiology and Public Health, Swiss Tropical and Public Health Institute, Socinstrasse 57, P.O. Box, CH-4002 Basel, Switzerland; [c] Department of Medical Parasitology and Infection Biology, Swiss Tropical and Public Health Institute, Socinstrasse 57, P.O. Box, CH-4002 Basel, Switzerland
* Department of Epidemiology and Public Health, Swiss Tropical and Public Health Institute, Socinstrasse 57, P.O. Box, CH-4002 Basel, Switzerland.
E-mail address: s.knopp@unibas.ch

Infect Dis Clin N Am 26 (2012) 341–358
doi:10.1016/j.idc.2012.02.006
0891-5520/12/$ – see front matter © 2012 Elsevier Inc. All rights reserved.

(more than half of the world's population) and the large amount of infected people (more than 1 billion), it is hard to understand why the diseases caused by intestinal nematodes are still widely neglected.[4] However, because of the increase in the tourist and food import industry, poverty-related crowding, and poor hygiene on one hand, and economic-, political-, and armed conflict-related migration on the other, nematode infections have recently gained renewed importance on the disease agenda in Europe and North America.[3,5–8]

The global burden attributable to common soil-transmitted helminthiasis (ascariasis, trichuriasis, and hookworm disease) is estimated at between 4.5 and 39 million disability-adjusted life years (DALYs).[9,10] For toxocariasis and trichinellosis no burden estimates are currently available.[11] Although these diseases can cause outbreaks and include severe manifestations with considerable fatality rates.[12]

This article reviews the epidemiology of intestinal nematode infections, including current distribution, life cycles, clinical features, and associated burden. Diagnostic approaches and treatment, and tools for prevention and control are discussed. Protective measures for travelers are highlighted (**Box 1**), and relevant information is given on vulnerable groups and case numbers in the United States (**Box 2**).

SOIL-TRANSMITTED HELMINTHS (*ASCARIS LUMBRICOIDES*, HOOKWORM, *STRONGYLOIDES STERCORALIS*, AND *TRICHURIS TRICHIURA*)
Life Cycle and Epidemiology

Common soil-transmitted helminths include the roundworm (*A lumbricoides*), 2 species of hookworm (*A duodenale* and *N americanus*), the whipworm (*T trichiura*), and the often neglected threadworm (*S stercoralis*).[2,13] The soil-transmitted helminths share many similarities in terms of transmission and epidemiology. For example, people become infected with *A lumbricoides* and *T trichiura* by ingesting fertilized eggs via consumption of contaminated food (eg, fruits and vegetables) or contact with contaminated hands. Worm larvae hatch in the intestine, and those of *A lumbricoides* penetrate the intestinal wall and migrate via the liver and heart to the lungs. From there, larvae are coughed up and swallowed, to re-enter the small intestine where they mature. Adult female *A lumbricoides* produce around 200,000 eggs per day (**Table 1**).[14–16] *T trichiura* develop in the intestine. Adult *T trichiura* attach to the mucosa of the large intestine. Females produce up to 5000 eggs per day.[2] The eggs of both species are excreted with the feces and undergo a maturation phase in the environment.

Hookworm and *S stercoralis* infections are acquired through skin penetration of the infective third-stage larvae (L_3), which are present in moist soil. Walking barefoot, playing on the ground, or farming and mining are known risk factors for acquiring these infections. Following host entry, the larvae undergo a journey through the vasculature, enter the airways, are swallowed, and finally reach the intestine, where hookworm larvae develop into adult male and female worms, whereas *S stercoralis* larvae mature into parthenogenetic egg-laying females.[8,17–19] Female *N americanus* produce between 9000 and 10,000 eggs per day and *A duodenale* between 25,000 and 30,000.[2] In contrast to the other soil-transmitted helminths, which do not reproduce within the host, *S stercoralis* infections are often perpetuated over long periods by autoinfection.[20] In that case, larvae hatch from eggs already in the gastrointestinal tract, develop into infective L_3, penetrate the intestinal mucosa, and migrate to the small intestine or to parenteral sites, eg, the lungs. *S stercoralis* can also enter a free-living nonparasitic life cycle ending in either infective L_3 (homogonic pathway)

Box 1
Protective measures against intestinal nematodes covered in this review

Ascaris lumbricoides and *Trichuris trichiura:*
- Avoid the ingestion of worm eggs
  - Peel or cook food
  - Boil drinking water
  - Wash hands with soap
  - Do not place small children directly on soil

Ancylostoma duodenale, Necator americanus, and *Strongyloides stercoralis:*
- Avoid skin penetration by larvae
  - Reduce skin contact with potentially infected soil
    - Wear closed shoes
    - Wear gloves for farming

Enterobius vermicularis
- Avoid the ingestion of worm eggs
  - Wash hands with soap
  - Regularly change and wash underwear with soap
  - Regularly change and wash towels, linen, and bed sheets with soap
  - Do not share linen and bed sheets; sleep in separate beds

Toxocara canis and *Toxocara cati*
- Avoid the ingestion of worm eggs
  - Wash hands with soap
  - Do not place small children directly on soil

Trichinella spp
- Avoid the ingestion of larvae
  - Do not eat raw or undercooked meat from domestic or sylvatic animals that has not been subjected to formal meat inspection

---

or free-living adults (heterogonic pathway) (**Fig. 1**), depending on environmental and genetic cues.[21]

Soil-transmitted helminth infections are particularly widespread in the tropical and subtropical regions of the world (**Table 2**). Indeed, social-ecological contexts govern the transmission of soil-transmitted helminths: warm and moist climate, which allow the development of helminth eggs and larvae, coupled with inappropriate hygiene, sanitation, and water.[25,26] The highest prevalence rates of soil-transmitted helminths occur in sub-Saharan Africa and southern and eastern Asia.[27,28] In general, school-aged children are at highest risk of infection with *A lumbricoides*, hookworm, and *T trichiura*.[29,30] Infection intensities of *A lumbricoides* and *T trichiura* peak in children aged 5 to 15 years, whereas hookworm infections may plateau in adulthood.[2] At highest risk of *S stercoralis* infections are individuals with altered cellular immunity, especially those receiving long-term steroid therapy, patients with lymphoma, kidney allograft recipients, travelers to endemic areas, and prisoners and other institutionalized people.[18] It is estimated that globally, more than 1.2 billion people are infected

Table 1
Characteristics of intestinal nematodes covered in the present review

	Infection Route	Adult Worm Location	Egg/Larvae Final Destination	No. of Eggs Shed by Female Worm Per Day	Life Span of Adult Worms	Intermediate Host/Vector	Time in Intermediate Host/until Eggs/Larvae become Infective
Ascaris lumbricoides	Ingestion of fertilized eggs	Small intestine	Eggs are passed with feces into soil	~200,000	~1 y	None	At least 8–10 d
Hookworms	Larvae penetrate skin	Small intestine	Eggs are passed with feces into soil and develop into infective larvae	*Necator americanus*: 9000–10,000 *Ancylostoma duodenale*: 25,000–30,000	5–7 y	None	~7 d
Trichuris trichiura	Ingestion of fertilized eggs	Large intestine	Eggs are passed with feces into soil	3000–5000	1.5–2 y	None	At least 12–15 d
Strongyloides stercoralis	Larvae penetrate skin; autoinfection	Small intestine	Larvae are passed with feces into soil	50	No number available	None	No number available
Enterobius vermicularis	Ingestion of fertilized eggs; autoinfection	Large intestine	Eggs attach to perianal skin and get into environment	16,000	~13 wk	None	~6 h
Toxocara canis and *Toxocara cati*	Ingestion of fertilized eggs	Small intestine	Eggs are passed with feces into soil	~200,000	~4 mo	Dog, cat	2–3 wk
Trichinella spp	Ingestion of encysted larvae contained in raw or undercooked meat	Small intestine	Larvae migrate to skeletal muscles and encyst	No number available	~4 wk	Mammals (particularly pigs), birds, reptiles	At least 18 d

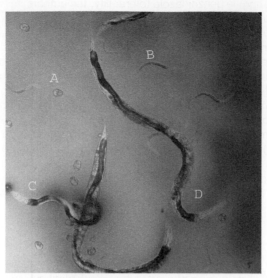

Fig. 1. *Strongyloides stercoralis* eggs (A), larvae (B), and free-living male (C) and female (D) adult worms on a Koga agar plate. (*Courtesy of* Hanspeter Marti, PhD, Swiss Tropical and Public Health Institute, Basel, Switzerland.)

with at least one soil-transmitted helminth species[2] and that more than half the world's population is at risk of infection.[14,22] In the developing world, particularly in rural settings, multiple-species soil-transmitted helminth infections are common.[31] In Europe, most infections are caused by *A lumbricoides* and *T trichiura* and occur in the poorest areas, mostly in Eastern and Southern Europe.[8] In the United States there is a high probability that ascariasis, trichuriasis, and strongyloidiasis are still important parasitic diseases (**Box 2**).[7] Parasitic gastrointestinal infections must also be considered in travelers, particularly in those returning from South America, sub-Saharan Africa, and South Asia.[39]

Clinical Features

Soil-transmitted helminths arguably are among the world's most important causes of physical and intellectual growth retardation.[2] The morbidity associated with soil-transmitted helminth infections depends on the intensity of infection, which is a function of the number of worms harbored in the human host. Common are intestinal symptoms such as abdominal pain, and general malaise and weakness. Heavy *A lumbricoides* infections can cause nutritional deficiencies and growth retardation as a result of lactose intolerance and malabsorption of vitamin A and possibly other nutrients.[2] In infected children partial intestinal obstruction can occur, which is typically associated with signs and symptoms of peritonitis. In adults, *A lumbricoides* worms can enter and block the ampullary orifice of the common bile duct, causing hepatobiliary and pancreatic disease symptoms. Fever tends to animate adult worms to move and emerge from the nasopharynx or anus. Adult worms might also enter the appendix, leading to acute appendicular colic and gangrene of the appendix tip. This process leads to symptoms similar to appendicitis, hence differential diagnosis is required.[2] An intense inflammatory response against *A lumbricoides* larval antigen in the lungs can result in verminous pneumonia.

Heavy chronic infection with *T trichiura* can cause inflammation and colitis. Chronic disease signs include diarrhea, impaired growth, anemia, and finger clubbing. The

Table 2
Epidemiology and burden of intestinal nematodes covered in the present review

	Geographic Distribution	No. of People at Risk	No. of Infected People (Million)	Global Burden (DALYs) (Year of Estimate)
Ascaris lumbricoides	Worldwide in at least 112 countries; particularly in sub-Saharan Africa, the Americas, South and East Asia	4.5 billion[14,22]	807–1221[2]	1,851,000 (2004)[23]
Hookworm			576–740[2]	1,092,000 (2004)[23]
Trichuris trichiura			604–795[2]	1,012,000 (2004)[23]
Strongyloides stercoralis	Worldwide in at least 70 countries; particularly in Southeast Asia, Latin America, sub-Saharan Africa, and parts of the southeastern United States	No number available	30–100[2]	No number available
Enterobius vermicularis	Worldwide	No number available	No number available	No number available
Toxocara canis and *T cati*	Worldwide	No number available	No number available	No number available
Trichinella spiralis	Worldwide	No number available	>10[24]	No number available

Box 2
Intestinal nematode infections in North America

Most nematode infections occur, yet are largely neglected, in the United States,[3] where prevalences are highest among poor people, ethnic minorities, women, and children.[32] The United States Gulf Coast, including Louisiana, Mississippi, and Alabama as well as neighboring regions of Texas and Florida, are considered most vulnerable in terms of neglected disease occurrence.[2,3,28,33]

Ascaris lumbricoides

- Appalachia, American South

- Refugees, Mexican-born migrant workers, African American populations

- <4 million cases[3,10,12,34]

Trichuris trichiura

- Appalachia, American South

- Refugees

- 13% of schoolchildren in Clay County (Eastern Kentucky)[35,36]

Hookworm *(Ancylostoma duodenale, Necator americanus)*

- Believed to be eliminated from the American South where in the early twentieth century highly endemic areas existed, but no large studies have been conducted since the 1970s[7]

- Refugees, Mexican-born migrant workers[3]

Strongyloides stercoralis

- Appalachia, American South

- Refugees, older white men with underlying chronic illnesses, poor white Appalachians

- 68,000 to 100,000 cases[3,14]

Enterobius vermicularis

- Most common worm infection in the United States

- Children younger than 18 years; people who take care of infected children; institutionalized people; no association with any particular socioeconomic level, ethnic group, or culture

- 42 million cases[37]

Toxocara canis and *Toxocara cati*

- Inner cities, American South (Mississippi Delta and the Cotton Belt), Appalachia

- Impoverished, socioeconomically disadvantaged children, rural children, inner-city children, Hispanics, African Americans

- 1.3 to 2.8 million cases[3]

- ~14% of the United States population has been infected (Centers for Disease Control and Prevention [CDC])

Trichinella spp

- Arctic Alaska, Canada

- Inuits, people from poor rural areas or tribal lands

- Between 2002 and 2007, an average of 11 cases per year were reported to CDC

- Incidence rate of Arctic trichinellosis (*Trichinella nativa*) in Alaska: 1.8 cases per 100,000 per year[38]

- Incidence rate of Arctic trichinellosis (*Trichinella nativa*) in the northernmost region of Canada: 11 cases per 100,000 per year[38]

most serious manifestation of heavy *T trichiura* infection is chronic dysentery and rectal prolapse.[40]

The attachment of hookworm to the intestinal mucosa and blood feeding causes bleeding, which can result in (iron-deficiency) anemia.[2] Of note, *A duodenale* take up larger amounts of blood than *N americanus*, which is explained by the larger size of the former hookworm species. Children and women of reproductive age, who have low iron reserves, are at particular risk of anemia. In pregnant women, severe iron deficiency can have a negative impact on the mother, fetus, and newborn baby.[41] The skin penetration of hookworm larvae results in ground itch, a local erythematous and papular rash accompanied by pruritus.[17] The lung passage of hookworm larvae results in less severe pneumonitis compared with that caused by *A lumbricoides* larvae.

S stercoralis infections might create cutaneous, gastrointestinal, or pulmonary symptoms. The extremely motile larvae may invade the skin in the perianal region (autoinfection), causing serpiginous, urticarial rashes termed larva currens (**Fig. 2**).[18,42] Hyperinfection and dissemination of *S stercoralis* can result in edema and infiltrates of the lung, whereas larvae penetrating the intestinal walls can carry enteral bacteria that are the cause of septicemia, meningitis, or pneumonia.[18,42]

Diagnosis and Treatment

As discussed in detail in the article by Rosenblatt and colleagues elsewhere in this issue, the diagnosis of soil-transmitted helminthiasis is based on the microscopic detection of eggs or larvae in fresh or fixed stool samples. The most widely used technique in epidemiologic surveys for the diagnosis of *A lumbricoides*, hookworm, and *T trichiura* is the Kato-Katz technique,[43,44] whereby a thick smear of a defined volume of stool (usually 41.7 mg) is stained and cleared with a malachite green or methylene blue and glycerol-soaked cellophane coverslip, and eggs are enumerated under a microscope by experienced laboratory technicians. The ether-concentration, McMaster, and FLOTAC techniques are also suitable for the diagnosis of soil-transmitted helminth infections.[45–47] *S stercoralis* larvae cannot be diagnosed with the aforementioned techniques. The Koga agar plate[48] and Baermann[49] methods allow the detection of *S stercoralis* larvae in fresh stool samples. Immunologic or serologic approaches for diagnosis have been investigated but are not widely used, as they are not able to distinguish past from present infections and suffer from considerable cross-reactivity between serum antibodies and antigens from different nematode species. Polymerase chain reaction (PCR) assays for the identification of molecular nematode markers in stool samples are very specific and sensitive, but are not yet

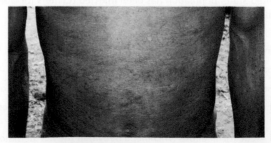

Fig. 2. *Strongyloides stercoralis* hyperinfection. (*Courtesy of* Hanspeter Marti, PhD, Swiss Tropical and Public Health Institute, Basel, Switzerland.)

routinely applied for individual patient management or in epidemiologic surveys because of technical constraints in resource-poor settings and their high costs.

The 2 benzimidazoles albendazole and mebendazole, and the macrocyclic lactone ivermectin, are the recommended drugs for soil-transmitted helminthiasis.[14,34,50] In preventive chemotherapy programs targeting ascariasis, trichuriasis, and hookworm disease, albendazole and mebendazole are used in single oral doses of 400 mg and 500 mg, respectively.[34,51] For trichuriasis, a randomized controlled trial performed in the People's Republic of China found high cure and egg reduction rates after triple-dose albendazole or mebendazole.[52] Indeed, 3-day courses of albendazole (400 mg per dose) or twice-daily mebendazole (100 mg per dose) is the recommended treatment scheme by physicians in special travel clinics in the North.[2,50] It was recently shown that a combination therapy of mebendazole (single oral dose of 500 mg) plus ivermectin (200 µg/kg) is more efficacious than single mebendazole and albendazole against *T trichiura*.[53] Ivermectin (200 µg/kg) is the treatment of choice against *S stercoralis*, but multiple doses of albendazole are also efficacious.[4,54]

Control and Prevention

Soil-transmitted helminthiasis control programs rely on the regular administration of anthelmintic drugs (mainly albendazole and mebendazole) to school-aged children or entire communities (when prevalence rates in the school-aged population are above a predefined threshold) to prevent morbidity. This strategy, termed preventive chemotherapy, also has an impact on transmission. Such programs have been implemented in many endemic countries following the 2001 World Health Assembly resolution 54.19, which urged all endemic member states to annually administer anthelmintic drugs to at least 75%, and up to 100% of all school-aged children at risk of morbidity by 2010.[4,55] However, in 2009 the global treatment coverage was estimated to be only 31%, far below the target set for 2010.[56] Besides these efforts, the community-wide administration of ivermectin or diethylcarbamazine (DEC) plus albendazole, in the context of programs to control lymphatic filariasis or onchocerciasis, has an impact on soil-transmitted helminths, including *S stercoralis*, but the effectiveness should be monitored more closely. Additional measures to prevent soil-transmitted helminth infections are the provision of improved sanitary infrastructure, safe water, abstaining from night-soil use for farming (commonly practiced in Southeast and East Asia), and adequate personal and food hygiene as well as wearing shoes. Results from a recent systematic review and meta-analysis suggest that people having access to sanitation have an approximately 50% lower risk of soil-transmitted helminth infection than those without.[26] Individuals can avoid *A lumbricoides* and *T trichiura* infections by peeling or cooking their food, boiling drinking water, and by consistent use of soap for hand washing (the mnemonic saying "cook it, peel it, or leave it") (see **Box 1**). Travelers should also be alerted to the risk of soil-transmitted helminth infections and the simple prevention measures. Hookworm and new *S stercoralis* infections (cave at: autoinfections are possible) can be prevented by reducing skin contact with potentially infected soil, for example by wearing closed shoes or gloves, and by placing infants on mats.

ENTEROBIASIS (*ENTEROBIUS VERMICULARIS*)
Life Cycle and Epidemiology

E vermicularis, also known as pinworm, is transmitted directly from person to person, but autoinfection is also possible. The most common ways of infection are via dust, food, hands, and water contaminated with eggs.[57] The adult worms live attached to the mucosa in the cecum and large intestine of humans. At night, female worms migrate out of the anus of their host and deposit their sticky eggs on the perianal skin. The eggs become infective within hours. If eggs are ingested, larvae hatch and mature to adult worms within 2 to 4 weeks[57] (see **Table 1**).

E vermicularis occur worldwide and infect millions of people, mainly children (see **Table 2**). Infections are most prevalent in temperate regions but also frequently occur in the tropics. It is the most common helminth infection in the United States.[58] Overcrowding in families, kindergartens, and schools as well as inadequate personal and community hygiene are the key risk factors for transmission. Children are at highest risk of infection; prevalences usually peak in children aged 5 to 10 years.

Clinical Features

E vermicularis infections are mostly asymptomatic. Reported symptoms include intense pruritus in the perianal area that can lead to insomnia, restlessness, and irritability.[57] In women, adult female pinworms can migrate to the genital tract, causing granulomas in the uterus, ovary, and the fallopian tubes, and pelvic peritoneum.

Diagnosis and Treatment

Pinworm infections are usually diagnosed using the adhesive-tape method for detection of ova, segments of adult worms, or intact worms (**Fig. 3**).[59] For this test, a transparent adhesive cellulose tape is placed on the subject's perianal area in the early morning before the individual showers or uses the toilet.[37] The tape is subsequently attached to a microscope slide for microscopic examination.[60] The eggs can be stained deep blue with lactophenol cotton blue, facilitating the detection and identification.[61] The threadlike, light-yellowish to white adult worms with a long, thin, sharply pointed tail may also be observed in the stool.[37]

Albendazole and mebendazole are efficacious against *E vermicularis*. Recommended regimens are single oral doses (mebendazole, 100–400 mg; albendazole, 100–400 mg) that are repeated after 1 week, to target worms that have developed from autoinfection.[57] Whether symptoms are present or not, it is advisable to treat all members in a household where an infection has occurred as family members are usually also infected with *E vermicularis*.[37]

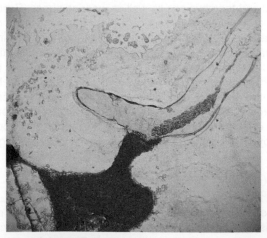

Fig. 3. *Enterobius vermicularis* adult female worm shedding countless eggs on an adhesive tape. (*Courtesy of* Tobias Schindler, BSc, Ifakara Health Center, Bagamoyo, Tanzania.)

Control and Prevention

In households or institutions where more than one individual is infected or repeated symptomatic infections occur, simultaneous treatment of all members along with a thorough cleaning of the rooms, towels, and bed linen is recommended. Individual and household hygiene, for example the regular washing of hands and linen, towels, and underwear with soap, is of major importance in preventing infections (see **Box 1**).

TOXOCARIASIS (*TOXOCARA CANIS* AND *TOXOCARA CATI*)
Life Cycle and Epidemiology

Toxocariasis is a zoonosis. The definitive hosts of *T canis* and *T cati* are dogs and cats, respectively. Humans are accidentally infected by ingesting *Toxocara* eggs containing infective L_3 or by eating raw or undercooked tissue with encapsulated L_3 of paratenic hosts such as cows, sheep, or chickens.[62] After egg ingestion the L_3 hatch in the small intestines, penetrate the intestinal wall, and are carried by the blood stream to the liver, and in some cases to the lungs, muscles, eyes, and/or the central nervous system. Humans are accidental hosts in which larvae fail to develop into reproducing adult worms but instead encapsulate in an arbitrary environment.

Similarly, in dogs and cats the L_3 encyst in tissues but can be reactivated in pregnant bitches, and reach their final destination in the dog's intestines either in the adult animal or after crossing the placenta, infecting fetuses. In the intestine of a definitive host, the female worm produces up to 200,000 eggs per day, shed with the feces[62] (see **Table 1**). In the environment, eggs embryonate and develop to L_3 within 2 to 3 weeks.

Toxocara infections occur wherever cats and dogs are kept. In the United States, toxocariasis is considered one of the most common human parasitic worm infections, while in developing countries it might pose an even greater public health problem.[63] However, the importance of toxocariasis in public health, including global and regional burden estimates, remains to be determined (see **Table 2**).[11]

Risk factors for infection include poverty, overcrowding, illiteracy, rural residence, and pica/geophagia.[64] Children playing on grounds contaminated with dog or cat feces and people having soil-related occupations are at particular risk of infection.[63,64]

Clinical Features

Toxocara infections in humans can remain asymptomatic, but larvae in tissues and organs can also cause severe local inflammatory reactions that result in both mechanical and immunopathologic damage, which are the basis of toxocariasis.[63,64] The 2 classic clinical syndromes in humans are (1) visceral larva migrans (systemic disease caused by larval migration through major organs) and (2) ocular larva migrans (disease is limited to the eyes and optic nerves). Larvae migrating through the liver and lungs are the cause of visceral larva migrans, which results in hepatitis and pneumonitis and might progress to hepatomegaly and pulmonary infiltrates or nodules accompanied by cough, wheezing, eosinophilia, lymphadenopathy, and fever. If larvae enter the central nervous system, they can cause meningoencephalitis and cerebritis, manifesting as seizures.[63] The migration of larvae through the eye (ocular larva migrans) results in inflammation and permanent ocular damage[63,64] Common and less severe symptoms known as covert and common toxocariasis in children and adults, respectively, resemble asthma and include wheezing, pulmonary infiltrates, and eosinophilia.

Diagnosis and Treatment

As no adult worms develop in the paratenic human host, no *Toxocara* eggs can be found in human feces, and hence the identification of infection relies on biopsies and, particularly, on serodiagnosis. The commercially available and most useful test for the diagnosis of visceral and ocular larva migrans caused by *T canis* and *T cati* is the enzyme immunoassay (EIA) using standardized *T canis* excretory-secretory (TES) antigens from infective-stage larvae.[63,65] A limitation of the indirect TES enzyme-linked immunosorbent assay (ELISA) for antibody detection is its cross-reactivity with other nematode infections. Hence, positive screening results from the ELISA should be confirmed by applying a TES Western blot, which visualizes *Toxocara*-specific low molecular weight bands (24–32 kDa).[11] Of note, antibody detection tests are not able to distinguish between past and present infections, because antibody titers can remain high in the absence of disease and after treatment, limiting their applicability. The detection of parasite DNA in humans is not very sensitive and reliable, because *Toxocara* does not replicate in the human host and larvae are encapsulated in tissue.[11] However, the detection of parasite DNA in soil samples and in definitive and paratenic animal hosts is possible with new PCR tests, and might be useful for the assessment of environmental contamination and the prevalence of infections in animals.[66,67]

Albendazole (500 mg given twice a day for 5 days) is the current first-line treatment for visceral larva migrans.[62] DEC has also been used to treat *Toxocara* infections. Indeed, DEC might be more effective than the benzimidazoles, but also more readily elicits major adverse reactions. Ocular toxocariasis should be treated in combination with steroids to reduce the inflammatory response.[11] Albendazole treatment (800 mg/d for adults and 400 mg/d for children) for 2 to 4 weeks kills persisting larvae.[68]

Control and Prevention

The public health importance of *Toxocara* infections remains to be elucidated, which will require national surveillance systems that are not yet in place in most countries. Measures to control transmission and prevent infections include: (1) sensitization of the general public, particularly pet owners, to raise awareness for the disease and its transmission; (2) regular deworming of puppies, adult dogs, and cats to reduce environmental contamination with *Toxocara* eggs; (3) improvements in the urban and rural sanitation structure to lower transmission between animals and humans; and (4) promotion of adequate personal hygiene (ie, hand washing), to prevent fecal-oral transmission of eggs (see **Box 1**).[11,63,64]

TRICHINELLOSIS (*TRICHINELLA* SPP)
Life Cycle and Epidemiology

Trichinellosis (trichinosis) is a zoonotic disease. The life cycle of the parasite includes an intestinal and a muscular phase. Humans, as well as pigs, rodents, and other animals, are infected by the ingestion of raw or undercooked meat containing encysted larvae.[69] During digestion, the *Trichinella* larvae are released into the stomach and subsequently penetrate the mucosa of the small intestine, where they develop into adult worms (see **Table 1**). Starting after 1 week and for a period of 3 to 4 weeks, adult female worms produce larvae, which cross the intestinal wall, spread via the blood vessels, and finally settle in striated skeletal muscles where they encyst after 4 to 5 weeks, but remain viable for several years.[69]

Trichinella infections occur worldwide (see **Table 2**). There are at least 8 *Trichinella* species, infecting a wide range of host species (mammals, birds, and reptiles), including humans. Among them, *Trichinella spiralis* is considered the most important in causing human trichinellosis.[70] Because approaches for the diagnosis and reporting of trichinellosis are not yet standardized, there is a lack of information on the global burden, current distribution, and incidence of trichinellosis in both animals and humans.[5,12] Estimates put forth more than 10 years ago suggest that globally, at least 10 million people are infected with *Trichinella*.[24] Autochthonous cases have been reported in 55 countries,[5] and accidental infections occur in areas and countries where people eat raw or undercooked meat that has not undergone testing for trichinellosis, and was imported from an endemic region.

Clinical Features

The clinical signs, symptoms, and course of disease vary between *Trichinella* species [69] and depend on the number of adult worms and larvae.[5] Trichinellosis includes a wide spectrum of clinical appearances ranging from asymptomatic to fatal.[5] In the acute phase of the disease, adult worms and particularly migrating larvae are responsible for the course of disease. The migration of larvae to their final destinations provokes acute immunologic, pathologic, and metabolic disturbances, which manifest as eosinophilia, increased levels of immunoglobulin E and muscle enzymes, diarrhea, abdominal pain, fever, myalgia, cutaneous rash, eyelid or facial edema, vasculitis, and intravascular thrombi.[5,69] In the acute infection, and because of the penetration and residency of larvae in the muscle, modifications of the cells and their environment are common.[5,69] More serious trichinellosis manifestations include cardiovascular, neurologic, ocular, respiratory, and digestive complications, which usually develop within 2 weeks after infection, and are more often seen in elderly and inappropriately treated people than in other population segments.[69] In pregnant women, *Trichinella* infections can cause abortion or premature delivery.[69]

Diagnosis and Treatment

The most reliable technique for diagnosing *Trichinella* infections is the ELISA, in combination with a Western blot.[69] Among the commercially available ELISA kits, only those showing no cross-reactions with other nematode antigens should be used.[69] However, anti-*Trichinella* antibodies usually cannot be detected at the onset of clinical signs. If a rapid confirmation of infection is required, counterimmunoelectrophoresis or latex agglutination tests can be applied which, though quick, are not commonly used because they are less sensitive and specific than ELISA. Trichinelloscopy allows determination of the intensity of infection (1000 larvae/g muscle tissue is considered a very heavy infection) and the species or genotype of the parasite. For this purpose, a small muscle sample is compressed between 2 microscope slides and examined under a light microscope at a magnification of 50× to 100×. However, this method is not very sensitive for detecting low-intensity infections. Additional diagnostic possibilities are the histologic examination of muscle tissue after hematoxylin-eosin staining, and the digestion of muscle tissue with pepsin (1%) and hydrochloric acid (1%) to detect early-stage larvae and late-stage (encapsulated) larvae, respectively. In general, as highlighted in the article by Rosenblatt and colleagues elsewhere in this issue, the diagnosis of trichinellosis in humans should be based on: (1) clinical picture (recognition of the signs and symptoms of trichinellosis); (2) laboratory findings (nonspecific laboratory parameters, ie, eosinophilia and muscle enzymes, antibody detection, and/or detection of larvae in a muscle biopsy); and (3) epidemiologic investigation (identification of source of infection and origin of meat, outbreak studies).[5,71]

Trichinellosis should ideally be treated at an early stage of infection to avoid serious complications. The anthelmintic drugs albendazole (400 mg twice daily for 8–14 days) and mebendazole (200–400 mg 3 times a day for 3 days, followed by 400–500 mg 3 times a day for 10 days) are recommended as first-line treatments.[5] Neither albendazole nor mebendazole are efficacious against all larval stages. Of note, mebendazole is particularly poorly absorbed in the gastrointestinal lumen and reaches only low plasma levels.[69] Severe symptoms should be treated with steroids, for example with prednisone (30–60 mg per day for 10–15 days).[5] Steroids must always be used in combination with anthelmintics, because they can increase the larval burden by delaying the expulsion of worms from the intestine.[69]

Control and Prevention

Trichinella infections in humans can be prevented at the individual level by avoiding the consumption of raw or undercooked meat and meat products from both domestic and sylvatic animals not tested for *Trichinella* larvae through formal meat inspection (see **Box 1**). At the population level, farming pigs under strict veterinary control and use of certified animal feed is important.[5]

In the United States and the European Union, there is a legal requirement to report trichinellosis cases. For example, the European Commission regulation no. 2075/2005 requires meat inspections for farmed and wild animal species that are susceptible to *Trichinella* infection (ie, domestic pigs, horses, and wild boars) and are slaughtered for consumption.[5] In the United States, a program to certify *Trichinella*-free pork production is being evaluated.[72] Despite these efforts, the movement of people (migrants and travelers), livestock, wildlife and, potentially, infectious food products increase the risk of spreading trichinellosis, illustrating the need for a rigorous testing and reporting system as well as good interaction between the public health and veterinary sector in affected countries.[5]

SUMMARY

Intestinal nematode infections, including soil-transmitted helminths, *E vermicularis*, *Toxocara* spp, and *Trichinella* spp inflict a considerable, yet underappreciated, public health burden not only on deprived populations in the tropics and subtropics but also in temperate and arctic areas of Europe and North America. The detection of light-intensity infections with the available diagnostic tools is generally not very sensitive and/or specific. Hence, the development of more accurate diagnostic methods, suitable for large-scale population screenings as well as for individual patient management, is essential for adequate surveillance and monitoring of the incidence and prevalence of disease in endemic countries, and in countries with a flourishing tourist and food import industry. The recognition and treatment of infections at an early stage can help avoid chronic morbid sequelae as infection progresses. While available anthelmintic drugs show moderate to good efficacy against some intestinal nematode species when administered at single oral doses within preventive chemotherapy programs (eg, albendazole and mebendazole),[73] other infections require multiple dosing or combination therapy and several disease outcomes cannot be inverted. Adopting preventive measures, first and foremost adequate food and personal hygiene, is hence key to the avoidance of infection and transmission of intestinal nematode infections.

REFERENCES

1. Hotez PJ, Yamey G. The evolving scope of PLoS Neglected Tropical Diseases. PLoS Negl Trop Dis 2009;3:e379.

2. Bethony J, Brooker S, Albonico M, et al. Soil-transmitted helminth infections: ascariasis, trichuriasis, and hookworm. Lancet 2006;367:1521–32.
3. Hotez PJ. Neglected infections of poverty in the United States of America. PLoS Negl Trop Dis 2008;2:e256.
4. WHO. Prevention and control of schistosomiasis and soil-transmitted helminthiasis: report of a WHO expert committee. WHO Tech Rep Ser 2002;912:1–57.
5. Gottstein B, Pozio E, Nockler K. Epidemiology, diagnosis, treatment, and control of trichinellosis. Clin Microbiol Rev 2009;22:127–45.
6. Hotez PJ, Gurwith M. Europe's neglected infections of poverty. Int J Infect Dis 2011;15:e611–9.
7. Hotez PJ. Neglected diseases and poverty in "The Other America": the greatest health disparity in the United States? PLoS Negl Trop Dis 2007;1:e149.
8. Hotez P. Neglected diseases amid wealth in the United States and Europe. Health Aff 2009;28:1720–5.
9. Hotez PJ, Molyneux DH, Fenwick A, et al. Incorporating a rapid-impact package for neglected tropical diseases with programs for HIV/AIDS, tuberculosis, and malaria. PLoS Med 2006;3:e102.
10. Utzinger J, Raso G, Brooker S, et al. Schistosomiasis and neglected tropical diseases: towards integrated and sustainable control and a word of caution. Parasitology 2009;136:1859–74.
11. Smith H, Holland C, Taylor M, et al. How common is human toxocariasis? Towards standardizing our knowledge. Trends Parasitol 2009;25:182–8.
12. Odermatt P, Lv S, Sayasone S. Less common parasitic infections in Southeast Asia that can produce outbreaks. Adv Parasitol 2010;72:409–35.
13. Olsen A, van Lieshout L, Marti H, et al. Strongyloidiasis—the most neglected of the neglected tropical diseases? Trans R Soc Trop Med Hyg 2009;103: 967–72.
14. Utzinger J, Keiser J. Schistosomiasis and soil-transmitted helminthiasis: common drugs for treatment and control. Expert Opin Pharmacother 2004;5:263–85.
15. Hotez PJ, Bottazzi ME, Franco-Paredes C, et al. The neglected tropical diseases of Latin America and the Caribbean: a review of disease burden and distribution and a roadmap for control and elimination. PLoS Negl Trop Dis 2008;2:e300.
16. Hotez PJ. Holidays in the sun and the Caribbean's forgotten burden of neglected tropical diseases. PLoS Negl Trop Dis 2008;2:e239.
17. Hotez PJ, Brooker S, Bethony J, et al. Hookworm infection. N Engl J Med 2004; 351:799–807.
18. Siddiqui AA, Berk SL. Diagnosis of *Strongyloides stercoralis* infection. Clin Infect Dis 2001;33:1040–7.
19. Warren KS. Helminthic diseases endemic in the United States. Am J Trop Med 1974;23:723–30.
20. Keiser PB, Nutman TB. *Strongyloides stercoralis* in the immunocompromised population. Clin Microbiol Rev 2004;17:208–17.
21. Ashton FT, Bhopale VM, Holt D, et al. Developmental switching in the parasitic nematode *Strongyloides stercoralis* is controlled by the ASF and ASI amphidial neurons. J Parasitol 1998;84:691–5.
22. Horton J. Global anthelmintic chemotherapy programs: learning from history. Trends Parasitol 2003;19:405–9.
23. WHO. The global burden of disease: 2004 update. Geneva (Switzerland): World Health Organization; 2008. p. 1–160.
24. Dupouy-Camet J. Trichinellosis: a worldwide zoonosis. Vet Parasitol 2000;93: 191–200.

25. Bartram J, Cairncross S. Hygiene, sanitation, and water: forgotten foundations of health. PLoS Med 2010;7:e1000367.
26. Ziegelbauer K, Speich B, Mäusezahl D, et al. Effect of sanitation on soil-transmitted helminth infection: systematic review and meta-analysis. PLoS Med 2012;9:e1001162.
27. de Silva NR, Brooker S, Hotez PJ, et al. Soil-transmitted helminth infections: updating the global picture. Trends Parasitol 2003;19:547–51.
28. Brooker S. Estimating the global distribution and disease burden of intestinal nematode infections: adding up the numbers—a review. Int J Parasitol 2010; 40:1137–44.
29. Woolhouse MEJ. Patterns in parasite epidemiology: the peak shift. Parasitol Today 1998;14:428–34.
30. Anderson RM, May RM. Helminth infections of humans: mathematical models, population dynamics, and control. Adv Parasitol 1985;24:1–101.
31. Steinmann P, Utzinger J, Du ZW, et al. Multiparasitism: a neglected reality on global, regional and local scale. Adv Parasitol 2010;73:21–50.
32. Hotez PJ, Stillwaggon E, McDonald M, et al. National summit on neglected infections of poverty in the United States [conference summary]. Emerg Infect Dis 2010;16:e1. Available at: http://www.cdc.gov/EID/content/16/5/e1.htm. Accessed February 7, 2012.
33. Hotez PJ. America's most distressed areas and their neglected infections: the United States Gulf Coast and the District of Columbia. PLoS Negl Trop Dis 2011;5:e843.
34. Hotez PJ, Molyneux DH, Fenwick A, et al. Control of neglected tropical diseases. N Engl J Med 2007;357:1018–27.
35. Walzer PD, Milder JE, Banwell JG, et al. Epidemiologic features of *Strongyloides stercoralis* infection in an endemic area of the United States. Am J Trop Med Hyg 1982;31:313–9.
36. Hotez PJ, Brindley PJ, Bethony JM, et al. Helminth infections: the great neglected tropical diseases. J Clin Invest 2008;118:1311–21.
37. Burkhart CN, Burkhart CG. Assessment of frequency, transmission, and genitourinary complications of enterobiasis (pinworms). Int J Dermatol 2005;44: 837–40.
38. Hotez PJ. Neglected infections of poverty among the indigenous peoples of the arctic. PLoS Negl Trop Dis 2011;4:e606.
39. Greenwood Z, Black J, Weld L, et al. Gastrointestinal infection among international travelers globally. J Travel Med 2008;15:221–8.
40. Bundy DAP, Cooper ES. *Trichuris* and trichuriasis in humans. Adv Parasitol 1989; 28:107–73.
41. Christian P, Khatry SK, West KP Jr. Antenatal anthelmintic treatment, birthweight, and infant survival in rural Nepal. Lancet 2004;364:981–3.
42. Grove DI. Human strongyloidiasis. Adv Parasitol 1996;38:251–309.
43. Katz N, Chaves A, Pellegrino J. A simple device for quantitative stool thick-smear technique in schistosomiasis mansoni. Rev Inst Med Trop São Paulo 1972;14: 397–400.
44. Speich B, Knopp S, Mohammed KA, et al. Comparative cost assessment of the Kato-Katz and FLOTAC techniques for soil-transmitted helminth diagnosis in epidemiological surveys. Parasit Vectors 2010;3:71.
45. Cringoli G, Rinaldi L, Maurelli MP, et al. FLOTAC: new multivalent techniques for qualitative and quantitative copromicroscopic diagnosis of parasites in animals and humans. Nat Protoc 2010;5:503–15.

46. Levecke B, De Wilde N, Vandenhoute E, et al. Field validity and feasibility of four techniques for the detection of *Trichuris* in simians: a model for monitoring drug efficacy in public health? PLoS Negl Trop Dis 2009;3:e366.
47. Utzinger J, Botero-Kleiven S, Castelli F, et al. Microscopic diagnosis of sodium acetate-acetic acid-formalin-fixed stool samples for helminths and intestinal protozoa: a comparison among European reference laboratories. Clin Microbiol Infect 2010;16:267–73.
48. Koga K, Kasuya S, Khamboonruang C, et al. A modified agar plate method for detection of *Strongyloides stercoralis*. Am J Trop Med Hyg 1991;45:518–21.
49. García LS, Bruckner DA. Diagnostic medical parasitology. 4th edition. Washington, DC: American Society for Microbiology; 2001. p. 1–791.
50. Keiser J, Utzinger J. The drugs we have and the drugs we need against major helminth infections. Adv Parasitol 2010;73:197–230.
51. WHO. Preventive chemotherapy in human helminthiasis: coordinated use of anthelminthic drugs in control interventions: a manual for health professionals and programme managers. Geneva (Switzerland): World Health Organization; 2006. p. 1–62.
52. Steinmann P, Utzinger J, Du ZW, et al. Efficacy of single-dose and triple-dose albendazole and mebendazole against soil-transmitted helminths and *Taenia* spp.: a randomized controlled trial. PLoS One 2011;6:e25003.
53. Knopp S, Mohammed KA, Speich B, et al. Albendazole and mebendazole administered alone or in combination with ivermectin against *Trichuris trichiura*: a randomized controlled trial. Clin Infect Dis 2010;51:1420–8.
54. Marti H, Haji HJ, Savioli L, et al. A comparative trial of a single-dose ivermectin versus three days of albendazole for treatment of *Strongyloides stercoralis* and other soil-transmitted helminth infections in children. Am J Trop Med Hyg 1996; 55:477–81.
55. Savioli L, Gabrielli AF, Montresor A, et al. Schistosomiasis control in Africa: 8 years after World Health Assembly Resolution 54.19. Parasitology 2009;136: 1677–81.
56. WHO. Soil-transmitted helminthiases: estimates of the number of children needing preventive chemotherapy and number treated, 2009. Wkly Epidemiol Rec 2011;86:257–68.
57. St Georgiev V. Chemotherapy of enterobiasis (oxyuriasis). Expert Opin Pharmacother 2001;2:267–75.
58. Rajamanickam A, Usmani A, Suri S, et al. Chronic diarrhea and abdominal pain: pin the pinworm. J Hosp Med 2009;4:137–9.
59. Jones JE. Pinworms. Am Fam Physician 1988;38:159–64.
60. WHO. Basic laboratory methods in medical parasitology. Geneva (Switzerland): World Health Organization; 1991. p. 1–121.
61. Parija SC, Sheeladevi C, Shivaprakash MR, et al. Evaluation of lactophenol cotton blue stain for detection of eggs of *Enterobius vermicularis* in perianal surface samples. Trop Doct 2001;31:214–5.
62. Rubinsky-Elefant G, Hirata CE, Yamamoto JH, et al. Human toxocariasis: diagnosis, worldwide seroprevalences and clinical expression of the systemic and ocular forms. Ann Trop Med Parasitol 2010;104:3–23.
63. Hotez PJ, Wilkins PP. Toxocariasis: America's most common neglected infection of poverty and a helminthiasis of global importance? PLoS Negl Trop Dis 2009; 3:e400.
64. Lee AC, Schantz PM, Kazacos KR, et al. Epidemiologic and zoonotic aspects of ascarid infections in dogs and cats. Trends Parasitol 2010;26:155–61.

65. de Savigny DH, Voller A, Woodruff AW. Toxocariasis: serological diagnosis by enzyme immunoassay. J Clin Pathol 1979;32:284–8.
66. Li MW, Lin RQ, Chen HH, et al. PCR tools for the verification of the specific identity of ascaridoid nematodes from dogs and cats. Mol Cell Probes 2007;21:349–54.
67. Borecka A, Gawor J. Modification of gDNA extraction from soil for PCR designed for the routine examination of soil samples contaminated with Toxocara spp. eggs. J Helminthol 2008;82:119–22.
68. Barisani-Asenbauer T, Maca SM, Hauff W, et al. Treatment of ocular toxocariasis with albendazole. J Ocul Pharmacol Ther 2001;17:287–94.
69. Dupouy-Camet J, Kociecka W, Bruschi F, et al. Opinion on the diagnosis and treatment of human trichinellosis. Expert Opin Pharmacother 2002;3:1117–30.
70. Pozio E, Murrell KD. Systematics and epidemiology of Trichinella. Adv Parasitol 2006;63:367–439.
71. Kociecka W. Trichinellosis: human disease, diagnosis and treatment. Vet Parasitol 2000;93:365–83.
72. Pyburn DG, Gamble HR, Wagstrom EA, et al. Trichinae certification in the United States pork industry. Vet Parasitol 2005;132:179–83.
73. Keiser J, Utzinger J. Efficacy of current drugs against soil-transmitted helminth infections: systematic review and meta-analysis. JAMA 2008;299:1937–48.

Nematode Infections: Filariases

Stefanie Knopp, PhD[a,b,*], Peter Steinmann, PhD[a,b],
Christoph Hatz, MD[a,c,d], Jennifer Keiser, PhD[a,e],
Jürg Utzinger, PhD[a,b]

KEYWORDS

- Filariasis • *Dracunculus medinensis* • *Loa loa* • *Mansonella perstans*
- *Onchocerca volvulus* • *Wuchereria bancrofti* • Epidemiology • Control

KEY POINTS

- More than 150 million people are affected by filarial infections that cause debilitating and irreversible disease outcomes; yet they belong to the "neglected tropical diseases."
- Filariae are not transmitted in Europe and North America, but travel clinics must be aware as infections might occur in immigrants, refugees, and long-term travelers.
- Available drugs reduce filariae transmission in endemic areas but do not mitigate disease symptoms.
- Current drugs can cause severe adverse reactions due to dying microfilariae, and must be applied with great care.
- Diagnostic tools to differentiate between pre-patent, patent, and post-patent infections are important for patient management and filariasis control with the ultimate goal of elimination.

Human diseases caused by filarial nematode infections are among the most debilitating and disfiguring ones described in the literature. Tens of millions of people are affected, yet they belong to the "neglected tropical diseases" and the "neglected infections of poverty."[1,2] One reason for this general neglect is that filarial nematodes

Funding: While preparing the current review, Stefanie Knopp was financially supported by the "Forschungsfonds" of the University of Basel. At present, Stefanie Knopp is financially supported by the University of Georgia Research Foundation Inc., which is funded by the Bill & Melinda Gates Foundation (SCORE project).
Conflict of interests: The authors have nothing to disclose.
[a] University of Basel, Petersplatz 1, CH-4003 Basel, Switzerland; [b] Department of Epidemiology and Public Health, Swiss Tropical and Public Health Institute, Socinstrasse 57, PO Box, CH-4002 Basel, Switzerland; [c] Department of Medical Services and Diagnostic, Swiss Tropical and Public Health Institute, Socinstrasse 57, PO Box, CH-4002 Basel, Switzerland; [d] Institute of Social and Preventive Medicine, University of Zurich, Hirschengraben 84, CH-8001 Zurich, Switzerland; [e] Department of Medical Parasitology and Infection Biology, Swiss Tropical and Public Health Institute, Socinstrasse 57, PO Box, CH-4002 Basel, Switzerland
* Department of Epidemiology and Public Health, Swiss Tropical and Public Health Institute, Socinstrasse 57, PO Box, CH-4002 Basel, Switzerland.
E-mail address: s.knopp@unibas.ch

Infect Dis Clin N Am 26 (2012) 359–381
doi:10.1016/j.idc.2012.02.005
0891-5520/12/$ – see front matter © 2012 Elsevier Inc. All rights reserved.

id.theclinics.com

are restricted to the tropics and subtropics, and are not transmitted in Europe and North America.[1] However, imported infections do occur in immigrants and refugees from endemic countries, and may occasionally be seen in long-term travelers and expatriates. Hence, clinics specialized in tropical and travel medicine must be aware of these diseases.[3]

Filariae larvae are transmitted by insect vectors. Adult worms live in defined areas of the body, specific for each filariae species. Several months or years after infection, either adult worms or their offspring (ie, microfilariae), cause disease-specific symptoms.[1] Among them are well-known disease outcomes, characterized by the emergence of a spaghetti-like worm (dracunculiasis), awfully enlarged extremities (elephantiasis), blindness and leopard skin (onchocerciasis), or small worms migrating through the eye (loiasis). Considerable progress has been made in the control and eventual elimination of filariae infections since the new millennium.[1,4,5] Mass drug administration (MDA) and large-scale vector control serve as the backbone of interventions.[6–9] While *Dracunculus medinensis* is close to being eradicated,[10] there are still an estimated 120 million people infected with lymphatic filariae (Wuchereria bancrofti, Brugia malayi, Brugia timori),[1] and 37 million people infected with *Onchocerca volvulus*.[1] Far fewer people are currently infected with *Loa loa* and *Mansonella perstans*, yet diseases caused by these filarial nematodes are of considerable public health importance.[11,12] At present, global burden of disease estimates are only available for lymphatic filariasis and onchocerciasis; they are as high as 5.9 million and 0.4 million disability-adjusted life years (DALYs), respectively.[2,13] Drugs, currently applied against filarial infections for mass treatment of at-risk populations, such as albendazole and ivermectin, are effective against larvae, but do not kill adult worms.[1,14] Hence, transmission can be reduced, but the diseases cannot be cured by drug intake and require other measures of mitigation.

This article describes the epidemiology of the most important filarial infections, including current distribution, life cycles, clinical features and associated burden, diagnostic approaches and treatment, and tools for prevention and control. Moreover, preventive measures for travelers are suggested (**Box 1**), and vulnerable groups and case numbers in North America identified (**Box 2**).

DRACUNCULIASIS OR GUINEA WORM DISEASE (*DRACUNCULUS MEDINENSIS*)
Life Cycle and Epidemiology

D medinensis, also known as the fiery serpent or guinea worm, is a memorable parasite. Humans become infected with guinea worm when drinking surface water that contains the intermediate host, a copepod of the genus *Cyclops*, which harbors infective third-stage larvae (L_3) (**Table 1**). Within the stomach, gastric juices kill the *Cyclops* and the guinea worm larvae are released. Those then migrate to the small intestine, penetrate the intestinal wall, and enter the abdominal cavity and retroperitoneal space. Male and female worms mate 60 to 90 days after infection. Within a year, fertilized female guinea worms grow and migrate to the skin surface, particularly of the lower limbs. The male worms die shortly after mating and are sometimes found calcified in different parts of the body (**Fig. 1**). Once the female worm reaches its final destination, it induces the formation of an aching blister and starts to emerge through the skin. Patients, who cool their aching legs in water, stimulate the female worm to release thousands of larvae. The larvae then live up to 3 days in the water or until they are ingested by *Cyclops*, in which, over a period of 2 weeks and 2 molts, they develop into infective larvae. The life cycle is completed when humans swallow infected *Cyclops*.[19,20] Dracunculiasis shows a strong seasonal pattern, and is associated

---

Box 1
Preventive measures against filarial infections for travelers

Dracunculus medinensis
- Avoid the ingestion of *Cyclops*
  - Do not drink unfiltered water from ponds or slow flowing rivers

Onchocerca volvulus
- Avoid bites of the day-active *Simulium* vector
  - Wear long clothes
  - Use insect repellents
  - Stay indoors
  - Ivermectin 150 µg/kg twice a year as preventive measure

Lymphatic filariae
- Avoid bites of the mosquito vectors
  - Wear long clothes
  - Use insect repellents
  - Sleep under a bednet (preferably long-lasting insecticide treated)

Loa loa
- Avoid bites of the day-active *Chrysops* vector
  - Wear long clothes
  - Use insect repellents
  - Diethylcarbamazine 300 mg/wk in long-term travelers to areas of high endemicity[3,15]

Mansonella perstans
- Avoid bites of the *Culicoides* vector
  - Wear long clothes
  - Use insect repellents

---

with either the rainy or dry seasons, whenever drinking from ponds or stagnant water sources becomes more likely and water bodies are of a size that favors transmission of the worm.

In 1986 guinea worm was still endemic in 20 countries of Africa and Asia, with an estimated 3.5 million people infected. The yearly incidence rate was 400,000 cases. In 1991, during the 44th World Health Assembly (WHA), member states endorsed the eradication of guinea worm disease.[21] In the meantime, great progress has been made in this regard thanks to concerted efforts spearheaded by the Carter Center (http://www.cartercenter.org/index.html). Indeed, in 2010 fewer than 2000 cases of guinea worm were reported in just a few very remote villages in only 6 African countries, namely Chad, Ethiopia, Ghana, Mali, Niger, and Sudan.[21–23] Provisional data for 2011 suggest that case numbers dropped to 1060, and that dracunculiasis only occurred in Chad, Ethiopia, Mali, and South Sudan. Nowadays, the greatest challenges to ultimately reach the goal of eradication are human migration, social and economic crisis, and armed conflict, particularly in areas of South Sudan where 97% of all registered cases occurred in 2011.[21]

Box 2
Filariasis in North America

Although filariases are not transmitted in North America, travel to endemic countries leads to exposure to filarial parasites and renders infections possible. In addition, imported cases are seen among recent immigrants from endemic countries. Currently, all presented filarial infections are listed as "rare disease" by the Office of Rare Diseases Research of the National Institutes of Health, and hence likely affect fewer than 200,000 people in the United States.

Dracunculus medinensis

- No case of dracunculiasis transmitted in the United States has ever been reported[16]

- Two cases (one in 1995 and one in 1997) were seen in the United States among refugees from Sudan[16]

Onchocerca volvulus

- Most infections seen in the United States occur in expatriate groups, such as missionaries, field scientists, and Peace Corps volunteers[17]

- Short-term travelers to endemic areas are at low risk of infection[17]

- Travelers who visit endemic areas for extended periods of time (generally >3 months; see first point) and live or work near blackfly habitats are at risk of infection[17]

- Between 1997 and 2004, a total of 81 cases detected among immigrants and people visiting friends or relatives were reported to the GeoSentinel Surveillance Network; an additional 20 cases were reported among travelers of nonendemic origin[18]

Lymphatic filariae

- Short-term travelers to endemic areas are at low risk of infection[17]

- Travelers who visit endemic areas for extended periods of time (generally >3 months) and who are intensively exposed to infected mosquitoes are at risk of infection[17]

- Between 1997 and 2004, a total of 49 *Wuchereria bancrofti* cases among immigrants and people visiting friends or relatives were reported to the GeoSentinel Surveillance Network; 18 cases were reported among travelers of nonendemic origin[18]

Loa loa

- Imported cases are observed occasionally in North America[18]

- Between 1997 and 2004, a total of 25 cases among immigrants and people visiting friends or relatives were reported to the GeoSentinel Surveillance Network; 43 cases were reported among travelers of nonendemic origin[18]

Mansonella perstans

- Imported cases are observed occasionally in North America[18]

Clinical Features and Associated Burden

Infections with guinea worm usually remain undiscovered until the painful blister develops as a result of an immunologic reaction to a few released larvae, and the female worm starts to emerge (**Box 3**). The closed blisters are sterile. Once open, the worm tracks caused by the emerging worm often become infected with bacteria. These secondary infections, if not disinfected and properly handled, can develop to painful inflammation of the surrounding tissue and finally the formation of abscesses. Development of tetanus, septic arthritis, or systemic sepsis may result. Despite dracunculiasis being rarely fatal and seldom causing permanent disability, the temporary morbidity negatively affects health and well-being, with considerable socioeconomic impact on patients and communities. Among other issues, there are negative

Table 1
Characteristics of filarial infections

	Infection by	Adult Worm Final Destination	Adult Worm Length (mm)	Egg/Larvae Final Destination	Number of Eggs/Larvae Shed by Female Worm per Day	Life Span of Adult Worms (Years)	Intermediate Host/Vector	Time in Vector/ Until Larvae are Infective
Dracunculus medinensis	Drinking water contaminated with water-flea (*Cyclops*)	Skin surface of lower limbs	Female: 600–1000 × 1.5–2.0 Male: 15–40 × 0.4	Larvae released into fresh water bodies	>1000 larvae	~1	Water-flea (*Cyclops*)	~2 wk
Onchocerca volvulus	Bite from blackfly (*Simulium*)	Subcutaneous worm bundles	Female: 350–700 × 0.4 Male: 20–50 × 0.2	Larvae found in upper dermis, nodules, and eyes	Up to 1500 larvae	~10	Blackfly (*Simulium*)	1–2 wk
Lymphatic filariae	Bite from mosquito (*Aedes, Anopheles, Culex*)	Lymphatic vessels	Female: 80–100 × 0.25 Male: 40 × 0.1	Larvae migrate in peripheral blood vessels	Up to 50,000 larvae	~10	Mosquito (*Aedes, Anopheles, Culex*)	At least 10–12 d
Loa loa	Bite from bloodsucking fly (*Chrysops*)	Worms migrate under skin in subcutaneous tissues	Female: 50–70 × 0.5 Male: 30–35 × 0.4	Larvae found in lung, peripheral blood, and in rare cases in urine, saliva, cerebrospinal and other body fluids	Several thousand larvae	Up to 17	Bloodsucking fly (*Chrysops*)	9–10 d
Mansonella perstans	Bite from midge (*Culicoides*)	Serous cavities, mesentery, and retroperitoneal tissues	Female: 70–80 × 0.1 Male: 35–45 × 0.06	Larvae found in blood stream	No number available	Unknown	Biting midge (*Culicoides*)	7–9 d

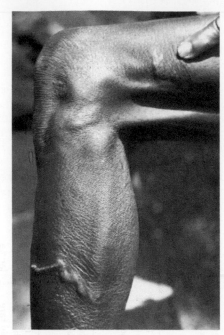

Fig. 1. Calcified guinea worm. (*Courtesy of* Peter J.T. Mayer, MD, Ringelai, Germany.)

educational consequences, as children might miss several weeks of schooling because they have difficulties to walk or have to take care of relatives with dracunculiasis. Similarly, adults with dracunculiasis often cannot work, and hence their subsistence agricultural activities are compromised. Because of the seasonal peak of dracunculiasis, many people in endemic villages are affected at the same time, further exacerbating the societal impact of the disease.[20]

Diagnosis and Treatment

The macroscopic diagnosis of a *D medinensis* infection is straightforward when the blister develops and the female worm starts to emerge. The detection of prepatent infections with immunodiagnostic methods has been a research topic[26,27] but has never reached broad application in the field.

The treatment of dracunculiasis is limited to the extraction of the worm by winding it around a stick, which, of note, is one explanation for the origin of the international sign of medicine and healing, the Asclepius rod. Pulling out the worm is painful and can take several days, because worms usually can be extracted only centimeter by centimeter. Massaging the skin and muscles, if not inflamed, and cooling with ice can accelerate the extraction and mitigate the pain (S. Knopp, personal observation in Togo; **Fig. 2**). To avoid secondary infections, an antibiotic ointment should be applied around the wound.[28] Anthelmintic drugs that are widely and effectively used against other nematode infections did not prove to have any direct effect on *D medinensis*,[20] and there is currently no vaccine available against dracunculiasis.[21]

Control and Prevention

There are several intervention points to control dracunculiasis: (1) the prevention of infection by filtering drinking water through a cloth filter; (2) vector control by killing

---

Box 3
Clinical manifestations of filarial worms

Cutaneous

    Dracunculus medinensis

    Onchocerca volvulus

    Loa loa

    Mansonella perstans

    Dirofilaria repens[a], *Dirofilaria immitis*[a]

Lymphatic

    Wuchereria bancrofti

    Brugia malayi, *Brugia timori*

Ocular

    Onchocerca volvulus

    Loa loa

    Dirofilaria repens[a], *Dirofilaria immitis*[a]

Pulmonary

    Dirofilaria repens[a], *Dirofilaria immitis*[a]

[a] *D repens* and *D immitis* are the heart worms of cats and dogs, respectively[24,25]: accidental infections of humans can occur in the Mediterranean but are not covered in this review devoted to tropical diseases.

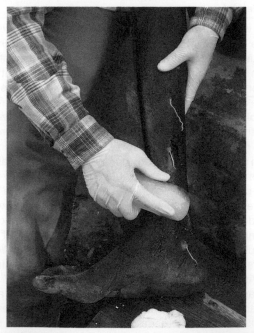

Fig. 2. Guinea worm extraction. (*Courtesy of* Stefanie Knopp, PhD, Swiss Tropical and Public Health Institute, Basel, Switzerland.)

Cyclops through treatment of open stagnant water bodies with a larvicide such as temephos (Abate); (3) educating patients with emerging worms to avoid contact with open water bodies; (4) treatment and care to safely extract the worm and disinfect and bandage the wounds; (5) infrastructure interventions to provide safe drinking water from boreholes or wells; (6) close surveillance of endemic villages and case containment; and (7) promotion of control efforts through local media, political leaders, and other champions.[29] Additional features that triggered the 1991 WHA declaration to eradicate guinea worm are the restricted potential of the intermediate host to spread to new habitats (*Cyclops* cannot fly or crawl out of water bodies), coupled with the seasonality of the disease.

Current efforts to control guinea worm disease are driven by the National Guinea Worm Elimination Programs of endemic nations, which work in close collaboration with the Global Guinea Worm Eradication Program championed by the Carter Center, Centers for Disease Control and Prevention (CDC), World Health Organization (WHO), and the United Nations Children's Fund (UNICEF). Since 1996, the WHO certifies countries to be free of dracunculiasis if they maintain adequate nationwide surveillance for at least 3 consecutive years and record no indigenous cases during this period.[30] In early 2012, 192 countries and territories had been certified to be free of or have eliminated dracunculiasis. However, the last steps toward eradication usually are the most difficult ones. As the original goal to eradicate guinea worm in 2009 was not achieved, in May 2011, during the 64th WHA, the call for dracunculiasis eradication has been reiterated (WHA resolution 64.16). Eventually achieving the goal of guinea worm eradication would constitute the first human parasitic infection to be eradicated even in the absence of a vaccine.

ONCHOCERCIASIS (*ONCHOCERCA VOLVULUS*)
Life Cycle and Epidemiology

People get infected with *O volvulus* when bitten by a blackfly of the genus *Simulium* containing the infective L_3 of the parasite. From the bite wound the larvae migrate to the subcutaneous tissues. After 2 molts, the larvae develop into adult worms that mate and encapsulate in fibrous tissues, which might clinically present as worm nodules mostly located over bony prominences (ie, chest, hips, shoulders, and head). Adult female worms have a life expectancy of 9-14 years, of which they reproduce during 9 to 11 years (see **Table 1**). Female worms are vivipar, and each fertilized female releases up to 1500 unsheathed microfilariae per day. The life span of microfilariae is about 2 years and they live mainly in the upper dermis and nodules, but are also often found in the eye where, on death, they induce an immune reaction eventually leading to blindness. From the dermis microfilariae can be sucked up by a blackfly while feeding from blood pools. In the blackfly, the first-stage larvae migrate from the gut to the thoracic muscles, molt twice, and develop into infective L_3 within 1 to 2 weeks. Larvae then migrate to the head and proboscis. People living in hyperendemic areas often carry multiple adult worms and have up to 2000 microfilariae per mg of skin, thus virtually guaranteeing the uptake and transmission of the parasite via the *Simulium* vector.

O volvulus is currently endemic in 27 countries of sub-Saharan Africa, Yemen, and 6 countries of Latin America. It is estimated that globally, some 37 million people are infected with the parasite, and that more than 102 million people are at risk of infection.[14,31–33] The transmission of *O volvulus* depends on the presence of the day-active blackfly *Simulium*, which breeds in fast-flowing rivers or streams.[34] Hence, people living in communities located in close proximity to rivers are at highest risk of infection and disease, reflected in the reference to the disease as "river blindness."

The prevalence and intensity of infection in humans increases with age, reaching a peak at an age of approximately 30 years. Overt morbidity such as depigmentation of the skin (leopard skin) and blindness are most common in people aged 40 years and older.[35]

Clinical Features and Associated Burden

Onchocerciasis includes an array of symptoms, mostly associated with immune reactions induced by dead microfilariae. Skin-related problems and blindness are primary symptoms and major causes of morbidity (see **Box 3**). Inflammation of the skin can result in intense itching, papular dermatitis, and lichenified onchodermatitis. Chronic *O volvulus* infections can lead to depigmentation of the skin (leopard skin) or its loss of elasticity and structure (lizard skin or hanging groin).[35] Hyperpigmentation (sowda) is rare and only appears in immunologic hyperactive individuals with severe chronic papular dermatitis. Whereas the microfilarial load is low in sowda patients, the immune response, and particularly the Th2 type response, is increased.[1,36] Blindness results from punctate keratitis, which develops around dead microfilariae and presents as a small white dot, followed by sclerosing keratitis, iridocyclitis and, finally, permanent visual impairment and blindness.[1] It has been hypothesized that the proinflammatory events leading to increased corneal opacity are stimulated not only by the parasite itself but also by endosymbiotic *Wolbachia* bacteria released by dying microfilariae.[33,37]

Blindness, visual impairment, and severe itching exert strong negative socioeconomic impacts on afflicted populations. It is estimated that in Africa alone, onchocerciasis caused a burden of 389,000 DALYs in 2004[13] (**Table 2**). Historically, the parasite has also blocked human settlement and land use in large swathes of fertile riverine land.

Diagnosis and Treatment

A still widely applied method for the point-of-care diagnosis of *O volvulus* infections is the skin snip, a biopsy of the upper dermis from the iliac crests or the scapulae. Tiny snips of the dermis are transferred into normal saline solution and examined under a microscope, enumerating the number of microfilariae. However, the sensitivity of the skin-snip test is low, particularly in low-endemicity areas. Moreover, the test is unpopular because of its painful invasiveness. Hence, the commercially available diethylcarbamazine (DEC)-based patch test has been developed.[40] For this test, body lotion containing DEC is applied to the skin, which locally kills dermal microfilariae. A papular rash 24 hours after application of the cream indicates an infection with *O volvulus*. Additional diagnostic methods, such as antigen or antibody detection tests, have been developed and show promising results, but are not yet routinely applied.[1,41] Rapid appraisal tools applied in onchocerciasis control programs involve estimating the proximity of communities to blackfly breeding sites and determining the nodule frequency in a sample of 50 men aged 20 years or older who had resided in endemic communities for a maximum of 10 years.[1,40]

The standard treatment against onchocerciasis is ivermectin (150–200 μg/kg oral dose), which is distributed to entire at-risk communities (pregnant women and children weighing <15 kg are ineligible) every 6 or 12 months.[1,3] The treatment does not kill adult worms but microfilariae, and hence does not clear infections but controls the disease and its transmission. Patients with high microfilarial load who are treated with ivermectin often experience severe skin disease caused by immune reactions to parasite antigen or endotoxins released by *Wolbachia* bacteria (**Fig. 3**). Suboptimal responses or resistance to ivermectin have not yet been unequivocally demonstrated for *O volvulus*.[41,42] DEC, which is used for MDA against lymphatic filariasis, should not be

Table 2
Epidemiology and burden of filarial infections

	Geographic Distribution	Population at Risk	Population Infected	Global Burden (DALY) (year)
Dracunculus medinensis	Six countries in Africa (2010)[23]	No number available	1797 (2010)[38]	No number available
Onchocerca volvulus	30 countries in Africa Yemen Six countries in Central and South America	>102 million in Africa[31]	37 million[32]	388,576 (2004)[13]
Lymphatic filariae	72 countries in Africa, Asia, the Western Pacific, parts of the Caribbean, and South America	1.39 billion[39]	120 million (2010)[39]	5,940,641 (2004)[13]
Loa loa	West- and Central Africa	No number available	No number available	No number available
Mansonella perstans	Central and South America At least 33 countries in Sub-Saharan Africa	No number available	At least 114 million in Africa (2010)[12]	No number available

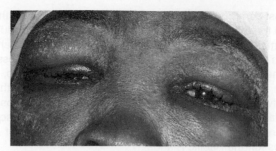

Fig. 3. Adverse reactions (swollen face and streaming eyes) after ivermectin treatment of an onchocerciasis patient. (*Courtesy of* Cornelia Mai, MSc, Tübingen, Germany.)

applied against *O volvulus*, or in areas where onchocerciasis is coendemic unless eye involvement of *O volvulus* is ruled out, because the death of microfilariae can induce strong local inflammation in the eyes. Moxidectin, a macrofilaricide, has been suggested as backup for ivermectin.[41] Suramin, previously applied to kill adult worms, has been abandoned because of its toxicity.[1,41] Doxycycline, an antibiotic active against the endosymbiotic *Wolbachia* bacteria that are essential for the development, embryogenesis, and survival of *O volvulus*, results in long-term sterilization of female worms and thus absence of microfilariae, if given over 6 weeks at 100 mg per day.[43] Considering the length of treatment, the anti-*Wolbachia* therapy is valuable for individual patient management but unsuitable for MDA in the context of onchocerciasis control programs.[1]

Control and Prevention

Large-scale control efforts targeting onchocerciasis commenced in the early 1970s. The Onchocerciasis Control Program (OCP) was set up in West Africa in 1974. Within the first 14 years, the OCP emphasized vector control in 11 countries, mainly spraying insecticides from helicopters and airplanes on blackfly breeding sites. Despite the initial success of reducing the risk of transmission among more than 30 million people, reinvasion of the blackfly in areas where transmission had been interrupted resulted in a recrudescence of infection.[36] From 1987 onwards, the focus shifted toward MDA, using ivermectin (Mectizan) given to entire at-risk communities. The drug was, and continues to be, donated by Merck.[44–46] In 1995, the African Program for Onchocerciasis Control (APOC) was initiated, aiming at the elimination of onchocerciasis as a disease of public health importance in Africa. This program is currently in the phasing-out period (2008–2015), and responsibility for sustained control will be taken over by national authorities. The control programs are also facing challenges because MDA using ivermectin in areas coendemic with *L loa* is contraindicated, as severe adverse reactions in *L loa* patients have been observed.[47,48] Further issues are ivermectin treatment in hypoendemic areas hitherto excluded from the APOC, sustainability of ivermectin distribution, postcontrol surveillance for recrudescence detection, surveillance for emergence of resistance, and decisions of when to stop MDA with ivermectin.[49]

LYMPHATIC FILARIASIS (*WUCHERERIA BANCROFTI, BRUGIA MALAYI,* AND *BRUGIA TIMORI*)
Life Cycle and Epidemiology

Lymphatic filariasis belongs to the oldest and most debilitating of the neglected tropical diseases.[50] Humans become infected with lymphatic filariae when mosquitoes carrying the L_3 take their blood meal. The larvae enter the skin and develop into adult worms, which most commonly reside in nests (lymphangiectasia) within the lymphatic vessels located in the extremities and male genitalia.[1] Over a reproductive life span of 5 to 8 years, a female filaria produces millions of sheathed microfilariae that periodically migrate from the lymphatic system to the peripheral blood vessels, where they are ingested by the feeding mosquito (see **Table 1**). In the mosquito, the microfilariae shed their sheath, penetrate the midgut wall, and migrate to the thoracic muscles, where they molt twice and finally migrate to the mosquito's proboscis, ready to be transmitted. Filarial worms are transmitted by a wide range of mosquitoes including *Culex* (in urban and semiurban areas), *Anopheles* (in rural areas of Africa and elsewhere), and *Aedes* (on the Pacific islands).

The 3 species causing lymphatic filariasis, namely *W bancrofti*, *B-malayi*, and *B timori*, are endemic in different tropical regions of the world and affect specific parts of the body. *W bancrofti* is the most widely distributed species and is responsible for 90% of the global number of cases. The distribution of *B malayi* is restricted to Southeast Asia, and the closely related *B timori* fills the niche in southeastern Indonesia.[1] Children living in endemic areas usually get infected within the first years of their life but then show no disease symptoms. The prevalence of lymphatic filariasis increases with age, and the disease becomes more overt in puberty and adulthood.[1,51]

Clinical Features and Associated Burden

Most infected people living in endemic areas present as asymptomatic carriers of microfilariae, but virtually all of them show subclinical damage of the lymphatic system and kidney, and have an altered immune system. It is widely assumed that filarial nematodes are able to modulate their host's immune system in such a way that it tolerates the long-term presence of the parasites without producing major disease signs.[52] However, about a third of infected people develop clinical signs attributable to damage of the lymphatic system, manifested mainly as lymphedema, hydrocele, and elephantiasis (see **Box 3**).[1,53] The most common acute manifestation is acute adenolymphangitis (ADL), which is characterized by fever attacks, painful swellings of the affected body area, and inflamed lymph nodes in the groin and axilla.[53] Episodes of ADL are caused by secondary infections due to bacteria that enter the body via skin lesions caused by fungal infections, injuries, eczema, insect bites, or other infections. Such infections are common on the affected limbs because normal immune defenses are impaired by the underlying lymphatic damage. Some episodes of local inflammation are also caused by the humans' immune response to adult worms that have been destroyed in the lymphatics, called acute filarial lymphangitis. The chronic manifestation of lymphatic filariasis is characterized by lymphedema (tissue swelling) or elephantiasis (skin/tissue thickening) of limbs and hydrocele (fluid accumulation) (**Figs. 4** and **5**).

Lymphatic filariasis is endemic in 72 countries, with an estimated 120 million people infected in 2010.[39] The disease is considered the second-largest cause of permanent and long-term disability (after mental illness) worldwide.[54] The visible effects of the disease result in social stigma, isolation, and psychological stress among affected individuals. In addition, ADL attacks may render affected individuals unable to work and require treatment, and hence lead to a considerable economic loss.[55] The global burden attributable to lymphatic filariasis was estimated at 5.9 million DALYs in 2004 (see **Table 2**).[13,56]

Diagnosis and Treatment

In the past, diagnosis of lymphatic filarial infections relied on clinical examination and on the microscopic detection of microfilariae in thick blood films, with samples

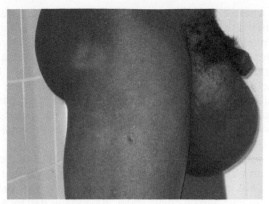

Fig. 4. Hydrocoele. (*Courtesy of* Thomas Fürst, PhD, Swiss Tropical and Public Health Institute, Basel, Switzerland.)

typically taken before midnight because of the predominantly nocturnal periodicity of *W bancrofti*.[1,57] The latter method is specific, inexpensive, and requires little infrastructure, and is still used as point-of-care diagnosis. However, it is not very sensitive and misses people with a low density of microfilariae in blood and those with a microfilaremic infections. In recent years, the diagnosis of filarial infection has been advanced, and several rapid and sensitive tests have been developed. Antigen detection from blood collected during day or night is sensitive for bancroftian filariasis diagnosis and also identifies latent infections. In 1997, a rapid immunochromatographic filariasis card test was introduced.[58] This test proved most useful, and hence is now

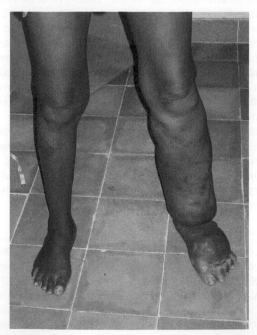

Fig. 5. Elephantiasis leg. (*Courtesy of* Thomas Fürst, PhD, Swiss Tropical and Public Health Institute, Basel, Switzerland.)

recommended by international authorities as the diagnostic method of choice.[57] Advantages are that the test is quick and easy to perform, and is only minimally invasive (100-μl finger-prick blood sample). Disadvantages are that it is not able to distinguish past from present infections, cannot detect *Brugia* infections, is still relatively costly, and might not be available in all endemic settings.[57] Other, less widely used diagnostic approaches include antibody detection to assess the level of contact with antigen in children, polymerase chain reaction (PCR) to detect filarial DNA in human blood samples (taken at night in areas with nocturnally periodic microfilariae), or molecular xenomonitoring (MX) to detect parasite DNA in pooled mosquitoes or human blood by PCR.[59–61]

The drugs of choice to treat lymphatic filariasis in individual patients are: (1) DEC (often combined with albendazole) given as single-dose treatment (6 mg/kg) if the patient continues to live in an endemic area or is younger than 9 years, or as 12-day course of 6 mg/kg per day; and (2) doxycycline, 200 mg per day for 4 weeks plus ivermectin (or without ivermectin because of the risk of serious adverse events in areas where *L loa* is coendemic). Drugs used in MDA campaigns are: (1) single-dose combinations of ivermectin (100–200 μg/kg) plus albendazole (400 mg) in Africa; and (2) DEC (6 mg/kg) plus albendazole (400 mg) in the remainder of the endemic regions, both distributed for at least 5 years.[1] Of note, DEC must not be applied in areas where onchocerciasis is coendemic because dying microfilariae can cause severe local inflammation in patients with ocular microfilariae.[1] Furthermore, DEC, and to a lesser extent ivermectin, can cause encephalopathy in *L loa*-endemic areas.[62]

DEC is effective against both microfilariae and adult worms.[53] However, a single dose usually does not clear all microfilariae and some adult worms survive. Treatment over 12 consecutive days results in complete microfilariae clearance.[1] Adverse events can occur and are mostly related to the death of adult worms and microfilariae, which can induce systemic inflammation due to the release of endosymbiotic *Wolbachia* bacteria. The adverse effects of ivermectin resemble those of DEC, but are milder because of the slower clearance of microfilariae.[53] Ivermectin and albendazole both effectively reduce the microfilarial load for several months after treatment, and the combination of both drugs prolongs the period of reduced peripheral microfilaremia. Anti-*Wolbachia* therapy using the antibiotic doxycycline results in long-term sterility and eventual death of adult bancroftian worms when administered daily at a 200 mg dose for 4 to 8 weeks.[63] It is also effective in reducing brugian microfilariae when given at 100 mg per day over 6 weeks.[64]

There is no cure for lymphedema, but a series of interventions is available to mitigate and prevent the progression of the swelling.[53] Such methods include keeping the affected limbs clean (to prevent secondary infections), bandaging, regular massage, and exercise and elevation while resting (to stimulate lymph circulation). At present, there are no drug interventions for hydrocele and hence surgery is the only intervention for this advanced form of chronic lymphatic filarial infection.

Control and Prevention

Traditionally, control of lymphatic filariasis was based on the selective treatment of infected individuals detected by mass screening of blood films.[63] In 2000, the Global Program to Eliminate Lymphatic Filariasis (GPELF) was initiated by the WHO as a response to WHA resolution 50.29, which encourages member states to eliminate lymphatic filariasis as a public health problem.[65] Today, the GPELF follows the strategy to (1) interrupt transmission through the annual administration of 2-drug combinations to at-risk communities in endemic areas for at least 5 years, and (2) to alleviate suffering and disease through the promotion of basic measures of hygiene and skin care to patients with lymphedema, and to provide surgery for men with hydrocele.[66] The GPELF is nowadays part of multi-intervention packages to control neglected tropical diseases by the integration of preventive chemotherapy, vector control, and morbidity management at global, national, and local levels. In 2010, MDA of DEC/ivermectin plus albendazole was implemented in 53 countries. Between 2000 and 2010, more than 3.4 billion treatments were delivered to a targeted population of 897 million people.[39] While the strategy of repeated rounds of MDA indeed resulted in the elimination of lymphatic filariasis in some countries,[39,67,68] others were less successful in halting transmission.[69] It remains to be determined which treatment coverage and duration of MDA (ideally combined with other control measures) are needed to achieve elimination, and to what extent the success of a program depends on the vector and parasite strains, endemicity level, and the drugs applied.[70] It is assumed that MDA must be applied for at least 4 to 6 years[71-73] depending on baseline infection prevalence and transmission intensity,[74] and that coverage should reach at least 80%.[54,75,76] An antigenemia prevalence of 0.1% is proposed as a target for indicating the interruption of lymphatic filariasis transmission by the GPELF.[77,78] Mathematical models are important tools in understanding transmission dynamics of parasitic diseases. Such models have been widely used for the planning and evaluation of control programs such as the GPELF,[70] and might underpin the global strategy to eventually reach elimination of lymphatic filariasis.[79] In a recent statement, the WHO urges its member states to adapt an integrated vector management approach against mosquitoes transmitting lymphatic filariae and malaria.[80] Furthermore, new guidelines on delivering treatment to whole communities, including a protocol for stopping MDA and conducting posttreatment surveillance, will be disseminated from 2012 onwards.[39]

LOIASIS (*LOA LOA*)
Life Cycle and Epidemiology

L loa infections are acquired when infective stages of the parasite actively migrate out of the mouthparts of the vector fly *Chrysops* and enter the biting wound while the fly takes a blood meal.[11]After maturing, the sheathed adult worms live freely in the subcutaneous tissues of humans. Daily, thousands of sheathed microfilariae produced by the gravid female worm are migrating via the lymphatic system to the lung, which serves as a reservoir (see **Table 1**). From there, microfilariae invade the peripheral blood, showing a diurnal periodicity. In rare cases, microfilariae are also found in urine, saliva, cerebrospinal fluid, and other body fluids.[11,81] The *Chrysops* vector is ingesting the microfilariae while taking a blood meal during the day. In the fly the larvae migrate from the gut to the thoracic muscles and from there to the head and proboscis of the fly.

L loa is endemic in the rainforest and some savannah areas of Central and West Africa, where several million people are infected.[81] The *Chrysops* flies live in and around forested and muddy areas, on the edges of water reservoirs, and in dying or rotting vegetation.[82] People at highest risk of infection are those living and working in such areas during the day, as *Chrysops* is day-biting. The prevalence of infection increases with age.[81]

Clinical Features and Associated Burden

As for other filarial infections, most people infected with *L loa* show no disease symptoms. A specific sign of *L loa* infection is the Calabar swelling, a subcutaneous edema of allergic type, often associated with localized, migrating or generalized itching (see

Box 3). Calabar swellings appear and disappear spontaneously at irregular intervals and can be observed on any part of the body, but typically occur in the limbs near the joints, which may render movement difficult and painful.[11] The swellings may be caused by antigenic material, for example, microfilariae released by adult female worms, or by larvae that migrate away from the biting wound after infection.[11,81] Other clinical signs can develop within a few months after infection but are often not overt for more than a decade. *L loa* is also known as the African eyeworm, because adult worms migrating under the skin are sometimes seen while passing the conjunctiva of the eye, often without other clinical symptoms. Migration of the adult worms may cause severe pain and inflammation in the eye and might result in blindness. Occasionally adult *L loa* have been detected in various other parts of the body including the testes, kidneys, and heart.[11] Although the burden of loiasis seems to be considerable in some areas of Central Africa, it has never been quantified, and hence no DALY figures are available (see **Table 2**).

Diagnosis and Treatment

L loa microfilariae can best be detected in blood samples taken between 10:00 and 14:00.[83,84] The classic method to determine infection and intensity is to count microfilariae in thin or thick blood films prepared from a defined volume of blood that has been stained with Giemsa. The sheath of *L loa* microfilariae stains only poorly with Giemsa. If microfilaremia is low, concentration techniques including sedimentation or filtration of blood may be required.[11] A PCR for species-specific DNA also exists, which is perhaps the most accurate technique for individual diagnosis of loiasis.[11] The interpretation of specific clinical signs, such as the Calabar swelling, or the detection of adult worms when they cross the subconjunctiva or sclera of the eye, is straightforward.

Adult *L loa* can be surgically extracted from the eye. For this purpose, the eye needs to be anesthetized and the worm extracted with forceps through a small incision in the conjunctiva.[81] To systemically kill adult worms and microfilariae, DEC administered at a dose of 8 to 10 mg/kg per day for 3 weeks is the standard treatment.[3] Caution is needed when administering the drug, because DEC can cause serious adverse reactions such as encephalitis and retinal hemorrhage, especially when the microfilarial load is high.[85] Alternatively, the anthelmintic drugs ivermectin, albendazole, and mebendazole have been shown to have microfilaricidal effects.[11,81] However, serious adverse events after ivermectin treatment have been reported: high *L loa* microfilaremia is statistically significantly associated with serious adverse reactions in people treated with ivermectin in the context of onchocerciasis control programs.[48] Observed adverse events include functional impairment for more than 1 week after treatment or microfilariae in the cerebrospinal fluid, causing coma. Occurrence of encephalopathy following albendazole treatment of highly filaremic *L loa* cases has been reported.[62,86] In patients presenting with high microfilarial load, anthelmintic treatment with albendazole (2 × 200 mg/d) for 21 days is recommended to slowly lower the microfilaremia.[3,62,86] Anti-*Wolbachia* (ie, doxycycline) treatment is ineffective against loiasis because *L loa* does not host the bacteria.[1]

Control and Prevention

There are currently no specific control programs targeting *L loa*. Onchocerciasis and lymphatic filariasis control programs cannot be implemented in regions in Central and West Africa where *L loa* is coendemic, because of the serious adverse reactions (namely encephalopathy) caused by ivermectin in patients coinfected with *L loa*.[87] For example, in onchocerciasis-endemic communities where more than 20% of the population also has loiasis, the risk of severe adverse reactions is considered to be unacceptably high. To predict whether loiasis is present at high levels in a community targeted for onchocerciasis control with ivermectin, the application of a simple questionnaire (Rapid Assessment Procedure for Loiasis, or RAPLOA) that assesses the history of visible worms moving in the lower part of the eye is recommended.[88,89]

MANSONELLOSIS (*MANSONELLA PERSTANS*)
Life Cycle and Epidemiology

M perstans filariasis is widespread in the tropics but still is one of the most neglected of the tropical diseases.[12] The larvae of *M perstans* are transmitted through the bite of tiny infected midges of the genus *Culicoides* (see **Table 1**). The larvae develop into adult worms that live in serous cavities and mesentery as well as retroperitoneal tissues. Unsheathed microfilariae released by the female adult parasites are carried through the blood stream; no periodic patterns of their presence in peripheral blood vessels have been observed.[90] Female midges ingest the microfilariae while taking their blood meal. In the vector, the larvae molt most likely twice before the infective stage is reintroduced into the human definitive host.

M perstans is endemic in rural populations living in sub-Saharan and in northern South America and the Caribbean, often in areas where *L loa*, *O volvulus*, and *W bancrofti* coexist. Infection prevalences are often very high (80–100%) in endemic areas, even among children.[12] In general, the prevalence and intensity of infection with *M perstans* increase with age, hence peak levels are observed in the adult population. Men usually are more likely to be infected than women.[12]

Clinical Features and Associated Burden

Little is known about the outcome of *M perstans* infections. As for other filarial infections, most infected people remain asymptomatic. The variety of symptoms attributed to *M perstans* infections include angioedema, arthralgia, fever, headache, pruritus, skin eruption, serositis, neurologic manifestations, ocular or palpebral pruritus, visual impairment, and chest pain (see **Box 3**).[90,91] Allergic reactions resembling the 'Calabar swellings' seen in *L loa* infections have been reported. The clinical outcomes are most likely related to the presence of adult worms in the serous body cavities and not to the microfilariae.[12]

Diagnosis and Treatment

Unsheathed microfilariae of *M perstans* can be detected by microscopic examination of peripheral blood samples taken at any time. When the microfilariae are present in high numbers, they can be easily detected and identified in thick or thin blood films stained with Giemsa.[12] Another technique for the quantitative detection of *M perstans* is the examination of fixed finger-prick blood samples in a counting chamber under a microscope.[92] However, because of the small size of the microfilariae and their unsheathed nature, they are more difficult to recognize than the larger sheathed microfilariae of other species.[12] Various concentration techniques have proved valuable for *M perstans* diagnosis in an experimental context.[12]

Drugs effective against other filariae such as DEC, ivermectin, albendazole, and mebendazole have limited efficacy against *M perstans*.[91] An effective, fast-acting, tolerable therapy that is easy to administer still needs to be identified.[12] In a recent trial, doxycycline, given at a daily dose of 200 mg for 4 to 8 weeks, was shown to be effective in reducing microfilaremia.[90] The therapy suppressed microfilariae for

36 months after treatment, suggesting that doxycycline has an effect on adult worms as well.[90]

Control and Prevention

Currently, there are no large-scale programs for the control of mansonellosis. Because of the insensitivity of *M perstans* to antifilarial drugs applied in onchocerciasis or lymphatic filariasis control programs, the species tends to persist in populations targeted by those programs. Data on the long-term impact of such programs on *M perstans* are conflicting.[12] A combination therapy of ivermectin plus albendazole, as used for MDA targeting lymphatic filariasis and onchocerciasis, failed to show marked decreases in *M perstans* microfilaremia.[92]

SUMMARY

Filarial infections can result in highly debilitating and irreversible disease outcomes, both physically and psychologically.[1,93,94] Despite filariae not being transmitted in Europe and North America, travel clinics must be aware of infections in patients who have spent an extended period of time in endemic areas, and handle cases carefully. With the exception of doxycycline, classically applied antifilarial drugs (DEC, ivermectin and albendazole) are able to kill microfilariae, but have only limited effects against adult worms.[33,43] These agents can thus reduce the transmission of the parasites in endemic areas but are not able to mitigate disease symptoms. Moreover, they often cause severe adverse reactions resulting from strong immune reactions to dying microfilariae, and must hence be applied with care.[1] Filariasis control programs targeting vectors and treating at-risk communities have successfully been implemented over the past decades in many endemic countries and have been able to reduce new or repeated infections.[1,33,36] However, continuous interventions and rigorous monitoring are still required in most (formerly) endemic places to avoid resurgence of transmission as well as physical damage and chronic disease. The development of diagnostic tools that reliably detect and differentiate prepatent, patent, and postpatent infections, as well as new, safe, and efficacious drugs that permanently sterilize or kill adult worms, are essential for progress in filariasis control and ultimately achieving the goal of elimination. The Bill & Melinda Gates–funded Death to Onchocerciasis and Lymphatic Filariasis (DOLF) project, commenced in 2010, aims at developing and validating improved treatments (new drugs and optimized treatment regimens) to eliminate onchocerciasis and lymphatic filariasis also in *L loa*–endemic areas. The ancillary benefit of repeated rounds of MDA using ivermectin and albendazole on soil-transmitted helminthiasis is also being evaluated. This program might become a pathfinder for operational research, paving the way from control towards integrated control and elimination of multiple neglected tropical diseases.

REFERENCES

1. Taylor MJ, Hoerauf A, Bockarie M. Lymphatic filariasis and onchocerciasis. Lancet 2010;376:1175–85.
2. Hotez PJ, Molyneux DH, Fenwick A, et al. Incorporating a rapid-impact package for neglected tropical diseases with programs for HIV/AIDS, tuberculosis, and malaria. PLoS Med 2006;3:e102.
3. Klion AD. Filarial infections in travelers and immigrants. Curr Infect Dis Rep 2008; 10:50–7.
4. Bockarie MJ, Molyneux DH. The end of lymphatic filariasis? BMJ 2009;338: b1686.

5. Cupp EW, Sauerbrey M, Richards F. Elimination of human onchocerciasis: history of progress and current feasibility using ivermectin (Mectizan®) monotherapy. Acta Trop 2011;120(Suppl 1):S100–8.
6. Molyneux DH, Bradley M, Hoerauf A, et al. Mass drug treatment for lymphatic filariasis and onchocerciasis. Trends Parasitol 2003;19:516–22.
7. Thylefors B, Alleman M. Towards the elimination of onchocerciasis. Ann Trop Med Parasitol 2006;100:733–46.
8. Ottesen EA. Lymphatic filariasis: treatment, control and elimination. Adv Parasitol 2006;61:395–441.
9. Ottesen EA, Hooper PJ, Bradley M, et al. The global programme to eliminate lymphatic filariasis: health impact after 8 years. PLoS Negl Trop Dis 2008;2: e317.
10. CDC. Progress toward global eradication of dracunculiasis, January 2010-June 2011. Morb Mortal Wkly Rep 2011;60:1450–3.
11. Boussinesq M. Loiasis. Ann Trop Med Parasitol 2006;100:715–31.
12. Simonsen PE, Onapa AW, Asio SM. *Mansonella perstans* filariasis in Africa. Acta Trop 2011;120(Suppl 1):109–20.
13. WHO. The global burden of disease: 2004 update. Geneva (Switzerland): World Health Organization; 2008. p. 1–160.
14. Hoerauf A, Pfarr K, Mand S, et al. Filariasis in Africa—treatment challenges and prospects. Clin Microbiol Infect 2011;17:977–85.
15. Nutman TB, Miller KD, Mulligan M, et al. Diethylcarbamazine prophylaxis for human loiasis. Results of a double-blind study. N Engl J Med 1988;319:752–6.
16. CDC. Imported dracunculiasis—United States, 1995 and 1997. Morb Mortal Wkly Rep 1998;47:209–11.
17. CDC. CDC health information for international travel 2012. The Yellow Book. Atlanta (GA): Centers for Disease Control and Prevention; 2011. p. 1–640.
18. Lipner EM, Law MA, Barnett E, et al. Filariasis in travelers presenting to the Geo-Sentinel Surveillance Network. PLoS Negl Trop Dis 2007;1:e88.
19. Greenaway C. Dracunculiasis (guinea worm disease). CMAJ 2004;170:495–500.
20. Cairncross S, Muller R, Zagaria N. Dracunculiasis (Guinea worm disease) and the eradication initiative. Clin Microbiol Rev 2002;15:223–46.
21. Richards FO, Ruiz-Tiben E, Hopkins DR. Dracunculiasis eradication and the legacy of the smallpox campaign: What's new and innovative? What's old and principled? (Presented at the Symposium on Smallpox Eradication: Lessons, Legacies & Innovations). Vaccine 2011, in press; doi: 10.1016/j.vaccine.2011.07.115.
22. CDC. Progress toward global eradication of dracunculiasis, January 2009-June 2010. Morb Mortal Wkly Rep 2010;59:1239–42.
23. WHO. Dracunculiasis eradication—global surveillance summary, 2010. Wkly Epidemiol Rec 2011;86:189–204.
24. Genchi C, Rinaldi L, Mortarino M, et al. Climate and *Dirofilaria* infection in Europe. Vet Parasitol 2009;163:286–92.
25. Pampiglione S, Rivasi F. Human dirofilariasis due to *Dirofilaria (Nochtiella) repens*: an update of world literature from 1995 to 2000. Parassitologia 2000;42: 231–54.
26. Bloch P, Simonsen PE. Immunoepidemiology of *Dracunculus medinensis* infections I. Antibody responses in relation to infection status. Am J Trop Med Hyg 1998;59:978–84.
27. Knopp S, Amegbo IK, Hamm DM, et al. Antibody and cytokine responses in *Dracunculus medinensis* patients at distinct states of infection. Trans R Soc Trop Med Hyg 2008;102:277–83.

28. Magnussen P, Yakubu A, Bloch P. The effect of antibiotic- and hydrocortisone-containing ointments in preventing secondary infections in guinea worm disease. Am J Trop Med Hyg 1994;51:797–9.

29. Ruiz-Tiben E, Hopkins DR. Dracunculiasis (Guinea worm disease) eradication. Adv Parasitol 2006;61:275–309.

30. WHO. Certification of dracunculiasis eradication; criteria, strategies, procedures—a practical guide. WHO/FIL/96.188 REV.1. Geneva (Switzerland): World Health Organization; 1996. p. 1–33.

31. WHO. African Programme for Onchocerciasis Control: meeting of national task forces, September 2011. Wkly Epidemiol Rec 2011;86:541–56.

32. APOC. Final communiqué of the 11th session of the Joint Action Forum (JAF) of APOC. Paris, Ouagadougou: African Programme for Onchocerciasis Control; 2005. p. 1–27.

33. Basáñez MG, Pion SD, Churcher TS, et al. River blindness: a success story under threat? PLoS Med 2006;3:e371.

34. WHO. Report from the 2009 InterAmerican Conference on Onchocerciasis: progress towards eliminating river blindness in the Region of the Americas. Wkly Epidemiol Rec 2010;85:312–28.

35. Murdoch ME, Asuzu MC, Hagan M, et al. Onchocerciasis: the clinical and epidemiological burden of skin disease in Africa. Ann Trop Med Parasitol 2002;96: 283–96.

36. Brattig NW. Pathogenesis and host responses in human onchocerciasis: impact of *Onchocerca* filariae and *Wolbachia* endobacteria. Microbes Infect 2004;6:113–28.

37. Saint Andre A, Blackwell NM, Hall LR, et al. The role of endosymbiotic *Wolbachia* bacteria in the pathogenesis of river blindness. Science 2002;295:1892–5.

38. WHO. Monthly report on dracunculiasis cases, January-December 2010. Wkly Epidemiol Rec 2011;86:81–92.

39. WHO. Global Programme to Eliminate Lymphatic Filariasis: progress report on mass drug administration, 2010. Wkly Epidemiol Rec 2011;86:377–88.

40. Molyneux DH. Filaria control and elimination: diagnostic, monitoring and surveillance needs. Trans R Soc Trop Med Hyg 2009;103:338–41.

41. Udall DN. Recent updates on onchocerciasis: diagnosis and treatment. Clin Infect Dis 2007;44:53–60.

42. Churcher TS, Pion SD, Osei-Atweneboana MY, et al. Identifying sub-optimal responses to ivermectin in the treatment of river blindness. Proc Natl Acad Sci U S A 2009;106:16716–21.

43. Hoerauf A. Filariasis: new drugs and new opportunities for lymphatic filariasis and onchocerciasis. Curr Opin Infect Dis 2008;21:673–81.

44. Collins K. Profitable gifts: a history of the Merck Mectizan Donation Program and its implications for international health. Perspect Biol Med 2004;47:100–9.

45. Peters DH, Phillips T. Mectizan Donation Program: evaluation of a public-private partnership. Trop Med Int Health 2004;9:4–15.

46. Thylefors B. The Mectizan Donation Program (MDP). Ann Trop Med Parasitol 2008;102:39–44.

47. Richard-Lenoble D, Kombila M, Rupp EA, et al. Ivermectin in loiasis and concomitant *O. volvulus* and *M. perstans* infections. Am J Trop Med Hyg 1988;39:480–3.

48. Gardon J, Gardon-Wendel N, Demanga N, et al. Serious reactions after mass treatment of onchocerciasis with ivermectin in an area endemic for *Loa loa* infection. Lancet 1997;350:18–22.

49. Boatin BA, Richards FO Jr. Control of onchocerciasis. Adv Parasitol 2006;61: 349–94.

50. Cox FEG. History of human parasitology. Clin Microbiol Rev 2002;15:595–612.
51. Witt C, Ottesen EA. Lymphatic filariasis: an infection of childhood. Trop Med Int Health 2001;6:582–606.
52. Hoerauf A, Satoguina J, Saeftel M, et al. Immunomodulation by filarial nematodes. Parasite Immunol 2005;27:417–29.
53. Palumbo E. Filariasis: diagnosis, treatment and prevention. Acta Biomed 2008; 79:106–9.
54. Gyapong JO, Kumaraswami V, Biswas G, et al. Treatment strategies underpinning the global programme to eliminate lymphatic filariasis. Expert Opin Pharmacother 2005;6:179–200.
55. Joseph A, Mony P, Prasad M, et al. The efficacies of affected-limb care with penicillin diethylcarbamazine, the combination of both drugs or antibiotic ointment, in the prevention of acute adenolymphangitis during bancroftian filariasis. Ann Trop Med Parasitol 2004;98:685–96.
56. WHO. Managing morbidity and preventing disability in the Global Programme to Eliminate Lymphatic Filariasis: WHO position statement. Wkly Epidemiol Rec 2011;86:581–8.
57. Weil GJ, Ramzy RM. Diagnostic tools for filariasis elimination programs. Trends Parasitol 2007;23:78–82.
58. Weil GJ, Lammie PJ, Weiss N. The ICT Filariasis Test: a rapid-format antigen test for diagnosis of bancroftian filariasis. Parasitol Today 1997;13:401–4.
59. Ramzy RM, Farid HA, Kamal IH, et al. A polymerase chain reaction-based assay for detection of Wuchereria bancrofti in human blood and Culex pipiens. Trans R Soc Trop Med Hyg 1997;91:156–60.
60. Williams SA, Laney SJ, Bierwert LA, et al. Development and standardization of a rapid, PCR-based method for the detection of Wuchereria bancrofti in mosquitoes, for xenomonitoring the human prevalence of bancroftian filariasis. Ann Trop Med Parasitol 2002;96:41–6.
61. Mladonicky JM, King JD, Liang JL, et al. Assessing transmission of lymphatic filariasis using parasitologic, serologic, and entomologic tools after mass drug administration in American Samoa. Am J Trop Med Hyg 2009;80:769–73.
62. Blum J, Wiestner A, Fuhr P, et al. Encephalopathy following Loa loa treatment with albendazole. Acta Trop 2001;78:63–5.
63. Taylor MJ, Makunde WH, McGarry HF, et al. Macrofilaricidal activity after doxycycline treatment of Wuchereria bancrofti: a double-blind, randomised placebo-controlled trial. Lancet 2005;365:2116–21.
64. Supali T, Djuardi Y, Pfarr KM, et al. Doxycycline treatment of Brugia malayi-infected persons reduces microfilaremia and adverse reactions after diethylcarbamazine and albendazole treatment. Clin Infect Dis 2008;46:1385–93.
65. WHO. Fiftieth World Health Assembly. Elimination of lymphatic filariasis as a public health problem. WHA50.29. Geneva (Switzerland): World Health Organization; 1997. p. 1–2.
66. WHO. Progress report 2000-2009 and strategic plan 2010-2020 of the global programme to eliminate lymphatic filariasis: halfway towards eliminating lymphatic filariasis. Geneva (Switzerland): World Health Organization; 2010. p. 1–93.
67. Mohammed KA, Molyneux DH, Albonico M, et al. Progress towards eliminating lymphatic filariasis in Zanzibar: a model programme. Trends Parasitol 2006;22:340–4.
68. Schlemper BR Jr, Steindel M, Grisard EC, et al. Elimination of bancroftian filariasis (Wuchereria bancrofti) in Santa Catarina state, Brazil. Trop Med Int Health 2000;5:848–54.

69. Agrawal VK, Sashindran VK. Lymphatic filariasis in India: problems, challenges and new initiatives. MJAFI 2006;62:359–62.
70. Stolk WA, de Vlas SJ, Habbema JDF. Advances and challenges in predicting the impact of lymphatic filariasis elimination programmes by mathematical modelling. Filaria J 2006;5:5.
71. Ottesen EA. The global programme to eliminate lymphatic filariasis. Trop Med Int Health 2000;5:591–4.
72. Ramzy RM, El Setouhy M, Helmy H, et al. Effect of yearly mass drug administration with diethylcarbamazine and albendazole on bancroftian filariasis in Egypt: a comprehensive assessment. Lancet 2006;367:992–9.
73. Molyneux DH. Elimination of transmission of lymphatic filariasis in Egypt. Lancet 2006;367:966–8.
74. Grady CA, de Rochars MB, Direny AN, et al. Endpoints for lymphatic filariasis programs. Emerg Infect Dis 2007;13:608–10.
75. Ramaiah KD, Vijay Kumar KN, Ravi R, et al. Situation analysis in a large urban area of India, prior to launching a programme of mass drug administrations to eliminate lymphatic filariasis. Ann Trop Med Parasitol 2005;99:243–52.
76. Michael E, Malecela-Lazaro MN, Kazura JW. Elimination of lymphatic filariasis. Lancet 2006;368:362–3.
77. WHO. Report of a WHO informal consultation on epidemiologic approaches to lymphatic filariasis elimination: initial assessment, monitoring and certification. WHO/FIL/99/196. Geneva (Switzerland): World Health Organization; 1998. p. 1–35.
78. Michael E, Malecela-Lazaro MN, Kabali C, et al. Mathematical models and lymphatic filariasis control: endpoints and optimal interventions. Trends Parasitol 2006;22:226–33.
79. Michael E, Gambhir M. Transmission models and management of lymphatic filariasis elimination. Adv Exp Med Biol 2010;673:157–71.
80. WHO. WHO position statement on integrated vector management to control malaria and lymphatic filariasis. Wkly Epidemiol Rec 2011;13:121–8.
81. Padgett JJ, Jacobsen KH. Loiasis: African eye worm. Trans R Soc Trop Med Hyg 2008;102:983–9.
82. Wanji S, Tendongfor N, Esum M, et al. Heterogeneity in the prevalence and intensity of loiasis in five contrasting bioecological zones in Cameroon. Trans R Soc Trop Med Hyg 2003;97:183–7.
83. Ridley JW. Parasitology for medical and clinical laboratory professionals. 1st edition. Florence (Italy): Delmar Cengage Learning; 2011.
84. Carbonez G, Van De Sompel W, Zeyen T. Subconjunctival Loa loa worm: case report. Bull Soc Belge Ophtalmol 2002;283:45–8.
85. Carme B, Boulesteix J, Boutes H, et al. Five cases of encephalitis during treatment of loiasis with diethylcarbamazine. Am J Trop Med Hyg 1991;44: 684–90.
86. Klion AD, Massougbodji A, Horton J, et al. Albendazole in human loiasis: results of a double-blind, placebo-controlled trial. J Infect Dis 1993;168:202–6.
87. Bradley M, Kumaraswami V. Essential tools—drugs and clinical drug trials. Am J Trop Med 2004;71:7–11.
88. Zouré HG, Wanji S, Noma M, et al. The geographic distribution of Loa loa in Africa: results of large-scale implementation of the Rapid Assessment Procedure for Loiasis (RAPLOA). PLoS Negl Trop Dis 2011;5:e1210.
89. WHO/TDR. Guidelines for rapid assessment of Loa loa. Geneva (Switzerland): World Health Organization and Special Programme for Research and Training in Tropical Diseases (TDR); 2002. p. 1–19.

90. Coulibaly YI, Dembele B, Diallo AA, et al. A randomized trial of doxycycline for *Mansonella perstans* infection. N Engl J Med 2009;361:1448–58.
91. Bregani ER, Rovellini A, Mbaidoum N, et al. Comparison of different anthelminthic drug regimens against *Mansonella perstans* filariasis. Trans R Soc Trop Med Hyg 2006;100:458–63.
92. Asio SM, Simonsen PE, Onapa AW. A randomised, double-blind field trial of ivermectin alone and in combination with albendazole for the treatment of *Mansonella perstans* infections in Uganda. Trans R Soc Trop Med Hyg 2009;103:274–9.
93. Person B, Bartholomew LK, Gyapong M, et al. Health-related stigma among women with lymphatic filariasis from the Dominican Republic and Ghana. Soc Sci Med 2009;68:30–8.
94. Babu BV, Mishra S, Nayak AN. Marriage, sex, and hydrocele: an ethnographic study on the effect of filarial hydrocele on conjugal life and marriageability from Orissa, India. PLoS Negl Trop Dis 2009;3:e414.

Schistosomiasis

Bruno Gryseels, MD, PhD

KEYWORDS

- Schistosomiasis • Bilharzia • *Schistosoma mansoni* • *Schistosoma haematobium*
- *Schistosoma japonicum* • Praziquantel • Neglected tropical diseases • Helminths

KEY POINTS

- Schistosomiasis is a tropical parasitic disease, caused by blood-dwelling, macroscopic worms of the genus *Schistosoma*, a trematode characterized by separate sexes.
- *Schistosoma mansoni* and *S japonicum* live in the mesenteric venules, *S haematobium* in the perivesical venules; the male worms holds the female in a permanent embrace.
- The worms excrete eggs that are excreted with the feces of urine, and release larvae (miracidiae) that can infect the intermediate hosts i.e. specific aquatic of amphibious snail species.
- Infection occurs through the skin during contact with surface water by secondary larvae (cercariae) that are released by the snails.
- *S mansoni* occurs in Africa and South America, *S haematobium* in Africa, *S japonicum* in South and East Asia; in endemic areas, prevalences can be very high especially among children.
- Eggs that are trapped in the tissues provoke immunogenic inflammatory, granulomatous and fibrotic reactions that cause intestinal, hepatosplenic or urinary disease which develops over many years.
- Most infected people show no, limited or non-specific symptoms. Severe disease develops in people with heavy, long-standing infections and probably unbalanced immune responses.
- Intestinal disease includes bloody or intermittent diarrhea, abdominal pain, colics, dysenteric syndromes, fatigue and anorexia.
- Hepatosplenic disease results in inflammatory and later fibrotic hepatomegaly and/or splenomegaly, portal hypertension, esophageal bleeding, ascites and cachexis.
- Urinary schistosomiasis presents with hematuria, dysuria, secondary infections, ureteral fibrosis and hydronephrosis.
- Schistosomiasis can be complicated by ectopic lesions especially in the central nervous system, the pulmonary system or in the genital area.
- Swimmers' itch can occur shortly after cercarial infection.
- Acute schistosomiasis is an allergic reaction occurring in the weeks after primary infection and presents as a flulike syndrome; it is a regular finding in travel clinics.
- The diagnosis of schistosomiasis relies on microscopic examination of stools or urine, serologic tests, PCR and imaging.
- Praziquantel is the drug of choice, active against all species in a single or oral dose. In some cases adjunct therapies may be useful.
- Current control strategies consist mainly of preventive therapy in communities or groups at risk. There is as yet no vaccine against schistosomiasis.
- On the long-term, only sanitation, water supply, education and socio-economic development can reduce and eliminate the transmission of schistosomiasis.

Institute of Tropical Medicine, Nationalestraat 155, B-2000 Antwerpen, Belgium
E-mail address: bgryseels@itg.be

Infect Dis Clin N Am 26 (2012) 383–397
doi:10.1016/j.idc.2012.03.004
0891-5520/12/$ – see front matter © 2012 Published by Elsevier Inc.

THE PARASITES

Adult schistosomes are macroscopically visible worms, with a white-grayish, cylindrical body approximately 1 to 1.5 cm in length.[1–3] Taxonomically, they belong to the class of Trematoda (flukes) and the phylum of Platyhelminthes (flatworms). The worms live in the bloodstream of the human host, where they can survive for up to 30 years with an average of 3 to 5 years. This is a remarkable evolutionary achievement, which requires intricate evasion mechanisms to all forms of innate and acquired immunity.

Schistosomes are also special by having separate genders, with the male holding the female in a continuous, monogamous embrace. The worms further feature two suckers, a complex tegument, a blind digestive tract, and reproductive organs (**Fig. 1**). They feed on blood cells and globulines, which they digest in a blind intestinal tract and the debris of which are regurgitated in the human bloodstream. The anaerobic metabolism serves mainly for the movements of the male schistosomes, and the egg production of the females.

TRANSMISSION

The transmission cycle of schistosomes is shown in **Fig. 2**. The female worms produce hundreds (*Schistosoma mansoni* and *S haematobium*) to thousands (*S japonicum*) of eggs per day, which are 100 to 180 μm in size and have a typical shape and spine that varies per species. Each egg contains one ciliated larva, the miracidium, which secretes enzymes that help the eggs to migrate from the blood vessels through the tissues into the lumen of the bladder (*S haematobium*) or the intestine (*S mansoni* and *S japonicum*). Most of the eggs are carried away with the bloodstream or trapped in tissues during this journey, but up to one-third are eventually excreted with urine or

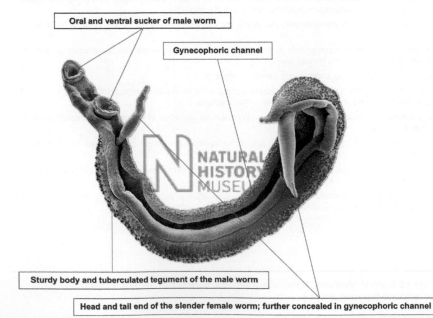

Fig. 1. The morphology of adult schistosomes. (Reproduced with permission of the Natural History Museum, London.)

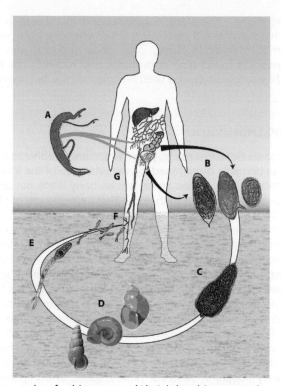

Fig. 2. Transmission cycle of schistosomes. (A) Adult schistosomes in small blood vessels around the intestines or bladder. (B) Schistosome eggs leave the body with excreta. Left-to-right: *S haematobium, S mansoni,* and *S japonicum.* (C) Miracidium hatches and swims freely in water. (D) Snail intermediate hosts are infected by miracidium. Left-to-right: *Oncomelania, Biomphalaria,* and *Biomphalaria.* (E) Cercariae hatch from snails 4 to 6 weeks later. (F) Cercariae infect humans through the skin. (G) Cercariae develop into schistosomula, which migrate with the bloodstream to the portal vein and mature into adult schistosomes, which mate and migrate to the destination. (*From* Gryseels B, Polman K, Clerinx J, et al. Human schistosomiasis. Lancet 2006;368:1106–18; with permission.)

feces. If an egg comes in contact with water, the miracidium escapes and uses its cilia to swim around in search for a suitable intermediate host.

The miracidium penetrates the snail and develops over a period of 4 to 6 weeks into multicellular sporocysts, which split into a multitude of secondary larvae. These "cercaria" consist of a large head with embryonic features of the adult schistosomes and a bifurcated tail. They leave the snail by the hundreds, under the stimulation of light. Cercarial shedding therefore occurs mainly between 10 AM and 4 PM, when the sun is high and human water contact most frequent.

The cercariae whirl around in the water for up to 72 hours. When they come in touch with human skin, they penetrate the dermis, shed their tail and migrate as "schistosomula" with the bloodstream to the heart, through the lungs, and into the liver and the portal veins. Here they mature in 4 to 6 weeks, mate, and migrate upstream to their final destination in the mesenteric veins, where the cycle starts again.

Each schistosome species can be transmitted only by a few specific snail species, belonging to the genus *Biomphalaria (S mansoni)*, *Bulinus (S haematobium)*, or *Oncomelania (S japonicum)*.[4,5] *Biomphalaria* and *Bulinus* are purely aquatic snails; *Oncomelania* are amphibian and spend part of their lives in the mud where they can survive low temperatures.[6] Therefore, *S japonicum* is found also in areas with cold winters but long, hot summers. *S japonicum* is furthermore a truly zoonotic infection, with a huge animal reservoir in cattle, pigs, dogs, rodents, and some 20 other mammals. *S mansoni* is found also in primates and rodents, but humans are the main reservoir. *S haematobium* can be bred in some rodents, but has no known animal host in nature.

DISTRIBUTION AND EPIDEMIOLOGY

Humans are host to six *Schistosoma* species, which are morphologically very similar. Their distribution is primarily determined by the presence of the intermediate hosts. The different location of the species in the human body leads not only to a different excretion path, but also to different pathology. Three species are of global or regional importance (**Fig. 3**): *S japonicum* (China and Southeast Asia) and *S mansoni* (Africa, Arabia, and South America) dwell in peri-intestinal venula, and cause intestinal and hepatosplenic schistosomiasis. *S haematobium* (Africa and Arabia) live in the perivesical plexus and causes urinary schistosomiasis of the bladder, ureters, and kidneys. *S intercalatum* (West and Central Africa), *S mekongi* (Mekong Delta), and *S malayensis* (Malaysia) are limited to a few local foci and of minor importance.[1–4,7,8] The World Health Organization estimates the number of infected people worldwide for decades at 200 million, and the number of deaths caused by schistosomiasis at 41,000 annually.[9] More than 90% of current cases occur in sub-Saharan Africa. Indeed, the number of cases in large historical foci as Brazil, Egypt, and China has been reduced to a few million. It is possible that global figures need to be reviewed downward. Transmission usually occurs in streams, ponds, lakes, and irrigation and drainage canals. Hydraulic development, human migration, and sanitary neglect have contributed greatly to the spread of schistosomiasis in rural areas, but increasingly also in urban slums.[1–3,10,11] Depending on local determinants, the epidemiology can vary strongly from one locality to another. Typically, prevalences and intensities of infection increase in young children to a peak around age 8 to 15 years, and then decrease to

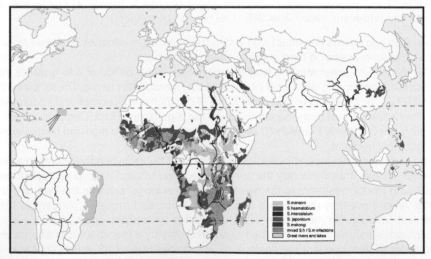

Fig. 3. World distribution map of schistosomiasis. (*From* Gryseels B, Polman K, Clerinx J, et al. Human schistosomiasis. Lancet 2006;368:1106–18; with permission.)

a plateau in adults.[1,3] Also within age groups, the distribution of parasites is strongly skewed so that a small part of the community is responsible for the largest part of egg output and most at risk for severe pathology. This predilection is thought to be determined by water contact patterns and immunogenetic factors.

ACUTE PATHOLOGY

Minutes after the cercarial infection, local urticaria may appear that usually last for a few hours but sometimes persist for days as more papulous lesions (**Fig. 4**). This "swimmers itch" is mainly seen after primary infections, especially in tourists and migrants. A similar syndrome can also be caused by animal trematodes in temperate climate zones, including North America and Europe.

One to four weeks after infection, the migrating and maturing schistosomula can cause a systemic hypersensitivity reaction. This acute form of schistosomiasis, also known as Katayama fever (after the marshy district in Japan where it was first described), starts as a flulike syndrome with protracted fever, fatigue, myalgia, headache, and dry cough.[1–3,12–14] Stool or urine examinations are still negative, but eosinophilia, positive serologic tests, and a history of tropical water contact usually indicate the diagnosis. The liver or spleen may be swollen and tender, and thorax radiography may reveal patchy infiltrates. Later, the migration and positioning of the mature worms to the mesenteric veins can lead to more pronounced abdominal symptoms, including intestinal cramps and diarrhea. Acute schistosomiasis can also be complicated by ectopic pathologies (discussed later).

Cercarial dermatitis and acute schistosomiasis caused by *S mansoni* or *S haematobium* are rarely seen in local people, probably because they have been desensitized at an early age but probably also because of underdiagnosis. Katayama fever is a frequent finding, however, among people being infected for the first time and thus also in western travel clinics. Most cases are tourists and travelers who have toured in sub-Saharan Africa. Typical sources of infection include the lakes Malawi, Victoria, and Volta; the Zambesi and Niger deltas; and some lake resorts in South Africa.[3,10] Many cases present in clusters of family members or tour groups.

Katayama fever caused by *S japonicum* is also common among local people, including adults who have been exposed for years, some even with a previous history of acute schistosomiasis.[6] The syndrome can be more severe and protracted than in

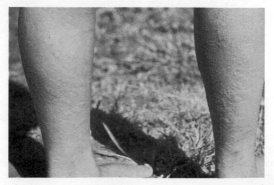

Fig. 4. Swimmers' itch. (*From* Topics in International Health Series: Schistosomiasis. Multimedia CD-ROM. New York: CABI Publishing, 1998. Copyright © The Trustee of The Wellcome Trust; with permission.)

other schistosome infections, and include also serious intestinal disease, outspoken splenomegaly and cachexia, or progress directly to advanced fibrotic pathology.

CHRONIC PATHOLOGY

Particularly in local populations, the main morbidity is caused by years of chronic infection in which not the worms but the eggs are the culprit.[1–3,15] As described, during their migration most eggs are trapped in tissues surrounding the intestinal or urinary systems, or in the liver and spleen after being evacuated by the bloodstream. The enzymes excreted to assist their penetration cause subsequently inflammatory and granulomatous immune reactions, characterized by eosinophilic infiltrations around the egg (**Fig. 5**). These reactions protect the human host against the foreign bodies and molecules, but if numerous and uncontrolled lead themselves to severe pathology. The nature of the symptoms is determined by the location of the worms and their eggs, and the severity by the intensity of infection and individual immune responses.

Urinary Schistosomiasis

Most *S haematobium* eggs are trapped in the vesical and ureteral walls, often in clusters (**Fig. 6**). Inflammatory and granulomatous reactions lead to ulcerations, micropolyps, and macropolyps and eventually fibrosis and calcification. The most typical symptom is hematuria, which in endemic areas is very common among children.

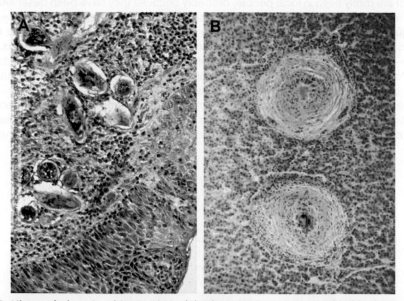

Fig. 5. Histopathology in schistosomiasis. (*A*) *S haematobium* eggs in a bladder biopsy, surrounded by granulomatous eosinophilic inflammation. (*B*) Eosinophilic granuloma around decaying egg of *S mansoni* in a portal sinusoid (hematoxylin-eosin stain, original magnification ×100). ([*A*] *Courtesy of* Erwin Vandenenden, Institute of Tropical Medicine, Antwerpen, Belgium; and [*B*] *From* Topics in International Health Series: Schistosomiasis. Multimedia CD-ROM. New York: CABI Publishing, 1998. Copyright © The Trustee of The Wellcome Trust; with permission.)

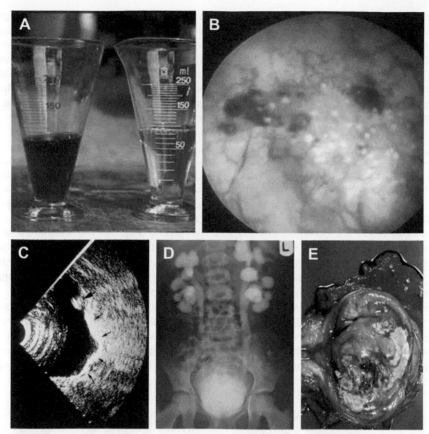

Fig. 6. Urinary schistosomiasis. (*A*) Hematuria. (*B*) Cystoscopy showing "sandy patches" lesions in bladder wall. (*C*) Irregular bladder wall (*small arrows*) and polyp (*large arrow*) on ultrasound. (*D*) Bilateral hydroureter and hydronephrosis on pyelography. (*E*) Squamous cell bladder carcinoma associated with chronic urinary schistosomiasis. ([*A*] *From* Gryseels B, Polman K, Clerinx J, et al. Human schistosomiasis. Lancet 2006;368:1106–18; with permission; and [*B–E*] *From* Topics in International Health Series: Schistosomiasis. Multimedia CD-ROM. New York: CABI Publishing, 1998. Copyright © The Trustee of The Wellcome Trust; with permission.)

In light forms the blood may only be microscopically detectable, or just visible in terminal urine. In more severe cases the entire urine can be dark-colored, and micturition painful and frequent.[1–3] Secondary bacterial infections and bladder stones may develop and exacerbate the symptoms. Although difficult to demonstrate or discern from the consequences of other poverty-related infections and conditions, schistosomiasis is believed to affect also the general well-being and productivity, translating into reduced work and school performance.[16]

The hematuria usually disappears after the age of 12 to 15 years, but the lesions may evolve to fibrosis or calcification of the bladder and lower ureters, unilateral or bilateral hydroureters, and hydronephrosis. Radiology or sonography may reveal frequent and impressive extensions in adults, but clinical morbidity often remains surprisingly limited. Hydronephrosis is mostly caused by compression rather than destruction of the parenchyma, although kidney failure may eventually develop. Direct mortality caused by urinary schistosomiasis has been rarely demonstrated.[3] Epidemiologic studies in Egypt and other foci point, however, to an association of chronic urinary schistosomiasis with squamous bladder cancer.[1–3,17] Although several carcinogenic pathways have been hypothesized, the causal relation is not yet and possibly never will be proved. Indeed, both diseases have dwindled simultaneously over the past decades, possibly as a combined result of successful schistosomiasis control programs. The schistosomiasis lesions may also have indirectly facilitated the impact of other mutagenic substrates, such as tobacco or industrial chemicals.[3]

Intestinal and Hepatosplenic Schistosomiasis

The eggs of S mansoni or S japonicum are trapped mainly in the wall and mesenterium of the large bowel and the rectum, much less in the small bowel. The surrounding granulomatous inflammation provokes microulcerations, pseudopolyps, muscular irritation, and microscopic bleeding. Abdominal pain, loss of appetite, and diarrhea with or without blood are common but atypical symptoms (**Fig. 7**). The frequency and severity of the symptoms is related to intensity of infection, and thus generally higher in children. Many people remain asymptomatic or have only intermittent complaints, but the same "subtle morbidity" as described previously is thought to have substantial impact on community health, especially in school-aged children.[16]

Hepatic schistosomiasis is initially caused by granulomatous inflammation around the eggs trapped in the liver, and in later stages by the resulting fibrosis that may aggregate to long fibrotic streaks, occluding the portal veins.[3] In children and adolescents the pathology is usually inflammatory and reversible, even if some mild fibrosis may be present. Typically, the left liver lobe is enlarged, extending a few to sometimes

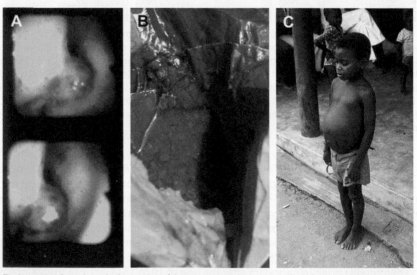

Fig. 7. Intestinal and early hepatic schistosomiasis (S mansoni). (A) Sigmoidal polyposis on endoscopy. (B) Severe bloody diarrhea caused by heavy infection. (C) Gross inflammatory hepatosplenomegaly in a young boy (see marks). ([A] From Topics in International Health Series: Schistosomiasis. Multimedia CD-ROM. New York: CABI Publishing, 1998. Copyright © The Trustee of The Wellcome Trust; with permission; and [B, C] From Gryseels B, Polman K, Clerinx J, et al. Human schistosomiasis. Lancet 2006;368:1106–18; with permission.)

15 cm below the costal arch (see **Fig. 7**). The spleen may be normal to grossly enlarged, because of increased portal blood pressure, hypersplenic reactions, or inflammation around locally deposited eggs. The organomegaly in children is strongly correlated with intensity of infection. In most cases, there is no apparent sign of hepatic dysfunction. Mild anemia may be associated with intestinal blood loss or hypersplenism, and may reinforce the general lack of well-being.

In older adolescents and young adults who have carried heavy infections over 5 to 10 years or more, the lesions become ever more fibrotic, larger, and irreversible (**Fig. 8**). Because only some heavily infected people develop such pathology, it is thought that some form of immunogenetic predisposition also needs to be present. The progression may also be more rapid in *S japonicum* infection, sometimes with little or no interval between acute and chronic disease.[1,6]

The fibrotic streaks, which take the pathognomonic form of "clay stem fibrosis," progressively occlude the portal veins, leading to portal hypertension, splenomegaly, portocaval shunting, and external or gastrointestinal varices. Liver enlargement is now typically discrete, hard, and nodular on palpation. Hepatocellular function remains usually preserved. However, ascites may occur but then usually has multiple causes.[3,18] The most dangerous, potentially fatal complication is gastroesophageal bleeding from the internal varices. Repeated or occult bleeding can lead to severe anemia and hypoalbuminemia. Advanced hepatosplenic schistosomiasis was a frequent cause of morbidity and mortality in Egypt, Sudan, Brazil, China, and the Philippines until the advent of modern schistosomicides.[1,3,10] Remarkably, advanced liver fibrosis caused by schistosomiasis has always been less frequent in all but a few areas in sub-Saharan Africa, which is attributed to ethnic and genetic factors.[3] Although cases have been described in long-term expatriates, it is not seen in accidentally infected tourists.

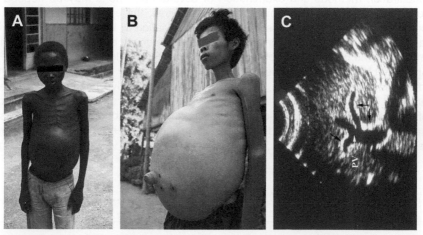

Fig. 8. Advanced hepatic schistosomiasis. (*A*) Chronic hepatic *S mansoni* with splenomegaly, moderate ascites, and growth retardation. (*B*) Advanced *S japonicum* in a young adult with splenomegaly, external varices, and severe ascites. (*C*) Ultrasound image of advanced periportal fibrosis (*black arrows*) and portal venodilatation (*white arrow*). ([*A*] *From* Gryseels B, Polman K, Clerinx J, et al. Human schistosomiasis. Lancet 2006;368:1106–18; with permission; and [*B, C*] *From* Topics in International Health Series: Schistosomiasis. Multimedia CD-ROM. New York: CABI Publishing, 1998. Copyright © The Trustee of The Wellcome Trust; with permission.)

Ectopic Schistosomiasis

In advanced hepatic schistosomiasis complicated by portal-caval shunting, pulmonary pathology can occur because of the deposition of eggs and subsequent granuloma formation in the lungs.[1,19] Initially, these give rise to bronchial symptoms. Eventually, fibrosis can develop followed by pulmonary hypertension and right heart disease. Glomerulonephritis caused by the deposition of immune complexes in the kidney has been described in long-standing S mansoni infections.[1,20] These complications have become rare in endemic areas where treatment is available, and are not common among travelers.

Eggs of S haematobium and S mansoni are easily transported to the genital and reproductive tract, where they give rise to hypertrophic or ulcerative lesions that may cause female infertility or facilitate the transmission of sexual infections, including HIV.[21] In men, inflammation of the epididymis, testicles, and prostate can be observed, also in travelers with light and recent infections. Sporadically, ectopic schistosomiasis lesions are also found in the skin, the peritoneum, or other organs.

Eggs or worms that are transported to the spinal cord or the brain can cause serious neurologic damage.[1,3,22,23] Neuroschistosomiasis caused by infection with S mansoni or S haematobium mainly leads to transverse myelitis, a syndrome that is sometimes also seen as a complication of acute schistosomiasis in travelers. Ectopic S japonicum infections have a tendency for the brain, leading to focal cerebral symptoms of an epileptic or paralytic nature.

DIAGNOSIS

The gold standard for the diagnosis of Schistosoma infection is the microscopic detection of eggs in stools or urine.[1–3,24] The typical size and shape allow an easy distinction from other helminth eggs, and among schistosome species (**Fig. 9**). Concentration methods and examination of several specimens may be needed to detect light infections.[25] For epidemiologic purposes, the eggs can be counted in a fixed amount of urine or feces, allowing an estimation of intensity of infection.[1–3] Quantitative measures are important to assess the intensity of transmission, the risk of morbidity, the need for control measures, and the evaluation of their impact.[26]

Antibody-based serologic assays are sensitive but may cross-react with other helminth infections and remain positive long after the active infection has disappeared.[1,26] Their main medical application is in travel clinics, where they are most useful in the diagnosis of acute schistosomiasis when microscopic examination is still negative.[14] An alternative is the detection of circulating antigens in serum or urine with labeled monoclonal antibodies, which, however, is not very sensitive for light

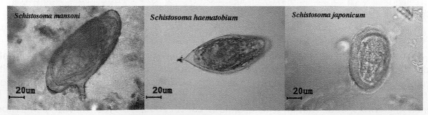

Fig. 9. Schistosome eggs under the microscope. Typical size, shape, and spine of S mansoni, S haematobium, and S japonicum. (*From* Gryseels B, Polman K, Clerinx J, et al. Human schistosomiasis. Lancet 2006;368:1106–18; with permission.)

infections, such as in tourists.[27] Recently, the detection by PCR of schistosome DNA in the sera of recently infected patients was shown to outperform parasitological and serological methods.[28]

In endemic areas, rapid assessment, indirect diagnosis, and population screening of urinary schistosomiasis can be done easily and cheaply with hematuria dipsticks or simple questionnaires.[29,30] Such tools are less readily available for S mansoni and S japonicum. The confirmation or assessment of organ complications requires radiologic, sonographic, or endoscopic methods by experienced specialists.[31] Calcifications of the urinary tract can easily be detected on direct radiographs. Contrast radiography is suitable to visualize other renal, urinary, and bladder pathology, and can also be applied for the diagnosis and measurement of portal vein distention or esophageal varices. For the latter, endoscopy is also suitable but must be handled carefully to avoid iatrogenic ruptures. In difficult cases, the assessment and differential diagnosis of hepatic fibrosis may require laparoscopy and wedge biopsy. Myelography and MRI can be useful for detailed imaging, especially for neuroschistosomiasis.

Ultrasonography has become a major tool for the diagnosis, assessment, and study of schistosomiasis pathology in hospital settings and in the field.[32] Urinary tract pathology and liver fibrosis or portal vein extension can be diagnosed and measured. Standardized protocols are available for epidemiologic studies and clinical applications.

TREATMENT

Until the 1970s, the treatment of schistosomiasis was almost as difficult and toxic as it still is today for trypanosomiasis and leishmaniasis.[10,33] Because pathology was limited in many cases, the decision to treat or not could be a real dilemma and wide-scale application for control purposes was a hazardous undertaking. In the early 1980s, praziquantel, an acylated quinoline–pyrazine active against all schistosome species in a single oral dose, came on the market.[33] It paralyzes and kills the worms within a few hours and adverse effects are usually few and limited to transient nausea or malaise. In heavy infections, transient colicky and bloody diarrhea can occur shortly after treatment, probably provoked by massive worm shifts. No long-term toxicity is known and praziquantel is safe for infants and pregnant women.[34]

The recommended doses range from 40 to 60 mg/kg according to the circumstances, species, and intensity. The lower dose is widely used in endemic areas and in control programs, where reduction of intensity of infection and risk of morbidity is the main objective, rather than absolute cure. In individual patients who are not exposed to reinfection, the dose may be increased to 60 mg/kg, in one or two takes with a 4-hour interval, and possibly repeated for 2 or 3 days.

Praziquantel does not kill eggs or schistosomula. Therefore, the etiologic treatment of acute schistosomiasis may have to be repeated or deferred until 2 to 3 months after the likely date of infection. In the meantime, symptomatic treatment can be given with standard analgesics and corticoids.[12–14]

Because eggs that are migrating through the tissues are not affected by praziquantel and may be excreted for weeks after the worms are killed, microscopic follow-up of treatment must be given sufficient time (ie, up to 4–6 weeks). In endemic areas, new infections may be contracted in that period, which may make it difficult to distinguish rapid reinfection from treatment failure.[35]

The organ pathology usually dissolves or decreases substantially in the weeks and months after treatment, as can be shown by radiographic or sonographic examination.[36] However, advanced liver fibrosis or severe nephropathy may be irreversible. The acute treatment of esophageal bleeding may require β-blockers, sclerotherapy, splenectomy, or portocaval shunting.[33] In the treatment of neuro-schistosomiasis, praziquantel should be associated with corticosteroids and possibly anticonvulsants, to avoid acute exacerbations after the death of ectopic worms.[23]

It has been shown that artemisinin and derivatives are active against schistosomula and, to a lesser extent, adult schistosomes.[37] Although they could be used as prophylaxis, this is not appropriate in malaria-endemic areas where artemisinin resistance in malaria must be avoided at all cost. Its curative use in acute schistosomiasis, in combination with praziquantel, is still being investigated.

Whereas some worrying results have been reported, and praziquantel tolerance can easily be induced in animal models, there is no clinical or epidemiologic evidence for the emergence of praziquantel resistance in the field.[35] Caution is needed, however, because there are no other multivalent schistosomicides available or in the development pipeline.

CONTROL

The control and prevention of schistosomiasis used to be largely based on the chemical destruction or environmental management of snail populations, a difficult, costly, and mostly inefficient method (**Fig. 10**).[1,3,10] Some countries, most notably Japan in the 1950s, have nevertheless been able to eliminate schistosomiasis by combining this approach with water supply, sanitation, and environmental interventions.[38] Nowadays, the emphasis has entirely shifted to preventive chemotherapy of communities and groups at risk.[39,40] Depending on the local epidemiology and resources, communities in endemic areas are either screened and treated if positive, or the entire population is treated regardless of individual infection status. This strategy especially targets school-aged children, who are most at risk and are easily accessible in schools. The drugs are distributed by special teams, local healthcare staff, community healthcare workers, or school teachers.

Although the primary objective of preventive chemotherapy is to control and prevent morbidity, it is also hoped that eventually transmission will be affected and even halted by sustained "mass drug administration." The dynamics of transmission are not linear, however, and eliminating schistosomiasis with drugs alone without additional measures in terms of sanitation, water supply, and education is unlikely to succeed.[3] In countries that are moving up the income and development ladder, such as Brazil, China, Egypt, and the Philippines, mass screening and treatment has resulted in quick advances that seem to be sustainable because of concurrent socioeconomic progress. In other areas, most notably sub-Saharan Africa, preventive chemotherapy has to be repeated at regular intervals for an as yet undetermined period to remain effective. Because logistical conditions are difficult and healthcare systems weak, this requires considerable resources and tenacity; the cost of the drug, actually at less than $ 0.15 per treatment, is no longer a limiting factor.

Recently, development agencies, global philanthropists, and pharmaceutical companies have teamed up in a massive effort to assist endemic countries with the introduction of preventive chemotherapy and mass drug administration for helminthic diseases, including schistosomiasis.[41] The stated objective is to eliminate these health problems and ensuing poverty by the year 2020. Critical issues are a balanced and sustainable integration in health service activities, appropriate adaptations of the global strategy to local priorities, circumstances and resources, and the avoidance of drug resistance.[3,42,43] The commitment and discipline must remain strong when

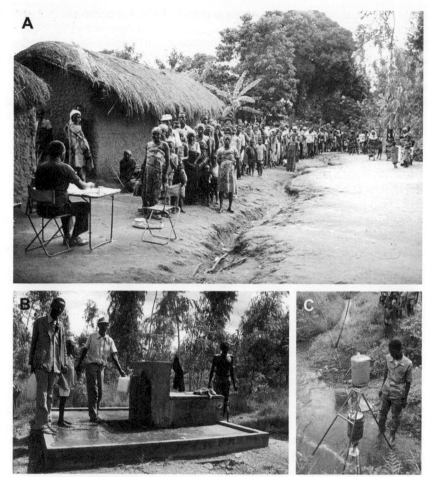

Fig. 10. Schistosomiasis control in the field. (*A*) Mass treatment with praziquantel in the community. (*B*) Safe water supply. (*C*) Snail control with molluscicides.

prevalences wane after a few treatment rounds. Most of all, the expected quick wins must be consolidated by the rapid improvement of living conditions, which can only be achieved by political and socioeconomic progress. Schistosomiasis remains a disease of poverty, and the one cannot be eradicated without the other.

REFERENCES

1. Jordan P, Webbe G, Sturrock FS. Human schistosomiasis. Wallingford (CT): CAB International; 1993.
2. Ross AG, Bartley PB, Sleigh AC, et al. Schistosomiasis. N Engl J Med 2002;346: 1212–20.
3. Gryseels B, Polman K, Clerinx J, et al. Human schistosomiasis. Lancet 2006;368: 1106–18.
4. Doumenge JP, Mott KE. Global distribution of schistosomiasis: CEGET/WHO Atlas. World Health Stat Q 1984;37:186–99.

5. Brown DS. Freshwater snails of Africa and their medical importance. 2nd edition. London: Taylor and Francis; 1994.

6. Ross AG, Sleigh AC, Li Y, et al. Schistosomiasis in the People's Republic of China: prospects and challenges for the 21st century. Clin Microbiol Rev 2001;14:270–95.

7. Chitsulo L, Engels D, Montresor A, et al. The global status of schistosomiasis and its control. Acta Trop 2000;77:41–51.

8. WHO Expert Committee. Prevention and control of schistosomiasis and soil-transmitted helminthiasis. Report of a WHO Expert Committee. World Health Organ Tech Rep Ser 2002;912:1–57.

9. Global burden of disease: update 2004. Geneva (Switzerland): World Health Organization; 2008.

10. Jordan P. From Katayama to the Dakhla Oasis: the beginning of epidemiology and control of bilharzia. Acta Trop 2000;77:9–40.

11. Steinmann P, Keiser J, Bos R, et al. Schistosomiasis and water resources development: systematic review, meta-analysis, and estimates of people at risk. Lancet Infect Dis 2006;6:411–25.

12. Jelinek T, Nothdurft HD, Loscher T. Schistosomiasis in travelers and expatriates. J Travel Med 1996;13:160–4.

13. Ross AG, Vickers D, Olds GR, et al. Katayama syndrome. Lancet Infect Dis 2007; 7:218–24.

14. Clerinx J, Van Gompel A. Schistosomiasis in travellers and migrants. Travel Med Infect Dis 2011;9:6–24.

15. Wilson MS, Mentink-Kane MM, Pesce JT, et al. Immunopathology of schistosomiasis. Immunol Cell Biol 2007;85:148–54.

16. King CH, Dickman K, Tisch DJ. Regauging the cost of chronic helminthic infection: meta-analysis of disability-related outcomes in endemic schistosomiasis. Lancet 2005;365:1561–9.

17. Vennervald BJ, Polman K. Helminths and malignancy. Parasite Immunol 2009;31: 686–96.

18. Strickland GT. Liver disease in Egypt: hepatitis C superseded schistosomiasis as a result of iatrogenic and biological factors. Hepatology 2006;43:915–22.

19. Schwartz E. Pulmonary schistosomiasis. Clin Chest Med 2002;23:433–43.

20. Barsoum R, Harrington JT, Mathew CM, et al. The changing face of schistosomal glomerulopathy. Kidney Int 2004;66:2472–84.

21. WHO. Report of an informal working group meeting on urogenital schistosomiasis and HIV transmission. Geneva (Switzerland): World Health Organization; 2010.

22. Carod-Artal FJ. Neuroschistosomiasis. Expert Rev Anti Infect Ther 2010;8: 1307–18.

23. Ross AG, McManus DP, Farrar J, et al. Neuroschistosomiasis. J Neurol 2012;259: 22–32.

24. Rabello A. Diagnosing schistosomiasis. Mem Inst Oswaldo Cruz 1997;92:669–76.

25. de Vlas SJ, Gryseels B. Underestimation of *Schistosoma mansoni* prevalences. Parasitol Today 1992;8:274–7.

26. Tsang VC, Wilkins PP. Immunodiagnosis of schistosomiasis. Immunol Invest 1997;26:175–88.

27. Van Lieshout L, Polderman AM, Deelder AM. Immunodiagnosis of schistosomiasis by determination of the circulating antigens CAA and CCA, in particular in individuals with recent or light infections. Acta Trop 2000;77:69–80.

28. Clerinx J, Bottieau E, Wichmann D, et al. Acute Schistosomiasis in a Cluster of Travelers From Rwanda: Diagnostic Contribution of Schistosome DNA Detection in Serum Compared to Parasitology and Serology. J Travel Med 2011;18:367–72.

29. Lengeler C, Utzinger J, Tanner M. Questionnaires for rapid screening of schisto-somiasis in sub-Saharan Africa. Bull World Health Organ 2002;80:235–42.
30. Tan H, Yang M, Wu Z, et al. Rapid screening method for *Schistosoma japonicum* infection using questionnaires in flood area of the People's Republic of China. Acta Trop 2004;90:1–9.
31. Palmer PE, Reeder CC. International Registry of Tropical Imaging. Radiology Department, Uniformed Services University USA 2011. Available at: http://tmcr.usuhs.mil. Accessed February 8, 2012.
32. Richter J, Hatz C, Haussinger D. Ultrasound in tropical and parasitic diseases. Lancet 2003;362:900–2.
33. Olds GR, Dasarathy S. Schistosomiasis. Curr Treat Options Infect Dis 2000;2: 88–99.
34. Dayan AD. Albendazole, mebendazole and praziquantel: review of non-clinical toxicity and pharmacokinetics. Acta Trop 2003;86:141–59.
35. Gryseels B, Mbaye A, de Vlas SJ, et al. Are poor responses to praziquantel for the treatment of *Schistosoma mansoni* infections in Senegal due to resistance? An overview of the evidence. Trop Med Int Health 2001;6:864–73.
36. Richter J. The impact of chemotherapy on morbidity due to schistosomiasis. Acta Trop 2003;86:161–83.
37. Utzinger J, Xiao SH, Tanner M, et al. Artemisinins for schistosomiasis and beyond. Curr Opin Investig Drugs 2007;8:105–16.
38. Minai M, Hosaka Y, Ohta N. Historical view of schistosomiasis japonica in Japan: implementation and evaluation of disease-control strategies in Yamanashi Prefec-ture. Parasitol Int 2003;52:321–6.
39. Molyneux DH, Hotez PJ, Fenwick A. "Rapid-impact interventions": how a policy of integrated control for Africa's neglected tropical diseases could benefit the poor. PLoS Med 2005;2:e336.
40. WHO. Preventive chemotherapy in human helminthiasis. Geneva (Switzerland): World Health Organisation; 2006.
41. Available at: http://www.gatesfoundation.org/press-releases/Pages/combating-10-neglected-tropical-diseases-120130.aspx. Accessed February 8, 2012.
42. Geerts S, Gryseels B. Drug resistance in human helminths: current situation and lessons from livestock. Clin Microbiol Rev 2000;13:207–22.
43. Mahmoud A, Zerhounic E. Neglected tropical diseases: moving beyond mass drug treatment to understanding the science. Health Aff (Millwood) 2009;28: 1726–33.

Trematode Infections
Liver and Lung Flukes

Thomas Fürst, MA[a,b], Urs Duthaler, PhD[a,c], Banchop Sripa, PhD[d],
Jürg Utzinger, PhD[a,b], Jennifer Keiser, PhD[a,c],*

KEYWORDS

- Trematode • Clonorchis sinensis • Opisthorchis viverrini • Fasciola hepatica
- Fasciola gigantica • Paragonimus spp

KEY POINTS

- Liver and lung fluke infections belong to the food-borne trematodiases that are transmitted through the consumption of contaminated undercooked aquatic food.
- Infections are most prevalent in Southeast Asia and Latin America, but might occur in North America due to international travel, human migration, and food trade.
- Clinical manifestations of liver and lung fluke infections are unspecific and, according to the parasites' location in the human host, comprise hepatobiliary and pleuropulmonary symptoms.
- Timely diagnosis and treatment are essential to avoid severe sequelae such as cholangiocarcinoma and ectopic complications as infections progress.
- Prevention and integrated control measures are essential to avoid transmission and include improved sanitation, food processing and inspection, ICE campaigns, and access to treatment.

Funding statement: Thomas Fürst is associated to the National Centre of Competence in Research (NCCR) North-South and received financial support through a Pro*Doc Research Module from the Swiss National Science Foundation (SNSF; project number PDFMP3-123185) and from the Freiwillige Akademische Gesellschaft (FAG) Basel. Jennifer Keiser acknowledges a personal career development grant from SNSF (projects no. PPOOA3–114941 and PPOOP3_135170).
Conflict of interests: The authors have nothing to disclose.

[a] University of Basel, Petersplatz 1, CH-4003 Basel, Switzerland; [b] Department of Epidemiology and Public Health, Swiss Tropical and Public Health Institute, P.O. Box, CH–4002 Basel, Switzerland; [c] Department of Medical Parasitology and Infection Biology, Swiss Tropical and Public Health Institute, P.O. Box, CH–4051 Basel, Switzerland; [d] Tropical Disease Research Laboratory, Department of Pathology, Khon Kaen University, Khon Kaen 40002, Thailand
* Department of Medical Parasitology and Infection Biology, Swiss Tropical and Public Health Institute, P.O. Box, CH–4002 Basel, Switzerland.
E-mail address: jennifer.keiser@unibas.ch

Infect Dis Clin N Am 26 (2012) 399–419
doi:10.1016/j.idc.2012.03.008
0891-5520/12/$ – see front matter © 2012 Elsevier Inc. All rights reserved.

id.theclinics.com

INTRODUCTION

Food-borne trematodiases are a cluster of mainly chronic diseases caused by parasitic worms of the class Trematoda.[1,2] Recent data suggest that food-borne trematodiases are an emerging public health problem, partially explained by the exponential growth of aquaculture (inland fish production) in Southeast Asia as well as intensified transport and trade of aquatic foodstuffs.[3] According to the final organs parasitized in the human host, food-borne trematodiases are grouped into liver, lung, and intestinal fluke infections.

This article focuses on the liver and lung flukes, the most prominent of which are *Clonorchis sinensis*, *Fasciola gigantica*, *Fasciola hepatica*, *Opisthorchis felineus*, and *Opisthorchis viverrini* (liver flukes), and *Paragonimus* spp (lung flukes).[1,2] These fluke infections together cause more than 85% of the global burden due to food-borne trematodiases.[4] The authors describe the epidemiology, including current distribution, global burden estimates, life cycle, and transmission; clinical signs and symptoms; diagnostic approaches for detecting infection and disease; and the present armamentarium for treatment and morbidity control. Measures for prevention and integrated control of the infections are discussed, and research needs are also emphasized.

EPIDEMIOLOGY

The epidemiology of liver and lung fluke infections, as well as other trematode and nematode infections, is governed by social-ecological contexts.[5–7] Nutrition-related behavior (ie, consumption of undercooked aquatic products such as freshwater fish, crabs, and water plants) and distribution networks of aquatic foodstuffs that are contaminated with metacercariae play important roles in liver and lung fluke infections.[1] The key risk factor for infection is the consumption of raw, undercooked, or pickled fish, crabs, and other aquatic products that are contaminated with the infectious stages of the parasites (ie, metacercariae). In Southeast Asia and the Americas, aquatic food dishes are often rooted in local traditions with high ethnic, cultural, and nutritional values. For example, culinary dishes that cause lung fluke infection in the people of the Republic of Korea include raw crab meat spiced with soy sauce (*kejang*). Liver fluke infections in the People's Republic of China (P.R. China) have been linked to the consumption of raw grass carp dishes and in Thailand and Lao People's Democratic Republic (Lao PDR) to the consumption of freshly prepared uncooked or fermented fish (*lab pla*, *koi pla*, *pla som*, and *pla ra*).[1,8] In Peru, *alfalfa* juice is consumed as a popular herbal medicine, but this habit has also been identified as a risk factor for *F hepatica* infection.[9] Food-borne trematodiases, in general, and liver and lung fluke infections, in particular, are rarely found in Africa, mainly explained by the tradition of cooking fish and other foodstuffs completely.[10]

Although eating habits are deeply rooted in local traditions and thus difficult to influence, the social-ecological systems in many endemic regions have changed over the past decades, which, in turn, also modified the epidemiologic patterns of food-borne trematodiases. For instance, in Asia, the changing demographic and economic situation and modified agricultural production systems and ecosystems, sometimes coupled with disease control and education efforts, resulted in a remarkable shift in the prevalence of paragonimiasis. Children living in poor rural setting who catch and eat raw crustaceans while playing or helping their parents in the fields are still at high risk for infection. However, an increasing number of better off, middle-aged, and usually male city dwellers enjoying delicacies such as freshwater crabs or undercooked meat of wild boars (*Sus scrofa leucomystax*), which may act as paratenic host for *Paragonimus westermani*, are at risk of infection during their participation at parties, festivals, and recreational visits to the countryside.[11] Similarly, foreign travelers tasting typical local delicacies during their journeys have been repeatedly diagnosed with liver and lung fluke infections after their return to their nonendemic home countries (**Box 1**). Hence, it remains to be seen how the underlying risk factors further influence the epidemiologic pattern of liver and lung fluke infections.[12]

DISTRIBUTION AND BURDEN

In mid-2007, Murray and colleagues[97] issued a call for experts and collaborators to reestimate the global burden of diseases, injuries, and risk factors, considering more than 175 conditions, with results to be presented in mid-2012, stratified for 20 regions of the world. The authors' group participated in this endeavor and was charged to estimate, for the first time, the global burden of human food-borne trematodiases. The group developed a broad-based computer-aided search and systematically examined not less than 11 electronic databases, adhering to a predefined protocol. This systematic review resulted in a comprehensive database, including literature of any language mainly published between January 1, 1980, and December 31, 2008.[4] While preparing this article, the authors updated their search, including additional relevant literature published between January 1, 2009, and the end of September 2011.

Probing this database for the current distribution and global burden of liver and lung fluke infections revealed the following: While *C sinensis* is endemic in East and Southeast Asia,[3,8,98] *O viverrini* mainly occurs in Southeast Asia.[3,8] The endemic area of *O felineus* expands further to the West, including parts of Central and Western Eurasia.[3,8] In contrast, the liver fluke *Fasciola* spp shows a worldwide distribution.[99] The lung fluke *Paragonimus* spp is endemic in Asia and Latin America and has also been reported from parts of North America and Africa.[3]

Fig. 1 shows the countries in which reports of autochthonous infections with the most important liver and lung flukes were identified in the reviewed literature. In brief,

---

Box 1

Liver and lung fluke infections in the United States, Canada, and nonendemic countries throughout the world

In the United States and Canada, autochthonous human cases of fascioliasis[13–16] and paragonimiasis[11,13,15,17,18] occur, but because there is no widespread tradition of eating raw aquatic products, the incidence of such cases remains very low. However, because of increasing international travel, migration, and trade, allochthonous cases of clonorchiasis,[19–31] opisthorchiasis,[19,24,26–28,32–34] fascioliasis,[19,32,35–40] and paragonimiasis[19,41–43] have been repeatedly diagnosed in travelers and immigrants in the United States and Canada. Furthermore, 3 reports on paragonimiasis also demonstrate the potential for human infection via imported contaminated food.[44–46] Autochthonous human infections with the widely neglected North American liver fluke *Metorchis conjunctus* have been reported from Canada and Greenland,[24,47–49] and metorchiasis caused by *Metorchis bilis* seems to be a seriously underestimated emerging disease in Russia.[50] The effect of globalization is also apparent by cases of allochthonous liver and lung fluke infections in the European countries, such as Czech Republic,[51,52] Denmark,[53] Finland,[54] France,[55–58] Germany,[59–62] Greece,[63] Netherlands,[64,65] Norway,[66] Romania,[67] Spain,[68–70] Switzerland,[71,72] and the United Kingdom.[73–75] Furthermore, allochthonous cases of clonorchiasis have been recorded from Brazil,[76,77] Egypt,[78] Japan,[79] Malaysia,[80,81] Surinam,[82] and Taiwan[83–86]; opisthorchiasis from Kuwait,[87] Malaysia,[80] and Taiwan[83–85,88,89]; fascioliasis from Israel,[90] Kuwait,[91] Pakistan,[92] and Saudi Arabia[93]; and paragonimiasis from Australia[94] New Zealand,[95] and Saudi Arabia.[96] The current listing of nonendemic countries with allochthonous cases is incomplete, and hence needs constant updating as new cases are reported in the peer-reviewed literature.

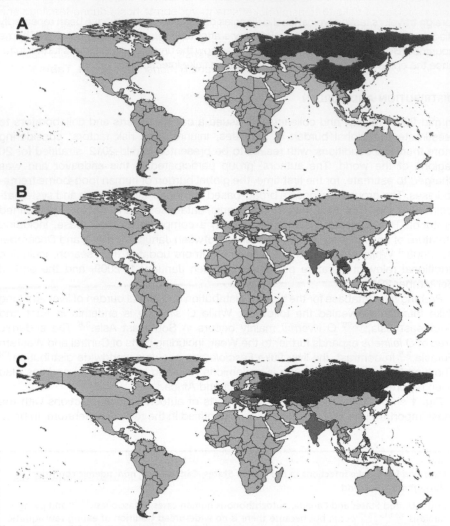

Fig. 1. Maps of the global distribution of autochthonous human cases of major liver and lung fluke infections reported in the literature. (*A*) *Clonorchis sinensis*, (*B*) *Opisthorchis viverrini*, (*C*) *Opisthorchis felineus*, (*D*) *Fasciola* spp, and (*E*) *Paragonimus* spp. Reported cases in the literature were carefully reviewed and efforts made to exclude allochthonous cases in returning travelers and migrants and cases infected via imported contaminated food. Bright colors indicate countries, where reliable national prevalence estimates on human infections after 1980 could be identified in the literature, and which were therefore included in the most recent global burden of disease estimates.[4] Pale colors indicate countries, where no reliable national prevalence estimates on human infections after 1980 could be identified in the literature, but where human cases were nevertheless reported.

autochthonous cases of *C sinensis* were reported in 10 countries (see **Fig. 1**A), *O viverrini* in 6 countries (see **Fig. 1**B), *O felineus* in 9 countries (see **Fig. 1**C), *Fasciola* spp in 81 countries (see **Fig. 1**D), and *Paragonimus* spp in 48 countries (see **Fig. 1**E). Truly autochthonous transmission is only possible in areas where suitable intermediate hosts are present for the parasites to fulfill their complex life cycles (see the next section on life cycles and transmission). However, because of increasing international

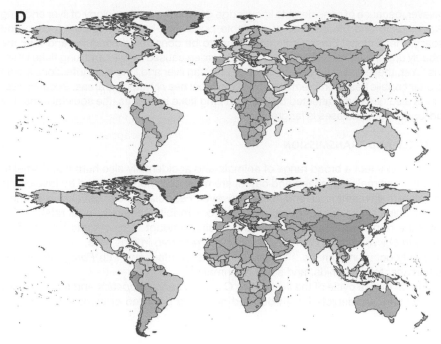

Fig. 1. (*continued*)

trade and travel as well as human migration (forced or unforced), liver or lung fluke infections may be diagnosed all over the world and the distinction between autochthonous and allochthonous infections is becoming increasingly difficult.

The case of fascioliasis offers an interesting historical example on the spread of liver fluke infection. In predomestication times, *F hepatica* occurred in the Near East. The postdomestication westwards spread of *F hepatica* to Europe began around 6000 years before Christ and continued during the Phoenician, Greek, and Roman eras. More recently, the export of European livestock during colonization facilitated the transoceanic spread of *F hepatica* to the New World, starting some 500 years ago. Intermediate host snails were most likely spread simultaneously in mud attached to the feet of the exported livestock, but *F hepatica* adapted quickly to new intermediate and definitive hosts. Because of its ability to proliferate in a wide range of different ecosystems, *F hepatica* is probably the vector-borne parasite species with the widest longitudinal, latitudinal, and altitudinal distribution nowadays.[99–101] However, most other liver and lung flukes and associated host species may not have the same colonization capacity as *F hepatica*.

In agreement with the endemic areas detailed above, an estimated 601 million people are at risk for infection with *C sinensis* in East and Southeast Asia; 67.3 million with *O viverrini* in Southeast Asia; 12.5 million with *O felineus* in Central and Western Eurasia; 91.1 million with *Fasciola* spp in Latin America, Middle East, and Europe; and 292.8 million with *Paragonimus* spp mainly in Asia and Latin America.[3] The authors' estimates for the year 2005 resulted in 15.3, 8.0, 0.4, 2.6, and 23.2 million people infected with *C sinensis*, *O viverrini*, *O felineus*, *Fasciola* spp, and *Paragonimus* spp, respectively. In terms of global burden, as expressed by disability-adjusted life years (DALYs), the corresponding numbers for infections with *C sinensis*, *O viverrini*, *O felineus*, *Fasciola* spp, and *Paragonimus* spp are 275,000, 74,000, less than 1000, 35,000, and 197,000 DALYs, respectively.

However, because of considerable knowledge gaps in the epidemiology of liver and lung fluke infection and the scarcity of available population-based data on infection and disease, these global burden estimates have to be considered carefully, and they are probably underestimates of the true disease burden caused by liver and lung fluke infections.[4] Yet, these first estimates confirm that human liver and lung fluke infections are an important public health problem in some of the most heavily affected areas. Because livestock is also negatively affected by liver and lung fluke infections, the societal impact of food-borne trematodiases is far greater.

LIFE CYCLE AND TRANSMISSION

Fasciola spp infect a broad range of animals and accidentally also humans. Domesticated farm animals (eg, sheep and cattle) are most commonly affected by fascioliasis and act as main mammalian end hosts. However, *Fasciola* spp can develop in a variety of wild animals (eg, deer, llamas, kangaroos, rabbits, beavers, and rats), which shows the remarkable capability of the parasite to adapt to new hosts.[102,103] Infections with *O viverrini* and *C sinensis* have been reported in pigs, rats, cats, and dogs but mainly occur in humans.[104] Definitive hosts of infections with *Paragonimus* spp are humans, felids, canids, and small mammals.[11]

In **Fig. 2**, the life cycle of the liver flukes *C sinensis* and *F hepatica* and the lung fluke *P westermani* are depicted, with detailed accounts provided elsewhere.[1,98] In brief,

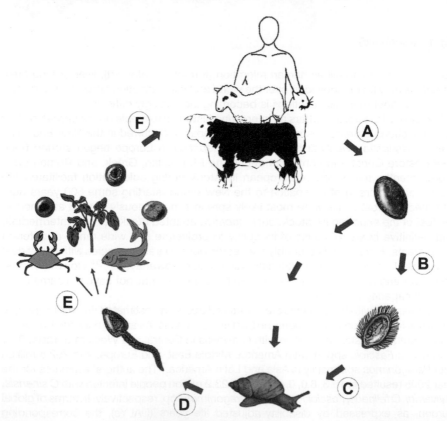

Fig. 2. Life cycle of major liver and lung flukes. (*Adapted from* Keiser J, Utzinger J. Food-borne trematodiases. Clin Microbiol Rev 2009;22:466–83.)

adult flukes produce eggs, which are released in the feces (liver flukes) or sputum (lung flukes) (see **Fig. 2**, A). Large numbers of fertilized eggs are typically released into the environment, so that transmission to new hosts is likely to occur. For example, an adult *F hepatica* fluke is able to produce as many as 20,000 eggs per day.[105] However, egg production is density-dependent, and hence varies according to worm burden. *F hepatica* eggs are oval with a large size from 130 to 145 μm in length and 70 to 90 μm in width. *P westermani* eggs range from 80 to 120 μm in length and 45 to 70 μm in width. For comparison, eggs of *C sinensis* are much smaller and measure only 25 to 35 μm in length and 15 to 17 μm in width.[104] Embryonated *F hepatica* and *P westermani* eggs release free-swimming miracidia (see **Fig. 2**, B), which invade the molluscan first intermediate hosts, species of *Lymnaea truncatula* (synonym *Galba truncatula*) (*F hepatica*), and Thiaridae and Pleuroceridae (*Paragonimus* spp) (see **Fig. 2**, C).[103,105] *C sinensis* and *Opisthorchis* spp eggs are typically ingested by *Bithynia* spp or *Parafossarulus* spp snails and miracidia are released directly in the gastrointestinal tract of the snail.[98] The miracidia multiply asexually within the snail and develop during several weeks into sporocyst, rediae, and cercariae (see **Fig. 2**, D).[1] For instance, a snail infected with a single *F hepatica* miracidium is able to produce around 4000 free-swimming cercariae.[106] Released cercariae either encyst on aquatic vegetation, such as watercress (*F hepatica*), or invade and encyst into the tissues of fish (*C sinensis*) or shellfish (*Paragonimus* spp) (see **Fig. 2**, E). Humans and other definitive hosts become infected by ingesting metacercariae through consumption of insufficiently cooked aquatic products or when drinking contaminated water (see **Fig. 2**, F).[13,98] After ingestion of the metacercariae, a juvenile worm is released, which migrates to the target organ, matures, and, after reaching sexual maturity, produces eggs (**Fig. 3**).

CLINICAL SIGNS AND SYMPTOMS

Chronic food-borne trematodiases are mainly asymptomatic. Regarding chronic clonorchiasis and opisthorchiasis, only few specific signs and symptoms occur, with the exception of an increased frequency of palpable liver, as revealed by community-based studies on physical examination.[107–111] Hematological and liver function tests are generally unremarkable, regardless of infection intensity. However, ultrasound examinations show high frequencies of left lobe liver and gallbladder enlargement, sludge and stones in the gallbladder, and poor hepatobiliary function also in asymptomatic cases.[111–114] Patients with symptomatic clonorchiasis and opisthorchiasis often present with pain in the right upper quadrant, weakness, lassitude, loss of appetite, diarrhea, indigestion, weight loss, ascites, and odema.[115,116] A particular feature of *O felineus* infection, not often reported for other liver fluke infections, is acute opisthorchiasis,[107] which is characterized by hepatosplenomegaly and tenderness, high levels of eosinophilia (up to 40%), and chills and fever. Acute opisthorchiasis occurs early in infection and may be associated with primary exposure to a large dose of metacercaria.

Clonorchis and *Opisthorchis* infection can lead to obstructive jaundice, cholangitis, cholecystitis, intra-abdominal mass, and, particularly in case of clonorchiasis, gallbladder or intrahepatic stones.[109,110,114,116] The most severe complication of Asian liver fluke infection is cholangiocarcinoma. Case-control studies in Thailand suggest a 5-fold increased risk of cholangiocarcinoma during *O viverrini* infection of any intensity, while heavily infected people may face a 15-fold higher risk.[117] With *O viverrini* antibody testing, even a 27-fold higher risk of cholangiocarcinoma has been determined.[118] Similarly, an elevated susceptibility to cholangiocarcinoma has been

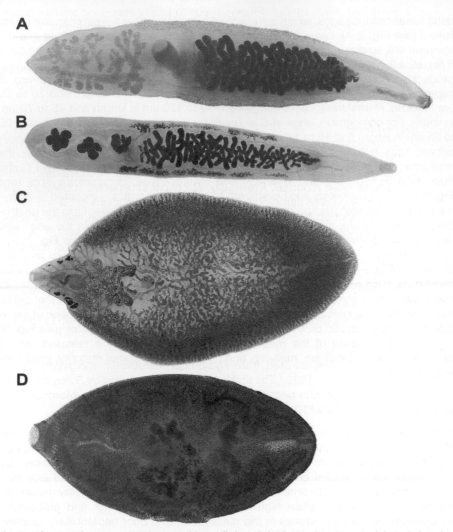

Fig. 3. Photos of major adult liver and lung flukes. (*A*) *Clonorchis sinensis*, (*B*) *Opisthorchis viverrini*, (*C*) *Fasciola hepatica*, and (*D*) *Paragonimus westermani*.

reported for *Clonorchis* infection.[108,109,119–121] In the most recently accomplished global burden estimation, meta-analyses were based on a broad literature review and revealed infection intensity–independent odds ratios of 4.4 with *O viverrini* and 6.1 with *C sinensis*.[4] Consequentially, both parasites have been designated as Group 1 carcinogen by the International Agency for Research on Cancer of the World Health Organization (WHO).[122]

As in case of the other liver flukes, human infections with *Fasciola* spp may proceed symptomatic or asymptomatic.[103] Symptoms usually occur 2 months after the ingestion of metacercariae and 1 to 2 months before the onset of egg excretion.[123–125] At the beginning of an infection, an acute phase may be caused by migration of the young developing fluke through the intestinal wall and the hepatic parenchyma before finally reaching the bile ducts. Manifestations of this acute phase include upper abdominal pain, prolonged fever, hepatomegaly, mild eosinophilia (early infection) or hypereosinophilia (mid or late acute infection), and multiple hypodense lesions seen on computed tomography (CT) scan.[103] In contrast, ultrasound examinations are mainly unremarkable.[126] Other symptoms included nausea, vomiting, anorexia, weight loss, lymphadenopathies, arthralgias, and cutaneous manifestations.[103,126] Rarely, *Fasciola* spp causes ectopic infections in the intestinal wall, lungs, pancreas, eye, brain, stomach wall, pharyngeal mucosa, skin, and other locations.[103,127–129]

The chronic phase of human fascioliasis begins after approximately 6 months, may last several years (>10 years), and is asymptomatic in about half of the cases.[130] In symptomatic cases, symptoms are more discrete and reflect intermittent biliary obstruction and inflammation caused by the adult fluke within the bile ducts. Manifestations comprise upper abdominal pain,[131] intermittent jaundice,[130] intrahepatic cystic abscesses with prolonged fever,[132] eosinophilic cholecystitis,[133] and extrahepatic cholestasis with increased levels of liver enzymes, mainly alanine aminotransferase, aspartate aminotransferase, total bilirubin, and γ-glutamyl transpeptidase (GGT).[134] In *Fasciola*-endemic areas, an increased level of GGT or alkaline phosphatase is a strong indicator of fascioliasis. In severe cases, ascites with blood and severe anemia may ensue. Because these signs and symptoms do not differentiate cholangitis and cholecystitis from other causes, the infection often goes unnoticed until worms are observed at surgery,[133] after laparoscopic cholecystectomy,[135] or during endoscopic retrograde cholangiopancreatography.[136] Gastrointestinal symptoms may persist even after treatment in about 2–4% of patients.[137] Eosinophilia may be absent in half of the chronic patients, so a normal eosinophil count does not rule out infection.[130,138]

Clinical manifestations of lung fluke infections show a wide spectrum. In fact, about 20% of patients with paragonimiasis were asymptomatic and identified accidentally by chest radiographic examination during routine health checks.[139] In pulmonary paragonimiasis, the common clinical symptom in the acute and subacute stage of infection is a chronic cough with rusty brown, blood-streaked, gelatinous, pneumonia-like sputum caused by the worms wandering in the pleural cavity. Furthermore, paragonimiasis cases may suffer from pleural effusion, pneumothorax, empyema from secondary bacterial infection, and, particularly in case of heavy physical exertion, hemoptysis. Leukocytosis is not prominent and eosinophilia (up to 20–25%) is characteristic in the acute and subacute phase of an infection but may return to normal in the chronic phase.[140] Pleurisy has also been described in infection with *P miyazakii*,[141] *P westermani*,[139,142,143] and *P heterotremus*.[144,145] Because of the similarity of the clinical manifestations, pulmonary paragonimiasis is frequently misdiagnosed as bronchial asthma, chronic bronchitis, bronchiectasis, and pulmonary tuberculosis.[146]

As the liver flukes *Fasciola* spp, the lung flukes *Paragonimus* spp may also occur in ectopic locations. Patients with extrapulmonary paragonimiasis may present with varying clinical manifestations depending on the exact location of the parasite in the human body. Cutaneous involvement is not uncommon and seen as painless, movable subcutaneous swellings most frequently on the abdomen or anterior chest wall. Immature worms are frequently found in surgically resected tissues. The subcutaneous manifestation has been reported in infections with *P skrjabini*, *P miyazakii*, *P westermani*,[147] and *P heterotremus*.[148] *Paragonimus* worms may also migrate into the central nervous system, thereby causing serious conditions and in rare cases even death.[141,149,150] The acute phase of central nervous system involvement can be seen as eosinophilic meningoencephalomyelitis. In chronic cases, the disease is characterized by convulsions, often associated with hemiplegia, and/or visual impairment with insidious onset.[151,152]

DIAGNOSIS

If inhabitants, migrants, or returning travelers from endemic areas present with any combination of the aforementioned, often diffuse clinical manifestations and particularly when they confirm the ingestion of undercooked aquatic food, liver and lung fluke infections should be listed as important differential diagnosis. Various techniques are available for the diagnosis of liver and lung fluke infections and associated disease, such as imaging techniques, detection of parasitic elements under a microscope, and immunologic and molecular methods.[1] However, these techniques differ considerably with regard to their diagnostic accuracy. Imaging techniques, such as ultrasonography or CT, for instance, are used to examine organ damage caused by chronic trematode infection and to monitor evolution and prognosis after treatment. Sensitivity and specificity are frequently insufficient for accurate disease diagnosis.[153,154]

The most widely used diagnostic approach is based on the direct detection of trematode eggs in biological samples, such as feces or bile aspirates for *C sinensis*, *Fasciola* spp, and *O viverrini*, or sputum for *Paragonimus* spp. Frequently used copromicroscopic techniques include the Kato-Katz method, or sedimentation, flotation, or an ether-concentration method of fixed stool samples.[155] A strength of these methods is that the infection intensity as expressed by the number of parasite eggs per gram of feces can be determined, which allows quantifying treatment outcomes in terms of not only cure rate but also egg reduction rate.[156] However, the sensitivity of these direct diagnostic tests, in particular for low-intensity infections, is frequently insufficient. Hence, multiple stool sampling or the combination of different diagnostic tests should be considered to enhance diagnostic accuracy.[155,157] Promising results have been obtained with a new multivalent flotation method (FLOTAC), which allows considerably larger amounts of feces to be examined than the Kato-Katz or the McMaster techniques.[158] Indeed, a single FLOTAC showed a considerably higher sensitivity than multiple Kato-Katz thick smears, McMaster, or sedimentation slides, including *F hepatica* diagnosis.[159]

Nevertheless, differential diagnosis of trematode species, such as *F hepatica* and *F gigantica*, or *C sinensis*, *O viverrini*, and various intestinal flukes (eg, *Haplorchis taichui* and *H pumilio*), using light microscopy poses problems because of the similarity of egg size, shape, and coloration.[155,160] Polymerase chain reaction (PCR) analysis allows identifying parasite species with high certainty.[1] Recently, PCR-based methods were developed, using species dissimilarities in mitochondrial and ribosomal DNA, eg, internal transcribed spacer 1/2 (ITS-1/2) regions, to discriminate between the above-mentioned trematodes.[161–164] PCR is an effective tool to detect the parasites at different development stages, such as metacercariae harbored in the second intermediate host (eg, fish and crabs) or DNA in biliary.[165–168] Recent studies have shown that real-time PCR methods were also able to quantitatively approximate the infection intensity because the threshold-cycle (DNA loads) and egg counts of *C sinensis* correlated.[169,170]

Early stage infections cannot be identified with diagnostic tests relying on the detection of parasite eggs. Consequently, copromicroscopy and PCR copying egg DNA may miss prepatent infections. Immunologic techniques, such as enzyme-linked immunosorbent assay (ELISA), which detect parasite antigens or antibodies in biofluids are applicable during all stages of the disease.[1,171] In general, ELISA techniques are more sensitive than copromicroscopy. Moreover, *F hepatica* infection can be diagnosed in bulk milk from dairy cows, which might be a valuable tool to monitor herd infections and consequently to set up appropriate intervention strategies.[172] Importantly, automation is easy to implement in the analysis process. Nonetheless, cross-reactions between parasite species and false-positive results owing to past infections might impair the method specificity, particularly, if the ELISA makes use of crude worm antigens rather than excretory-secretory antigens.[173]

TREATMENT

Praziquantel is the only drug available for the treatment of infections with *C sinensis* and *O viverrini*. The recommended treatment schedule of both liver fluke infections, according to guidelines put forward by WHO is oral administration of praziquantel at a dose of 25 mg/kg 3 times a day for 2 days.[13] This treatment schedule shows high efficacy and is also recommended for infections in travelers. Complete cure of all patients was achieved in 3 studies against *C sinensis* and 2 studies against *O viverrini*.[174] However, national treatment guidelines might slightly differ. For example, in Lao PDR 3 times 25 mg/kg praziquantel are administered for 1 day only.[175] In preventive chemotherapy programs, that is, the large-scale administration of anthelmintic drugs to at-risk populations without prior diagnosis,[176] a single dose of 40 mg/kg praziquantel is commonly used. Cure rates observed with 40 mg/kg praziquantel are somewhat lower. For example, an overall cure rate of 76% was obtained from 5 studies in *C sinensis*–infected patients.[174] Praziquantel is also efficacious against infections with *Paragonimus* spp and for this lung fluke infection, the WHO recommendation is to use doses of 25 mg/kg praziquantel 3 times a day for 2 days.[13] An overall cure rate of 94% was obtained in 6 studies in patients with *Paragonimus* infection who followed this treatment schedule.[174]

Because of the general neglect of food-borne trematodiases, the good safety and efficacy profile of praziquantel against most fluke infections, and no signs of parasite strains developing resistance to praziquantel, there has been little incentive to develop novel trematocidal drugs.[177] Nevertheless, the opisthorchicidal and clonorchicidal activity of 2 anthelmintics, albendazole and tribendimidine, have been explored in clinical trials. Albendazole is a benzimidazole drug that is widely used in community-based preventive chemotherapy and individual patient management against intestinal nematode infections (*Ascaris lumbricoides*, hookworm, and *Trichuris trichiura*)[5] and lymphatic filariasis.[7] Albendazole also shows activity against Asian liver flukes when given over a period of several days and at multiple doses. Treatment of *O viverrini*–infected patients with 400 mg albendazole twice daily for 3 and 7 days resulted in cure rates of 40% and 63%, respectively.[178] Complete cure was achieved in *C sinensis*–infected patients treated with 10 mg/kg albendazole twice daily for 7 consecutive days.[179]

Recently, the opisthorchicidal activity of tribendimidine, an anthelmintic marketed in P.R. China since 2004[180] has been tested in an exploratory phase 2 trial. In contrast to albendazole requiring multiple doses, high activity was observed with a single oral dose of tribendimidine (200 mg for children younger than 14 years and 400 mg for individuals aged 14 years and older). Nineteen of 24 *O viverrini*–infected patients treated with tribendimidine were cured (79%) and a very high egg reduction rate (99%) was determined.[181] Further studies with tribendimidine, including finding the right dose and pharmacokinetic investigations in *O viverrini*–infected patients, and a proof-of-concept study in *C sinensis*–infected patients have been initiated.

Triclabendazole is an alternative drug used for treating patients infected with *Paragonimus* spp and standard treatment of patients infected with *Fasciola* spp. A single oral dose of 10 mg/kg triclabendazole is recommended against these infections. In the case of treatment failures, the dosage can be increased to 20 mg/kg administered in 2 divided doses. Treatment with triclabendazole is highly efficacious and well tolerated. However, there are concerns that triclabendazole resistance, which already occurs in veterinary medicine,[182] will infringe on human health. No alternatives to triclabendazole are currently in sight because the drug development pipeline is empty.[177] A recent study in *Fasciola*-infected patients in Egypt has shown that the antimalarial drug artemether, administered according to doses previously used in the treatment of malaria, only has little effect against this liver fluke.[183]

PREVENTION

Chemotherapy is the current mainstay for morbidity control due to liver and lung fluke infections. However, control programs should be holistically designed and consider the root behavioral, ecological, and social causes of food-borne trematodiases.[1] Truly integrated strategies include setting-specific combinations of control measures, such as information, communication, and education (ICE) campaigns, improved sanitation, and control of intermediate, reservoir and paratenic hosts. The main aim of ICE campaigns is to change human behavior and particularly the dissuasion of people from eating raw or insufficiently cooked aquatic food. Travelers should be alerted that consumption of these food products poses a risk for infection. Improved food processing and food inspections further decrease the risk for human infections. Improved sanitation not only lowers the risk for humans to ingest parasite metacercariae but also helps to avoid that fertilized parasite eggs reach the environment where suitable intermediate hosts proliferate. Considering the wide range of animal intermediate, reservoir, paratenic, and definitive hosts, integrated approaches are the only way to ultimately interrupt disease transmission. Because the aquatic and livestock production sector is also negatively affected by liver and lung fluke infections, these sectors would greatly benefit from the aforementioned interventions.[1,13,127]

All government agencies concerned (eg, ministries of health, education, agriculture, and environment), the food industry, farmers, consumers, local communities, and nongovernmental organizations should get involved in the implementation and monitoring of such integrated control strategies. Intersectoral collaboration and (partial) integration in existing programs would not only help to ensure the commitment of all stakeholders but also improve cost-efficiency as control efforts go to scale.[13,184]

SUMMARY

Liver and lung fluke infections as well as other food-borne trematodiases are underappreciated emerging diseases. Although being important public health problems in some of the most heavily affected areas, they should be carefully observed in regions previously considered as nonendemic. Furthermore, they are also of growing importance for travel clinics in Europe and North America. However, accurate diagnosis and general neglect of these parasitic worm infections still pose problems.

The complex life cycle of these fluke infections and the epidemiology is strongly influenced by social-ecological systems factors. Human and animal infections can result in severe morbidity and, in rarer cases, even death. At present, safe and efficacious drugs against liver and lung fluke infections are available, but there is a pressing need to develop new trematocidal drugs to reduce the dependence on praziquantel and triclabendazole and provide additional options in case of emerging resistance. Considering behavioral factors and the social-ecological contexts that govern the complex life cycles and epidemiology of liver and lung fluke infections, the authors are convinced that integrated approaches are essential for sustainable control of these parasitic worm infections.

REFERENCES

1. Keiser J, Utzinger J. Food-borne trematodiases. Clin Microbiol Rev 2009;22: 466–83.
2. Sripa B, Kaewkes S, Intapan PM, et al. Food-borne trematodiases in Southeast Asia: epidemiology, pathology, clinical manifestation and control. Adv Parasitol 2010;72:305–50.
3. Keiser J, Utzinger J. Emerging foodborne trematodiasis. Emerg Infect Dis 2005; 11:1507–14.
4. Fürst T, Keiser J, Utzinger J. Global burden of human food-borne trematodiasis: a systematic review and meta-analysis. Lancet Infect Dis 2012;12:210–21.
5. Knopp S, Steinmann P, Keiser J, et al. Nematode infections—soil-transmitted helminths and *Trichinella*. Infect Dis Clin North Am 2012.
6. Utzinger J, N'Goran EK, Caffrey CR, et al. From innovation to application: social-ecological context, diagnostics, drugs and integrated control of schistosomiasis. Acta Trop 2011;120:S121–37.
7. Knopp S, Steinmann P, Keiser J, et al. Nematode infections: filariasis. Infect Dis Clin North Am 2012.
8. Sripa B, Bethony JM, Sithithaworn P, et al. Opisthorchiasis and *Opisthorchis*-associated cholangiocarcinoma in Thailand and Laos. Acta Trop 2011;120: S158–68.
9. Marcos L, Maco V, Samalvides F, et al. Risk factors for *Fasciola hepatica* infection in children: a case-control study. Trans R Soc Trop Med Hyg 2006;100: 158–66.
10. Traoré SG, Odermatt P, Bonfoh B, et al. No *Paragonimus* in high-risk groups in Côte d'Ivoire, but considerable prevalence of helminths and intestinal protozoon infections. Parasit Vectors 2011;4:96.
11. Blair D, Agatsuma T, Wang W. Paragonimiasis. In: Murrell KD, Fried B, editors. World class parasites, vol. 11. Dordrecht (The Netherlands): Springer; 2007. p. 117–50.
12. Li T, He S, Zhao H, et al. Major trends in human parasitic diseases in China. Trends Parasitol 2010;26:264–70.
13. WHO. Control of foodborne trematode infections. Report of a WHO study group. World Health Organ Tech Rep Ser 1995;849:1–157.
14. Esteban JG, Barguesa MD, Mas-Coma S. Geographical distribution, diagnosis, and treatment of human fascioliasis: a review. Res Rev Parasitol 1998;58:13–42.
15. Fried B, Abruzzi A. Food-borne trematode infections of humans in the United States of America. Parasitol Res 2010;106:1263–80.
16. MacLean JD, Graeme-Cook FM. Case records of the Massachusetts General Hospital. Weekly clinicopathological exercises. Case 12-2002. A 50-year-old man with eosinophilia and fluctuating hepatic lesions. N Engl J Med 2002; 346:1232–9.
17. Lane MA, Barsanti MC, Santos CA, et al. Human paragonimiasis in North America following ingestion of raw crayfish. Clin Infect Dis 2009;49:e55–61.
18. CDC. Human paragonimiasis after eating raw or undercooked crayfish: Missouri, July 2006–September 2010. Morb Mortal Wkly Rep 2010;59:1573–6.
19. Lee MB. Everyday and exotic foodborne parasites. Can J Infect Dis 2000;11: 155–8.
20. O'Leary MJ, Berthiaume JT, Sakbun V. Treatment of *Clonorchis sinensis* in Hawaii's Laotian population—experience with praziquantel. Hawaii Med J 1985; 44:63–4.

21. Lewin MR, Weinert MF. An eighty-four-year-old man with fever and painless jaundice: a case report and brief review of Clonorchis sinensis infection. J Travel Med 1999;6:207–9.
22. Yellin AE, Donovan AJ. Biliary lithiasis and helminthiasis. Am J Surg 1981;142: 128–36.
23. Buchwald D, Lam M, Hooton TM. Prevalence of intestinal parasites and association with symptoms in Southeast Asian refugees. J Clin Pharm Ther 1995;20: 271–5.
24. Chai JY, Murrell KD, Lymbery AJ. Fish-borne parasitic zoonoses: status and issues. Int J Parasitol 2005;35:1233–54.
25. Schwartz DA. Cholangiocarcinoma associated with liver fluke infection: a preventable source of morbidity in Asian immigrants. Am J Gastroenterol 1986;81:76–9.
26. Skeels MR, Nims LJ, Mann JM. Intestinal parasitosis among Southeast Asian immigrants in New Mexico, USA. Am J Public Health 1982;72:57–9.
27. Woolf A, Green J, Levine JA, et al. A clinical study of Laotian refugees infected with Clonorchis sinensis or Opisthorchis viverrini. Am J Trop Med Hyg 1984;33: 1279–80.
28. Stauffer WM, Sellman JS, Walker PF. Biliary liver flukes (opisthorchiasis and clonorchiasis) in immigrants in the United States: often subtle and diagnosed years after arrival. J Travel Med 2004;11:157–9.
29. Kantrowitz M, Wall I, Braha J, et al. Clonorchiasis causing biliary obstruction 15 years after immigration to the United States. Am J Gastroenterol 2010;105:S210.
30. Shamah S, Rahmani R, Nakkala K, et al. A rare case of cholangitis secondary to severe clonorchiasis 20 years after migration. Am J Gastroenterol 2011;106:S211.
31. Naidu P. Partial common bile duct (CBD) obstruction with live Clonorchis sinensis; a case report. Can J Infect Dis Med Microbiol 2010;21:42A.
32. Wong RK, Peura DA, Mutter ML, et al. Hemobilia and liver flukes in a patient from Thailand. Gastroenterology 1985;88:1958–63.
33. Hoffman SL, Barrett-Connor E, Norcross W, et al. Intestinal parasites in Indochinese immigrants. Am J Trop Med Hyg 1981;30:340–3.
34. Lalezari D, Simmons T. A rare case of human liver fluke with a sequel of oriental cholangitis, obstructive hepatopathy and mirizzi syndrome. Am J Gastroenterol 2010;105:S206.
35. Alatoom A, Sheffield J, Gander RM, et al. Fascioliasis in pregnancy. Obstet Gynecol 2008;112:483–5.
36. Graham CS, Brodie SB, Weller PF. Imported Fasciola hepatica infection in the United States and treatment with triclabendazole. Clin Infect Dis 2001;33:1–6.
37. Noyer CM, Coyle CM, Werner C, et al. Hypereosinophilia and liver mass in an immigrant. Am J Trop Med Hyg 2002;66:774–6.
38. Price TA, Tuazon CU, Simon GL. Fascioliasis: case reports and review. Clin Infect Dis 1993;17:426–30.
39. Badalov NL, Anklesaria A, Torok A, et al. Fasciola hepatica causing acute pancreatitis complicated by biliary sepsis. Gastrointest Endosc 2009;70:386–7.
40. Keshishian J, Brantley SG, Brady PG. Biliary fascioliasis mimicking sphincter of oddi dysfunction. South Med J 2010;103:366–8.
41. Wall MA, McGhee G. Paragonimiasis. Atypical appearances in two adolescent Asian refugees. Am J Dis Child 1982;136:828–30.
42. Collins MS, Phelan A, Kim TC, et al. Paragonimus westermani: a cause of cavitary lung disease in an Indochinese refugee. South Med J 1981;74: 1418–20.

43. Johnson JR, Falk A, Iber C, et al. Paragonimiasis in the United States. A report of nine cases in Hmong immigrants. Chest 1982;82:168–71.
44. Meehan AM, Virk A, Swanson K, et al. Severe pleuropulmonary paragonimiasis 8 years after emigration from a region of endemicity. Clin Infect Dis 2002;35: 87–90.
45. Wright RS, Jean M, Rochelle K, et al. Chylothorax caused by *Paragonimus westermani* in a native Californian. Chest 2011;140:1064–6.
46. Boland JM, Vaszar LT, Jones JL, et al. Pleuropulmonary infection by *Paragonimus westermani* in the United States: a rare cause of eosinophilic pneumonia after ingestion of live crabs. Am J Surg Pathol 2011;35:707–13.
47. Behr MA, Gyorkos TW, Kokoskin E, et al. North American liver fluke (*Metorchis conjunctus*) in a Canadian aboriginal population: a submerging human pathogen? Can J Public Health 1998;89:258–9.
48. MacLean JD, Ward BJ, Kokoskin E, et al. Common-source outbreak of acute infection due to the North American liver fluke *Metorchis conjunctus*. Lancet 1996;347:154–8.
49. Naiman HL, Sekla L, Albritton WL. Giardiasis and other intestinal parasitic infections in a Manitoba Canada residential school for the mentally retarded. Can Med Assoc J 1980;122:185–8.
50. Mordvinov VA, Yurlova NI, Ogorodova LM, et al. *Opisthorchis felineus* and *Metorchis bilis* are the main agents of liver fluke infection of humans in Russia. Parasitol Int 2012;61:25–31.
51. Ditrich O, Sterba J, Giboda M. The morphology of the eggs of *Paragonimus westermani* (Trematoda). Angew Parasitol 1988;29:101–5 [in German].
52. Skracikova J, Straka S, Galikova E. Findings of intestinal parasites in foreigners and persons being in work contact with them. Prac Lek 1986;8:192–4 [in Czech].
53. Moller A, Settnes OP, Jensen NO, et al. A case of cerebral paragonimiasis in Denmark. Case report. APMIS 1995;103:604–6.
54. Siikamaki HM, Kivela PS, Sipila PN, et al. Fever in travelers returning from malaria-endemic areas: don't look for malaria only. J Travel Med 2011;18:239–44.
55. Ambroise-Thomas P, Peyron F, Goullier A, et al. Praziquantel in the treatment of opisthorchiasis in Southeast Asian refugees. Evaluation of 153 cases. Bull Soc Pathol Exot Filiales 1985;78:492–9 [in French].
56. Malvy D, Ezzedine KH, Receveur MC, et al. Extra-pulmonary paragonimiasis with unusual arthritis and cutaneous features among a tourist returning from Gabon. Travel Med Infect Dis 2006;4:340–2.
57. Luong Dinh Giap G, Lam Tan B, Faucher P, et al. Hepatic distomatosis caused by *Clonorchis/Opisthorchis* spp. in refugees from South-East Asia - effects of treatment with praziquantel. Med Trop (Mars) 1983;43:325–30 [in French].
58. Couturier F, Hiar I, Hansmann Y, et al. Place of triclabendazole in the treatment of human hepatic fascioliasis. Med Mal Infect 1999;29:753–7 [in French].
59. Schwacha H, Keuchel M, Gagesch G, et al. *Fasciola gigantica* in the common bile duct: diagnosis by ERCP. Endoscopy 1996;28:323.
60. Metter K, Gloser H, von Gaisberg U. Fascioliasis after a stay in Turkey. Dtsch Med Wochenschr 2000;125:1160–3 [in German].
61. Löscher T, Nothdurft HD, Prüfer L, et al. Praziquantel in clonorchiasis and opisthorchiasis. Tropenmed Parasitol 1981;32:234–6.
62. Tappe D, Triefenbach R. Histopathological diagnosis of opisthorchiasis in an immigrant. Am J Trop Med Hyg 2010;83:734–5.
63. Tselepatiotis E, Mantadakis E, Papoulis S, et al. A case of *Opisthorchis felineus* infestation in a pilot from Greece. Infection 2003;31:430–2.

64. van Daele PL, Madretsma GS, van Agtmael MA. Stomach ache and fever after consumption of watercress in Turkey: fascioliasis. Ned Tijdschr Geneeskd 2001; 145:1896–9 [in Dutch].

65. Cats A, Scholten P, Meuwissen SG, et al. Acute *Fasciola hepatica* infection attributed to chewing khat. Gut 2000;47:584–5.

66. Jensenius M, Flaegstad T, Stenstad T, et al. Fascioliasis imported to Norway. Scand J Infect Dis 2005;37:534–7.

67. Lazar L, Nackechbandi AM. Prevalence of parasitic diseases among refugees and immigrants in Romania. Am J Trop Med Hyg 2003;69:259–60.

68. Ananos G, Trilla A, Graus F, et al. Paragonimiasis and pulmonary tuberculosis. Med Clin (Barc) 1992;98:257–9 [in Spanish].

69. Requena A, Dominguez MA, Santin M. An African-born man with chronic recurrent hemoptysis. Clin Infect Dis 2008;46:319–20.

70. Esteban-Gutierrez G, Rojo-Marcos G, Cuadros-Gonzelez J, et al. Eosinophilia in a patient from Thailand and Laos. Enferm Infecc Microbiol Clin 2011;29:629–30 [in Spanish].

71. Andresen B, Blum J, von Weymarn A, et al. Hepatic fascioliasis: report of two cases. Eur Radiol 2000;10:1713–5.

72. Nuesch R, Gremmelmaier D, Hirsch HH, et al. Chest pain after air travel. Lancet 2005;365:1902.

73. Chand MA, Herman JS, Partridge DG, et al. Imported human fascioliasis, United Kingdom. Emerg Infect Dis 2009;15:1876–7.

74. Green EW, Partridge DG, Green ST, et al. Increasing prevalence of human fascioliasis (and an association with khat usage) in Sheffield, UK: a clinical and epidemiological case series. J Infect 2009;59:S449.

75. Behar JM, Winston JS, Borgstein R. Hepatic fascioliasis at a London hospital— the importance of recognising typical radiological features to avoid a delay in diagnosis. Br J Radiol 2009;82:e189–93.

76. Dias RM, Mangini AC, Torres Domingas MA, et al. The occurrence of *Clonorchis sinensis* in East Asian immigrants in Brazil and the suspension of laboratorial examination to get the permanent visa. Rev Bras Anal Clin 1992;24:29–30 [in Portuguese].

77. Leite OH, Higaki Y, Serpentini SL, et al. Infection by *Clonorchis sinensis* in Asian immigrants in Brazil. Treatment with praziquantel. Rev Inst Med Trop São Paulo 1989;31:416–22 [in Portuguese].

78. Morsy AT, al-Mathal EM. *Clonorchis sinensis* a new report in Egyptian employees returning back from Saudi Arabia. J Egypt Soc Parasitol 2011;41: 221–5.

79. Onodera S, Saito K, Saito T, et al. Clonorchiasis complicated with duodenal papillary cancer in a visitor from China. Nippon Shokakibyo Gakkai Zasshi 2007;104:213–8 [in Japanese].

80. Shekhar KC. Epidemiological assessment of parasitic zoonoses in Malaysia. Southeast Asian J Trop Med Public Health 1991;22:337–9.

81. Kan SK, Chong EL. An imported case of *Clonorchis sinensis* in Sabah, Malaysia. Ann Trop Med Parasitol 1980;74:267–9.

82. Oostburg BF, Smith SJ. Clonorchiasis in Surinam. Trop Geogr Med 1981;33: 287–9.

83. Cheng HS, Haung ZF, Lan WH, et al. Epidemiology of *Blastocystis hominis* and other intestinal parasites in a Vietnamese female immigrant population in southern Taiwan. Kaohsiung J Med Sci 2006;22:166–70.

84. Wang LC. Parasitic infections among Southeast Asian labourers in Taiwan: a long-term study. Epidemiol Infect 1998;120:81–6.
85. Wang LC. Changing patterns in intestinal parasitic infections among Southeast Asian laborers in Taiwan. Parasitol Res 2004;92:18–21.
86. Lu CT, Sung YJ. Epidemiology of *Blastocystis hominis* and other intestinal parasites among the immigrant population in northeastern Taiwan by routine physical examination for residence approval. J Microbiol Immunol Infect 2009;42:505–9.
87. Hira PR, al-Enizi AA, al-Kandari S, et al. Opisthorchiasis in Kuwait: first report of infections in Thai migrant workers in the Arabian Gulf. Ann Soc Belg Med Trop 1987;67:363–8.
88. Cheng HS, Shieh YH. Investigation on subclinical aspects related to intestinal parasitic infections among Thai laborers in Taipei. J Travel Med 2000;7:319–24.
89. Peng HW, Chao HL, Fan PC. Imported *Opisthorchis viverrini* and parasite infections from Thai labourers in Taiwan. J Helminthol 1993;67:102–6.
90. Dan M, Lichtenstein D, Lavochkin J, et al. Human fascioliasis in Israel: an imported case. Isr J Med Sci 1981;17:430–2.
91. al-Mekhaizeem K, al-Mukhaizeem F, Habib MA. *Fasciola hepatica* infestation presenting as biliary obstruction 11 years after open cholecystectomy and CBD exploration. Kuwait Med J 2004;36:293–5.
92. Shah SA, Khan MY, Ahmad J. Fascioliasis - a cause of obstructive jaundice: a case report. J Postgrad Med Inst 2010;24:332.
93. el-Mathal EM, Fouad MA. Human fascioliasis among immigrant workers in Saudi Arabia. J Egypt Soc Parasitol 2005;35:1199–207.
94. Hughes AJ, Biggs BA. Parasitic worms of the central nervous system: an Australian perspective. Intern Med J 2002;32:541–53.
95. McManus TE, Thomas M, Rogers D, et al. Pleuropulmonary paragonimiasis. Intern Med J 2009;39:203–4.
96. al-Mohaya SA, al-Sohaibani M, Bukhari H, et al. Pulmonary paragonimiasis presenting as a hemorrhagic pleural effusion. Eur J Respir Dis 1987;71:314–6.
97. Murray CJL, Lopez AD, Black R, et al. Global burden of disease 2005: call for collaborators. Lancet 2007;370:109–10.
98. Lun ZR, Gasser RB, Lai DH, et al. Clonorchiasis: a key food-borne zoonosis in China. Lancet Infect Dis 2005;5:31–41.
99. Mas-Coma S, Valero MA, Bargues MD. *Fasciola*, lymnaeids and human fascioliasis, with a global overview on disease transmission, epidemiology, evolutionary genetics, molecular epidemiology and control. Adv Parasitol 2009;69:41–146.
100. Mas-Coma S. Human fascioliasis: epidemiological patterns in human endemic areas of South America, Africa and Asia. Southeast Asian J Trop Med Public Health 2004;35:1–11.
101. Mas-Coma S. Human fascioliasis. In: Cotruvo JA, Dufour A, Rees G, et al, editors. Waterborne zoonoses: identification, causes and control. London: IWA Publishing; 2004. p. 305–22.
102. Robinson MW, Dalton JP. Zoonotic helminth infections with particular emphasis on fasciolosis and other trematodiases. Philos Trans R Soc Lond B Biol Sci 2009; 364:2763–76.
103. Mas-Coma S, Bargues MD, Valero MA. Fascioliasis and other plant-borne trematode zoonoses. Int J Parasitol 2005;35:1255–78.
104. Sithithaworn P, Yongvanit P, Tesana S, et al. Liver flukes. In: Murrell KD, Fried B, editors. World class parasites, vol. 11. Dordrecht (The Netherlands): Springer; 2007. p. 3–52.

105. Andrews SJ. The life cycle of *Fasciola hepatica*. In: Dalton JP, editor. Fasciolosis. Wallingford (United Kingdom): CAB International; 1999. p. 1–29.
106. Krull WH. The number of cercariae of *Fasciola hepatica* developing in snails infected with a single miracidium. In: Christie JR, editor. Proceedings of the Helminthological Society of Washington. Washington, DC: The Helminthological Society of Washington; 1941. p. 55–8.
107. Bronshtein AM. Opisthorchiasis and diphyllobothriasis morbidity in the native population of the Kyshik settlement, Khanty-Mansi Autonomous Okrug. Med Parazitol (Mosk) 1986;44–8 [in Russian].
108. IARC. Infection with liver flukes (*Opisthorchis viverrini*, *Opisthorchis felineus* and *Clonorchis sinensis*). IARC Monogr Eval Carcinog Risks Hum 1994;61:121–75.
109. Rim HJ. The current pathobiology and chemotherapy of clonorchiasis. Korean J Parasitol 1986;24:1–141.
110. Upatham ES, Viyanant V, Kurathong S, et al. Relationship between prevalence and intensity of *Opisthorchis viverrini* infection, and clinical symptoms and signs in a rural community in north-east Thailand. Bull World Health Organ 1984;62: 451–61.
111. Elkins DB, Mairiang E, Sithithaworn P, et al. Cross-sectional patterns of hepatobiliary abnormalities and possible precursor conditions of cholangiocarcinoma associated with *Opisthorchis viverrini* infection in humans. Am J Trop Med Hyg 1996;55:295–301.
112. Choi MS, Choi D, Choi MH, et al. Correlation between sonographic findings and infection intensity in clonorchiasis. Am J Trop Med Hyg 2005;73:1139–44.
113. Pungpak S, Viravan C, Radomyos B, et al. *Opisthorchis viverrini* infection in Thailand: studies on the morbidity of the infection and resolution following praziquantel treatment. Am J Trop Med Hyg 1997;56:311–4.
114. Mairiang E, Laha T, Bethony JM, et al. Ultrasonography assessment of hepatobiliary abnormalities in 3359 subjects with *Opisthorchis viverrini* infection in endemic areas of Thailand. Parasitol Int 2012;61:208–11.
115. Rim HJ. Clonorchiasis: an update. J Helminthol 2005;79:269–81.
116. Pungpak S, Riganti M, Bunnag D, et al. Clinical features in severe opisthorchiasis viverrini. Southeast Asian J Trop Med Public Health 1985;16:405–9.
117. Haswell-Elkins MR, Mairiang E, Mairiang P, et al. Cross-sectional study of *Opisthorchis viverrini* infection and cholangiocarcinoma in communities within a high-risk area in northeast Thailand. Int J Cancer 1994;59:505–9.
118. Honjo S, Srivatanakul P, Sriplung H, et al. Genetic and environmental determinants of risk for cholangiocarcinoma via *Opisthorchis viverrini* in a densely infested area in Nakhon Phanom, northeast Thailand. Int J Cancer 2005;117: 854–60.
119. Lim MK, Ju YH, Franceschi S, et al. *Clonorchis sinensis* infection and increasing risk of cholangiocarcinoma in the Republic of Korea. Am J Trop Med Hyg 2006; 75:93–6.
120. Shin HR, Lee CU, Park HJ, et al. Hepatitis B and C virus, *Clonorchis sinensis* for the risk of liver cancer: a case-control study in Pusan, Korea. Int J Epidemiol 1996;25:933–40.
121. Choi D, Lim JH, Lee KT, et al. Cholangiocarcinoma and *Clonorchis sinensis* infection: a case-control study in Korea. J Hepatol 2006;44:1066–73.
122. Bouvard V, Baan R, Straif K, et al. A review of human carcinogens—part B: biological agents. Lancet Oncol 2009;10:321–2.
123. Gutierrez Y. Diagnostic parasitology of parasitic infections with clinical correlations. Philadelphia: Lea & Febiger; 1990.

124. Hardman EW, Jones RL, Davies AH. Fascioliasis—a large outbreak. BMJ 1970; 3:502–5.

125. Chen MG. *Fasciola hepatica* infection in China. In: Cross JH, editor. Emerging problems in food-borne parasitic zoonosis: impact on agriculture and public health. Bangkok (Thailand): Thai Watana Panich Press; 1991. p. 356–60.

126. Fica A, Dabanch J, Farias C, et al. Acute fascioliasis—clinical and epidemiological features of four patients in Chile. Clin Microbiol Infect 2012;18:91–6.

127. Sithithaworn P, Sripa B, Kaewkes S, et al. Food-borne trematodes. In: Cook GC, Zumla AI, editors. Manson's tropical diseases. London: W. B. Saunders; 2009. p. 1461–76.

128. Xuan LT, Hung NT, Waikagul J. Cutaneous fascioliasis: a case report in Vietnam. Am J Trop Med Hyg 2005;72:508–9.

129. Le TH, De NV, Agatsuma T, et al. Molecular confirmation that *Fasciola gigantica* can undertake aberrant migrations in human hosts. J Clin Microbiol 2007;45: 648–50.

130. Marcos Raymundo LA, Maco Flores V, Terashima Iwashita A, et al. Clinical characteristics of chronic infection by *Fasciola hepatica* in children. Rev Gastroenterol Peru 2002;22:228–33 [in Spanish].

131. Rana SS, Bhasin DK, Nanda M, et al. Parasitic infestations of the biliary tract. Curr Gastroenterol Rep 2007;9:156–64.

132. Aroonroch R, Worawichawong S, Nitiyanant P, et al. Hepatic fascioliasis due to *Fasciola hepatica*: a two-case report. J Med Assoc Thai 2006;89:1770–4.

133. Umac H, Erkek AB, Ayaslioglu E, et al. Pruritus and intermittent jaundice as clinical clues for *Fasciola hepatica* infestation. Liver Int 2006;26:752–3.

134. el-Shazly AM, Soliman M, Gabr A, et al. Clinico-epidemiological study of human fascioliasis in an endemic focus in Dakahlia Governorate, Egypt. J Egypt Soc Parasitol 2001;31:725–36.

135. Bulbuloglu E, Yuksel M, Bakaris S, et al. Diagnosis of *Fasciola hepatica* cases in an operating room. Trop Doct 2007;37:50–2.

136. Fullerton JK, Vitale M, Vitale GC. Therapeutic endoscopic retrograde cholangiopancreatography for the treatment of *Fasciola hepatica* presenting as biliary obstruction. Surg Innov 2006;13:179–82.

137. Rondelaud D, Dreyfuss G, Vignoles P. Clinical and biological abnormalities in patients after fasciolosis treatment. Med Mal Infect 2006;36:466–8.

138. Torres GB, Iwashita AT, Vargas CM, et al. Human fasciolasis and gastrointestinal compromise: study of 277 patients in the Cayetano Heredia National Hospital (1970-2002). Rev Gastroenterol Peru 2004;24:143–57 [in Spanish].

139. Nakamura-Uchiyama F, Mukae H, Nawa Y. Paragonimiasis: a Japanese perspective. Clin Chest Med 2002;23:409–20.

140. Nakamura-Uchiyama F, Onah DN, Nawa Y. Clinical features of paragonimiasis cases recently found in Japan: parasite-specific immunoglobulin M and G antibody classes. Clin Infect Dis 2001;32:e151–3.

141. Miyazaki I. An illustrated book of helminthic zoonoses. Tokyo: International Medical Foundation of Japan; 1991.

142. Jeon K, Koh WJ, Kim H, et al. Clinical features of recently diagnosed pulmonary paragonimiasis in Korea. Chest 2005;128:1423–30.

143. Mukae H, Taniguchi H, Matsumoto N, et al. Clinicoradiologic features of pleuropulmonary *Paragonimus westermani* on Kyusyu Island, Japan. Chest 2001;120: 514–20.

144. Devi KR, Narain K, Bhattacharya S, et al. Pleuropulmonary paragonimiasis due to *Paragonimus heterotremus*: molecular diagnosis, prevalence of infection and

clinicoradiological features in an endemic area of northeastern India. Trans R Soc Trop Med Hyg 2007;101:786–92.

145. Vidamaly S, Choumlivong K, Keolouangkhot V, et al. Paragonimiasis: a common cause of persistent pleural effusion in Lao PDR. Trans R Soc Trop Med Hyg 2009;103:1019–23.

146. Liu Q, Wei F, Liu W, et al. Paragonimiasis: an important food-borne zoonosis in China. Trends Parasitol 2008;24:318–23.

147. Dainichi T, Nakahara T, Moroi Y, et al. A case of cutaneous paragonimiasis with pleural effusion. Int J Dermatol 2003;42:699–702.

148. Clyti E, Kheosang P, Huerre M, et al. Cutaneous paragonimiasis with flare up after treatment: a clinical case from Laos. Int J Dermatol 2006;45:1110–2.

149. Yokogawa M. *Paragonimus* and paragonimiasis. Adv Parasitol 1969;7:375–87.

150. Lv S, Zhang Y, Steinmann P, et al. Helminth infections of the central nervous system occurring in Southeast Asia and the Far East. Adv Parasitol 2010;72:351–408.

151. Jaroonvesama N. Differential diagnosis of eosinophilic meningitis. Parasitol Today 1988;4:262–6.

152. Nishimura K, Hung T. Current views on geographic distribution and modes of infection of neurohelminthic diseases. J Neurol Sci 1997;145:5–14.

153. Chen MG, Mott KE. Progress in assessment of morbidity due to *Fasciola hepatica* infection: a review of recent literature. Trop Dis Bull 1990;87:R1–38.

154. WHO. Report of the WHO informal meeting on use of triclabendazole in fascioliasis control. Geneva (Switzerland): WHO; 2006.

155. Johansen MV, Sithithaworn P, Bergquist R, et al. Towards improved diagnosis of zoonotic trematode infections in Southeast Asia. Adv Parasitol 2010;73:171–95.

156. Wood IB, Amaral NK, Bairden K, et al. World Association for the Advancement of Veterinary Parasitology (W.A.A.V.P.) second edition of guidelines for evaluating the efficacy of anthelmintics in ruminants (bovine, ovine, caprine). Vet Parasitol 1995;58:181–213.

157. Bergquist R, Johansen MV, Utzinger J. Diagnostic dilemmas in helminthology: what tools to use and when? Trends Parasitol 2009;25:151–6.

158. Cringoli G, Rinaldi L, Maurelli MP, et al. FLOTAC: new multivalent techniques for qualitative and quantitative copromicroscopic diagnosis of parasites in animals and humans. Nat Protoc 2010;5:503–15.

159. Duthaler U, Rinaldi L, Maurelli MP, et al. *Fasciola hepatica*: comparison of the sedimentation and FLOTAC techniques for the detection and quantification of faecal egg counts in rats. Exp Parasitol 2010;126:161–6.

160. Haswell-Elkins MR, Levri E. Food-borne trematodes. In: Cook GC, Zumla AI, editors. Manson's tropical diseases. London: W. B. Saunders; 2003. p. 1471–86.

161. Ai L, Dong SJ, Zhang WY, et al. Specific PCR-based assays for the identification of *Fasciola* species: their development, evaluation and potential usefulness in prevalence surveys. Ann Trop Med Parasitol 2010;104:65–72.

162. Lovis L, Mak TK, Phongluxa K, et al. PCR diagnosis of *Opisthorchis viverrini* and *Haplorchis taichui* infections in a Lao community in an area of endemicity and comparison of diagnostic methods for parasitological field surveys. J Clin Microbiol 2009;47:1517–23.

163. Rokni MB, Mirhendi H, Mizani A, et al. Identification and differentiation of *Fasciola hepatica* and *Fasciola gigantica* using a simple PCR-restriction enzyme method. Exp Parasitol 2010;124:209–13.

164. Sato M, Thaenkham U, Dekumyoy P, et al. Discrimination of *O. viverrini, C. sinensis, H. pumilio* and *H. taichui* using nuclear DNA-based PCR targeting ribosomal DNA ITS regions. Acta Trop 2009;109:81–3.

165. Cai XQ, Yu HQ, Bai JS, et al. Development of a TaqMan based real-time PCR assay for detection of *Clonorchis sinensis* DNA in human stool samples and fishes. Parasitol Int 2012;61:183–6.

166. Caron Y, Righi S, Lempereur L, et al. An optimized DNA extraction and multiplex PCR for the detection of *Fasciola* spp. in lymnaeid snails. Vet Parasitol 2011;178:93–9.

167. Chen MX, Ai L, Zhang RL, et al. Sensitive and rapid detection of *Paragonimus westermani* infection in humans and animals by loop-mediated isothermal amplification (LAMP). Parasitol Res 2011;108:1193–8.

168. Jang JS, Kim KH, Yu JR, et al. Identification of parasite DNA in common bile duct stones by PCR and DNA sequencing. Korean J Parasitol 2007;45:301–6.

169. Kim EM, Verweij JJ, Jalili A, et al. Detection of *Clonorchis sinensis* in stool samples using real-time PCR. Ann Trop Med Parasitol 2009;103:513–8.

170. Rahman SM, Bae YM, Hong ST, et al. Early detection and estimation of infection burden by real-time PCR in rats experimentally infected with *Clonorchis sinensis*. Parasitol Res 2011;109:297–303.

171. Löscher T. Progress in immunodiagnosis and chemotherapy of helminthiases. Internist 1983;24:610–8 [in German].

172. Duscher R, Duscher G, Hofer J, et al. *Fasciola hepatica* – monitoring the milky way? The use of tank milk for liver fluke monitoring in dairy herds as base for treatment strategies. Vet Parasitol 2011;178:273–8.

173. Choi MH, Park IC, Li S, et al. Excretory-secretory antigen is better than crude antigen for the serodiagnosis of clonorchiasis by ELISA. Korean J Parasitol 2003;41:35–9.

174. Keiser J, Utzinger J. The drugs we have and the drugs we need against major helminth infections. Adv Parasitol 2010;73:197–230.

175. Ministry of Health. Diagnosis and treatment at the district. A diagnosis and treatment guideline for the district hospital in Lao PDR. Vientiane (Lao PDR): Ministry of Health; 2004.

176. WHO. Preventive chemotherapy in human helminthiasis: coordinated use of anthelminthic drugs in control interventions. A manual for health professionals and programme managers. Geneva (Switzerland): WHO; 2006.

177. Keiser J, Utzinger J. Advances in the discovery and development of trematocidal drugs. Expert Opin Drug Discov 2007;2:S9–23.

178. Pungpark S, Bunnag D, Harinasuta T. Albendazole in the treatment of opisthorchiasis and concomitant intestinal helminthic infections. Southeast Asian J Trop Med Public Health 1984;15:44–50.

179. Liu YH, Wang XG, Gao P, et al. Experimental and clinical trial of albendazole in the treatment of clonorchiasis sinensis. Chin Med J 1991;104:27–31.

180. Xiao SH, Wu HM, Tanner M, et al. Tribendimidine: a promising, safe and broad-spectrum anthelmintic agent from China. Acta Trop 2005;94:1–14.

181. Soukhathammavong P, Odermatt P, Sayasone S, et al. Efficacy and safety of mefloquine, artesunate, mefloquine-artesunate, tribendimidine, and praziquantel in patients with *Opisthorchis viverrini*: a randomised, exploratory, open-label, phase 2 trial. Lancet Infect Dis 2011;11:110–8.

182. Fairweather I. Triclabendazole progress report, 2005–2009: an advancement of learning? J Helminthol 2009;83:139–50.

183. Keiser J, Sayed H, el-Ghanam M, et al. Efficacy and safety of artemether in the treatment of chronic fascioliasis in Egypt: exploratory phase-2 trials. PLoS Negl Trop Dis 2011;5:e1285.

184. WHO WPRO. Informal consultation on novel approaches in the prevention and control of neglected tropical diseases in the Western Pacific region. Manila (Philippines): WHO WPRO; 2011.

Cestode Infestations
Hydatid Disease and Cysticercosis

Enrico Brunetti, MD[a],*, A. Clinton White Jr, MD[b]

KEYWORDS

- Tapeworms • Cestodes • Cystic echinococcosis • Alveolar echinococcosis
- Cysticercosis • Neurocysticercosis

KEY POINTS

- The most relevant forms of human disease caused by cestode larvae are echinococcosis, caused by Echinococcus granulosus (cystic echinococcosis) and Echinococcus multilocularis (alveolar echinococcosis), and cysticercosis, caused by Taenia solium.
- These infections occur worldwide, but their relevance is particularly high in developing countries, where poor hygiene conditions facilitate the transmission of the parasites.
- The therapeutic approach is often complex, requiring surgery and/or chemotherapy and, in the case of cystic echinococcosis, percutaneous treatments.

Cestodes (commonly known as tapeworms) have different stages of life cycle in intermediate and definitive hosts. Humans can serve as definitive hosts for the adult tapeworms and as intermediate hosts during the larval stages. The adult tapeworms that most commonly infect humans include the pork tapeworm (*Taenia solium*), the beef tapeworm (*Taenia saginata*), the fish tapeworm (*Diphyllobothrium latum*), and the dwarf tapeworm (*Hymenolepis nana*). Humans can serve as both definitive host and intermediate hosts for 2 species, *T solium* and *H nana*. In the case of *H nana*, both stages develop in the intestines of the infected person (the cysticercoid in the intestinal wall and the tapeworm in the lumen). In the case of *T solium*, the pork tapeworm, humans are the obligate host for the adult tapeworm stage but can also harbor the larvae in tissue as cysts. Ingestion of *T solium* ova results in dissemination of larvae that encyst in various tissues, muscles, and organs, resulting in cysticercosis in humans.

The 2 most relevant forms of human disease caused by the tapeworm *Echinococcus* spp are cystic echinococcosis or hydatidosis caused by *E granulosus* and alveolar echinococcosis caused by *Echinococcus multilocularis*. The adult tapeworms live in the

The authors declare no conflicts of interest.

[a] Division of Infectious and Tropical Diseases, San Matteo Hospital Foundation, WHO Collaborating Centre for Clinical Management of Cystic Echinococcosis, University of Pavia, Pavia 27100, Italy; [b] Infectious Diseases Division, Department of Internal Medicine, University of Texas Medical Branch, 301 University Boulevard, Route 0435, Galveston, TX 77555-0435, USA
* Corresponding author.
E-mail address: enrico.brunetti@unipv.it

Infect Dis Clin N Am 26 (2012) 421–435
doi:10.1016/j.idc.2012.02.001
0891-5520/12/$ – see front matter © 2012 Elsevier Inc. All rights reserved.

id.theclinics.com

intestine of their definitive hosts, the canines, particularly dogs and foxes. The tapeworm ova are excreted in the canine feces, and when ingested by suitable intermediate animal hosts while grazing, they develop into cysts into the animals' organs. Humans can become accidentally infected by ingestion of eggs, and the larvae that hatch from these ova develop mainly in the liver and in the lungs, but may be located in any organ.

CYSTIC ECHINOCOCCOSIS

Echinococcal cysts comprise the host-derived pericyst, which surrounds the parasite endocyst. The endocyst includes an outer acellular laminated layer and an inner germinative layer. The germinative layer gives rise to brood capsules and protoscolices. Early-stage cysts are filled with clear fluid. With nonsurgical treatments, or sometimes spontaneously, the cystic structures can degenerate (see classification). When ingested by canines, the protoscolices convert to tapeworms. After the rapture of cyst in the abdomen, the protoscolices can seed the peritoneum producing new cysts (secondary echinococcosis).

Epidemiology

E granulosus species occur on all continents, in areas where sheep are reared. The highest prevalence is found in parts of Eurasia, Africa, Australia, and South America. Within the endemic zones, the prevalence of the parasites varies from sporadic to high, but only a few countries can be regarded as being free of *E granulosus* (**Fig. 1**). *E granulosus* comprises several different species and genotypes that may affect the epidemiology, pathology, and control of cystic echinococcosis (CE). Ten distinct genotypes (G1–G10) have been identified till date. Some distinct species have been identified (*Echinococcus equinus*, *Echinococcus ortleppi*). Most *E granulosus* isolates from human patients thus far have been of the sheep genotype (G1).[1]

The exact incidence of CE is unknown because of the slow rate of growth and variable clinical presentation. Early cyst are clinically silent and no case of acute CE has ever been reported. Most epidemiologic reports were based on hospital-based surveys, which underestimate the actual rates of infection, especially in low socio-economic groups with limited resources. With the advent of portable ultrasound scanners,

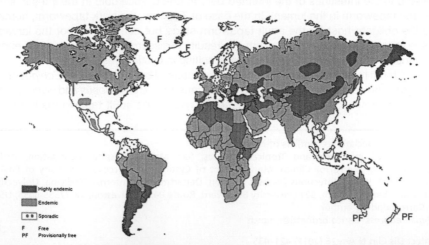

Fig. 1. Geographic distribution of *Echinococcus granulosus*. (*Courtesy of* J. Eckert; © Institute of Parasitology, University of Zurich (J. Eckert, F. Grimm & H. Bucklar.) Used with permission.)

however, community-based surveys have been conducted even in remote areas.[2] These studies uncovered population infection rates of up to 6.6%.

Clinical Manifestations

Clinical manifestations of cestode infestations range from asymptomatic infection to severe, potentially fatal disease. Hydatid cysts may be found incidentally in ultrasonography, chest radiograph, or body scanning. Patients may seek medical attention when a large cyst has some mechanical effect on organ function or when rupture of a cyst causes acute hypersensitivity reactions. The liver is the primary location of echinococcal cysts, including nearly 70% of cases. The lungs are the second most common location. However, CE can also rarely occur in other organs. Upper abdominal discomfort and pain, poor appetite, and a mass in the abdomen are common symptoms with cysts that reach a certain size. In these cases physical examination may reveal hepatomegaly, a palpable mass if on the surface of the liver or other organs, and abdominal distension. Manifestations of complicated cysts may include jaundice, coliclike pains, portal hypertension, ascites, and compression of the inferior vena cava. If pulmonary cysts rupture, symptoms may include intense cough and vomiting of hydatid material and cystic membranes. Patients may present with chest pain, chronic cough, pneumothorax, eosinophilic pneumonitis, pleural effusion, pulmonary embolism, hemoptysis, or biliptysis. Cysts in the heart can cause a cardiac mass, pericardial effusion, and embolism. Cysts in the breast may be confused with neoplasms. Patients with cysts in the spine and in the brain present with neurologic symptoms, including paralysis and seizures.

Diagnosis

Imaging studies, especially ultrasonography and chest radiography are the main diagnostic tests for CE. Serologic tests, such as enzyme-linked immunosorbent assay (ELISA), indirect hemagglutination (IHA), and immunoblotting are used to aid the diagnosis. Most routine laboratory tests are nonspecific. Eosinophilia is low grade or absent and if present may reflect fluid leakage from cyst. Rapture of cyst into the biliary tree causes an increase in the level of alkaline phosphatase, sometimes in association with hyperamylasemia and eosinophilia (up to 60%).

Ultrasonography is the most common procedure for diagnosing asymptomatic CE in the liver and is also useful for monitoring the response to treatment or monitoring cyst growth rate. The World Health Organization Informal Working Group on Echinococcosis (WHO-IWGE) developed a standardized ultrasound classification (**Fig. 2**).[3] Cysts are assigned one of 6 stages in 3 clinical groups. Unilocular (CE1) or multivesicular with daughter cysts (class CE2) are classified as active and usually are viable. Class CE3 contains cysts that are thought to be degenerating (Transitional group). There are 2 types of CE3: CE3a, featuring the water-lily sign for floating membranes, and CE3b, predominantly solid with daughter cysts. CE3a and CE3b respond differently to percutaneous treatment and albendazole (ABZ), which are generally effective for CE3a and ineffective for CE3b.[4] Nuclear magnetic resonance spectroscopy demonstrated that CE3a and CE3b have different metabolic characteristics.[5] Classes CE4 and CE5 are considered inactive. By ultrasonography they are pseudosolid (echogenic) with increasing degrees of calcification and are nearly always nonviable.

Computed tomography (CT) allows the inspection of any organ, detection of smaller cysts located outside the liver, and a more accurate topography of the cyst. CT can sometimes differentiate parasitic from nonparasitic cysts. Magnetic resonance imaging (MRI) may have some advantages over CT, in the evaluation of biliary fistulas, postsurgical residual lesions, recurrences, and selected extrahepatic infections.[6]

WHO-IWGE CLASSIFICATION OF ULTRASOUND IMAGES OF CYSTIC
ECHINOCOCCOSIS CYSTS

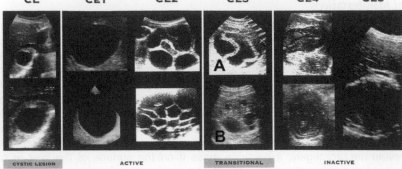

Fig. 2. (*A, B*) World Health Organization Informal Working Group on Echinococcosis (WHO-IWGE) standardized classification of Echinococcal cysts. (*From* World Health Organization, 2001. PAIR: Puncture, Aspiration, Injection, Re-Aspiration. An option for the treatment of Cystic Echinococcosis. WHO/CDS/CSR/APH/2001.6.)

Plain radiographs are useful when cysts occur in the lungs, bone, and muscle as well as to detect calcified cysts.

Serology
Serologic tests, such as ELISA, IHA, and Western Blot, are used to confirm presumptive imaging diagnoses. However, they are not standardized and the sensitivity varies with the location of the cysts.[7] Serologic tests are more often positive with hepatic cysts than pulmonary, brain, or splenic cysts. Serologic tests are more often positive when the cyst is in active (CE2) and transitional (CE3a and b) stages. Serologic tests are often negative in patients with inactive cysts. However, there are many exceptions to this rule, and the interpretation of serologic test may be puzzling even to an experienced clinician. Titers tend to only decrease slowly as the cyst becomes inactive (CE4, CE5) or after radical surgery. Titers may remain positive after conservative surgery, in which the germinal layer is not completely removed. Antibody titers usually increase transiently after medical or percutaneous treatments, which may be due to antigen release.

Other diagnostic procedures
Fine-needle aspiration (FNA) biopsy of the cyst performed under ultrasonographic guidance, under anthelmintic coverage can be used to differentiate CE, malignancy, abscesses, and nonparasitic cysts. The procedure should only be performed if personnel are available to manage the rare anaphylactic reaction.

Treatment
The appropriate treatment depends on cyst characteristics (for hepatic cysts, size and stage are the most important criteria), the therapeutic resources available, and the physician's preference. The level of evidence supporting one therapeutic modality over the other is low because only few prospective, randomized studies comparing different treatments are available.[7]

Surgery has been the traditional approach for the treatment of CE. During recent decades, chemotherapy, percutaneous procedures, and a watch-and-wait approach have been successfully introduced. These alternatives have replaced surgery as the treatment of choice in many cases.[8]

Surgery
Surgery remains the therapy of choice in complicated cysts (ie, rupture, biliary fistula, compression of vital structures, superinfection, hemorrhage), or large cysts with many daughter vesicles (CE3b) that are not suitable for percutaneous treatments.

   Traditional approaches have included radical resectioning including pericystectomy or more conservative techniques. Laparoscopic surgery has emerged as an alternative to open procedures in some cases. The relative advantages of the different approaches have not been clearly established. Thus, there remains controversy regarding the safest and most effective technique.[9] In all cases, perioperative ABZ prophylaxis, from at least 1 week before surgery to at least 4 weeks postoperatively, is recommended as a cautionary measure to minimize the risk of fluid spillage and consequent secondary echinococcosis from seeding of protoscoleces in the abdominal cavity. Although praziquantel is used by some in addition to ABZ, there is no clear evidence of its effectiveness.[10]

Percutaneous treatments
Percutaneous techniques aim either to destroy the germinal layer with scolicidal agents or to evacuate the entire endocyst. The most popular method in the first group is PAIR (puncture, aspiration, injection of a scolicidal agent, and reaspiration). Modified catheterization techniques have been used for cysts, which are difficult to drain or tend to relapse after PAIR, such as CE2 and CE3b cysts.

   Among nearly 6000 cysts that have been punctured for diagnosis or therapy, 99 patients developed anaphylaxis which was fatal in 2 cases.[11] ABZ should always be administered for at least 30 days after puncture. PAIR usually induces permanent solidification of CE1 and CE3a cysts. By contrast, multivesicular cysts (ie, CE2 and CE3b) tend to relapse after PAIR.[12,13]

Chemotherapy
Antiparasitic drugs are playing an increasing role in the management of CE. ABZ, 10 to 15 mg/kg/d, should be administered continuous without interruption. ABZ usually causes solidification of small- and medium-sized CE1 and CE3a cysts (**Fig. 3**). By contrast, it is usually ineffective for larger (diameter more than 10 cm) CE1 and CE3a cysts. Chemotherapy alone has no permanent effect on CE2 and CE3b cysts.[14]

   The adverse effects of benzimidazole antiparasitic drugs include hepatotoxicity, cytopenia, and alopecia. Increased level of aminotransferases may be noted because of drug-related toxicity or from killing the parasites. Benzimidazoles should be avoided

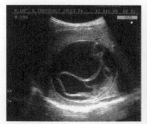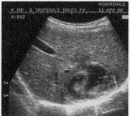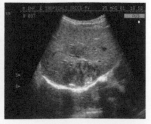

Fig. 3. Progressive decrease in size and solidification of a CE3a cyst after treatment with Albendazole over 2 years. The cyst goes from CE3a to CE4 stage. (*From* Busilacchi P, Rapaccini L, editors. Ecografia clinica. Napoli (Italy): Idelson-Gnocchi; 2006; with permission.)

during pregnancy, if possible, because of potential teratogenicity. Instead, treatment should be delayed in most cases until after delivery.[7]

Watch and wait

Some studies have suggested that inactive cysts in the liver that are free of complications can be safely monitored without being treated.[15] Prospective studies need to be performed to confirm the safety of this option.

Follow-up

CE can relapse for years after treatment. Follow-up for at least 5 years is required to evaluate local recurrences. FNA should be performed to ascertain the viability of the cyst contents in cases that are unclear from imaging and serologic studies (**Fig. 4**).

ALVEOLAR ECHINOCOCCOSIS (E MULTILOCULARIS)

Tissue larvae of E multilocularis cause alveolar echinococcosis. In the liver, E multilocularis produces a multivesiculated mass that may liquefy centrally and grows by infiltrating the surrounding tissues. Canines, including foxes and dogs, are the usual definitive hosts. Rodents are the usual intermediate hosts. Humans are incidental intermediate hosts, infected from eggs shed in the environment by the final hosts (eg, dogs).

Epidemiology

E multilocularis is endemic to the northern hemisphere, with especially high endemicity in western China, Tibet, and central Asia; the Jura mountains in Central Europe; and arctic areas.[16–18] E multilocularis has recently been reported in northern areas of Europe including the Baltic regions.

Clinical Manifestations and Diagnosis

E multilocularis infection in humans almost always invades the liver, as a tumorlike mass, gradually expanding over decades. Right upper quadrant discomfort and swelling are the main symptoms in about one-third of patients. Imaging studies demonstrate a lesion that may be misdiagnosed as a primary or metastatic liver tumor. The etiologic confirmation remains difficult and is based on histopathology, supported by serology.

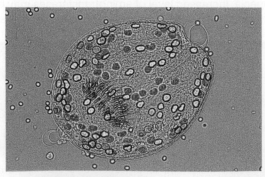

Fig. 4. Viable protoscolex in the cystic fluid aspirated with PAIR seen at light microscopy (unstained, ×20).

Treatment

Unlike CE, surgery remains the main modality of treatment of E multilocularis infection. Infected tissues should be completely removed if possible. Even cases apparently cured should be treated with a 2-year course of ABZ to decrease the rate of relapse. However, most cases are not amenable to surgery, and in those cases ABZ therapy can be extended indefinitely to suppress growth of the lesion, which may result in an almost normal life expectancy.[19] Some cases have been managed, as a last resort, with liver transplantation.[20]

CYSTICERCOSIS

Definitions

Cysticercosis is caused by infection with the larval stage of T solium. Humans are the obligate definitive host for the intestinal tapeworm. The mature segments termed proglottids produce the ova, which infect pigs (the normal intermediate host) (**Fig. 5**). In the pig, the ova hatch, release the invasive larvae, which mature into cysticercus within the tissues. The cysticercus consists of a translucent bladder and a mural nodule containing the invaginated scolex. When ingested in undercooked pork, the scolex evaginates, attaches to the intestines, and forms the tapeworm. The tapeworm carriers shed the infectious ova, which are sticky and attach to the hands of the tapeworm carrier. The ova are typically transmitted by close contacts, including infecting the carrier himself. Ingested ova release the invasive larvae, which migrate through the bloodstream to tissues, where they form cysts (cysticercosis). Neurocysticercosis refers to the presence of cysticerci in the central nervous system, including cysticerci in the brain parenchyma (parenchymal neurocysticercosis), the ventricles, the subarachnoid space, spine, or eye (extraparenchymal neurocysticercosis).

Epidemiology

Cysticercosis has a global distribution in all areas where pigs are raised under conditions in which they can ingest human fecal material (**Fig. 6**).[21] The total number of persons infected is unknown, but estimates suggest more than 50 million people.

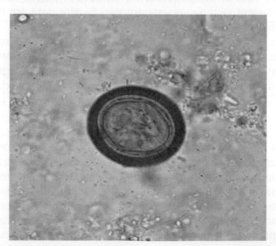

Fig. 5. *Taenia* spp egg in unstained wet mount. (*From* Centers for Disease Control. DPDx Parasite Image Library. Available at: http://www.dpd.cdc.gov/dpdx/HTML/ImageLibrary/S-Z/Taeniasis/body_Taeniasis_il1.htm.)

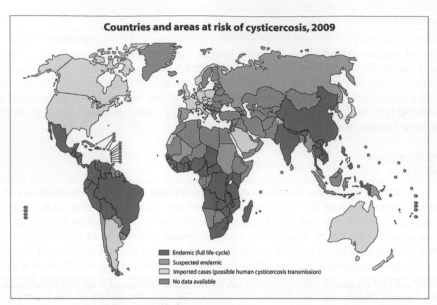

Fig. 6. Global distribution of cysticercosis. (*Data from* World Health Organization. Map Production: Control of Neglected Tropical Diseases (NTD). World Health Organization.) (*Adapted from* World Health Organization Map Production. Control of neglected tropical diseases. Geneva: World Health Organization, 2010; with permission. Copyright © 2010, all rights reserved. Available at: http://gamapserver.who.int/mapLibrary/Files/Maps/Global_cysticercosis_2009.png.)

Data on the prevalence and incidence of disease are limited by the requirement for neuroimaging studies. However, in studies from endemic areas, approximately 30% of cases with seizure disorders have evidence of neurocysticercosis on imaging studies.[21–26] High prevalence rates have been documented throughout much of Latin America including areas in Mexico, Guatemala, Honduras, Ecuador, Peru, Brazil, and Bolivia. More than 10% of the population in endemic villages have neuroimaging abnormalities consistent with neurocysticercosis. Similar data are being developed in sub-Saharan Africa.[27–29]

Cysticercosis is widespread in South and Southeast Asia. Neurocysticercosis is a common cause of seizures in India, with many patients presenting with single enhancing lesions on CT scan. Cysticercosis is also frequently diagnosed in nonendemic areas. For example, approximately 2000 cases are diagnosed each year in the United States.[30,31]

Pathobiology

The pathogenesis of neurocysticercosis varies significantly with the location of the parasite and the associated host inflammatory response. Studies in immigrants from endemic areas suggest that there is a period of several years between infection and onset of symptoms.[30] During that period, the cysts are thought to effectively suppress the host response. The cysticerci eventually lose their ability to modulate the host inflammatory response and are attached by a granulomatous response, which gradually degrades the parasite. Inflammation in the brain parenchyma is linked to seizures.[31]

In some cases, the degenerating parasite forms a calcified granuloma. These calcified granulomas may be intermittently associated with edema and/or contrast enhancement on MRI (suggesting inflammation) and may cause chronic epilepsy.[31–33]

Cysticerci within the ventricles can cause obstructive hydrocephalus. Subarachnoid cysticercosis is characterized by a significant inflammatory reaction. This inflammatory arachnoiditis may lead to vasculitis and stroke, communicating hydrocephalus, or basilar meningitis. Some subarachnoid cysticerci enlarge to more than 5 cm, and the cysticerci or associated edema may cause mass effect.

Clinical Manifestations

The clinical manifestations of neurocysticercosis are extremely pleomorphic varying with the location of the parasite and the host response **(Figs. 7–10)**.[31] Headaches are common in all forms of disease. Seizures are typically associated with cysticerci or inflammation in the brain parenchyma. By contrast, the symptom of extraparenchymal disease (eg, ventricular and subarachnoid cysticercosis) is increased intracranial pressure.

Parenchymal neurocysticercosis

The main clinical manifestation of parenchymal neurocysticercosis is seizures. It is common for patients evaluated for seizures in endemic areas to have a single enhancing lesions due to cysticercus **(Fig. 8)**. The seizures can be focal, generalized, or focal with secondary generalization. Some may have a single seizure. The seizures are typically seen during the period in which the cysticercus is degenerative. Complete radiographic resolution is also often associated with resolution of the seizures. When cyst degeneration is accompanied by formation of calcified lesions, there is a substantial risk factor for recurrent seizures. Patients with multiple lesions also present with seizures. Seizures are more likely to recur in patients with multiple lesions than in patients with single lesions.

Calcified parenchymal lesions

Degeneration of the parasites often leads to formation of intracerebral calcifications **(Fig. 9)**. Calcified lesions are associated with recurrent seizures and chronic epilepsy.

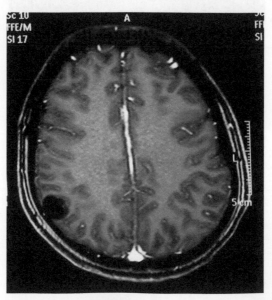

Fig. 7. MRI scan showing a viable cysticercus in the right brain.

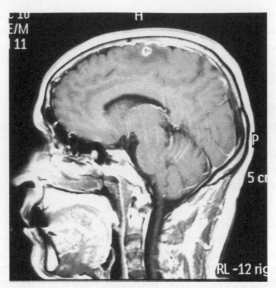

Fig. 8. MRI scan showing a cystic lesion with ring enhancement in the superior parietal lobe.

Extraparenchymal cysticerci

Patients with cysticerci in the ventricles typically present with symptoms caused by obstructive hydrocephalus, mainly headache, nausea and vomiting, dizziness, or altered mental status. Patients may have papilledema with altered vision. There is marked variability in the acuity of presentation from mild symptoms noted intermittently for years to rapid decompensation over a period of a few hours. Obstructive

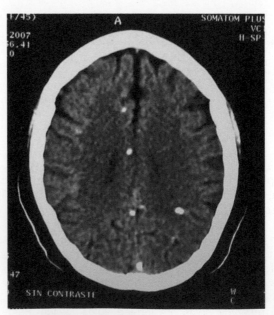

Fig. 9. CT scan showing multiple nodular calcifications.

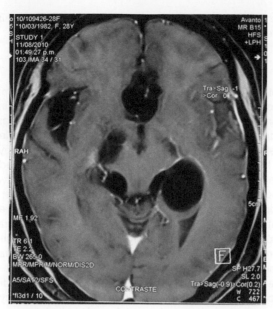

Fig. 10. MRI scan showing multiple cystic lesions in the subarachnoid space.

hydrocephalus is a medical emergency and is frequently fatal if not treated appropriately.

Subarachnoid cysticerci in the basilar cisterns cause one of the more severe forms of neurocysticercosis (**Fig. 10**). Patients often have multiple cysticerci in the brain parenchyma, ventricles, spine, or eye. Cysticerci in the basilar cisterns often cause arachnoiditis, which may lead to vascular involvement with strokes, meningeal signs, or communicating hydrocephalus.

Diagnosis

Neuroimaging studies (eg, CT and MRI scans) are the mainstay of diagnosis for neuro-cysticercosis.[31,34] CT scans are more sensitive at identifying calcified lesions, which appear as 2- to 5-mm nodules (see **Fig. 9**). Parenchymal cysticerci or obstructive hydrocephalus are also usually visible in CT scan, but cysts in the ventricles or subarachnoid space are less easily recognized because the cyst fluid is usually iso-dense with cerebrospinal fluid (CSF). MRI scans are better at identifying the cystic lesions, especially in the ventricles and subarachnoid space. The cysticerci are typi-cally round, 1 to 2 cm in diameter (see **Fig. 8**). The walls of viable cysticerci are usually thin and difficult to visualize. Symptomatic patients often display enhancement of the cyst walls or surrounding tissues and associated edema. The scolex may appear as a 1- to 2-mm solid nodule, cylinder, or spiral, on the side of the cystic lesions. The presence of a scolex inside a cystic lesion is a diagnostic of cysticercosis. In patients in whom the scolex is not visualized, serologic tests can be used to confirm the diag-nosis. The enzyme-linked immunotransfer blot (EITB) is an immunoblot assay using semipurified membrane glycoproteins. The demonstration of antibody by EITB is highly specific for cysticercosis.[35] Although the sensitivity is excellent in cases with extraparenchymal or multiple parenchymal cysticerci, the sensitivity is suboptimal in those with single enhancing lesions or just calcifications.[36] Antigen-detection assays are thought to be more specific for viable cases and are increasingly available.[37] However, there are also problems with sensitivity.[38]

TREATMENT

Optimal treatment of neurocysticercosis often includes symptomatic therapy for seizures and hydrocephalus and specific therapy for the parasites (including antiparasitic drugs or surgical removal).[31,34,39] Antiepileptic drugs, such as phenytoin and carbamazepine, are used to control the seizures. Newer antiepileptic drugs may also be at least effective. Neurosurgery is the mainstay of therapy for obstructive hydrocephalus.[40] Most cysticerci in the ventricles can be managed by endoscopic removal of the cysticerci, which is associated with less postoperative morbidity than either open procedures or nonoperative approaches. The main alternative approach is cerebrospinal diversion via a ventriculoperitoneal shunt accompanied by chronic steroids and/or antiparasitic drugs to decrease the rate of shunt failure. Although there are anecdotes of patients being successfully treated with antiparasitic drugs without surgical procedures, retrospective case series have demonstrated substantial morbidity and mortality with this approach.[40,41] Patients with just calcified lesions do not have viable cysticerci and do not benefit from antiparasitic drugs.

In randomized-controlled trials, patients with parenchymal neurocysticercosis have demonstrated more rapid resolution of parenchymal cystic lesions with fewer generalized seizures when treated with corticosteroids and ABZ (15 mg/kg/d in 2 daily doses usually for 7–8 days) compared with placebo.[42–44] Praziquantel (50–100 mg/kg/d in 3 daily doses) may also be used, but its benefits are less well defined. Patients with single enhancing lesions do well with or without antiparasitic therapy, but studies have demonstrated a slightly more rapid radiologic resolution and fewer seizures when treated with steroids and/or antiparasitic drugs.[43] However, the effects were not significant in a meta-analysis.[45]

Subarachnoid cysticercosis is associated with significant morbidity and mortality. However, there are no data from controlled trials on management. In retrospective analyses, courses of the antiparasitic regimens used for parenchymal disease are associated with poor efficacy.[41] Most experts recommend treatment with prolonged courses of antiparasitic drugs (eg, ABZ for >28 days) and chronic antiinflammatory medications (eg, prednisone 1 mg/kg/d).[34,39] A combination of praziquantel with ABZ may have enhanced activity in some cases.[46,47] Methotrexate has been used as a steroid-sparing agent. Communicating hydrocephalus should be treated with CSF diversion (eg, ventriculoperitoneal shunting). Endoscopic debulking has been used in some cases.

OTHER LARVAL CESTODE INFECTIONS

Sparganosis refers to tissue infection with the larval (plerocercoid) stage of *Spirometra mansonoides*. Sparganosis is acquired from exposure of skin to infected flesh (eg, poultices of infected frogs, birds, or fish) or by ingestion. The plerocercoids develop in tissues, causing subcutaneous or central nervous system nodules or larva migrans. Treatment usually requires surgical removal of the nodule.[48]

Coenurosis is a rare infection caused by the human infection of *Taenia serialis or Taenia multiceps* at the larval stage, which are canine tapeworms. After invasion, the larvae form a cystic lesion containing multiple scolices (the coenurus), most frequently identified in brain, eye, or soft tissues. The usual approach to treatment is surgical removal.[49]

ACKNOWLEDGMENTS

The authors are grateful to Prof Peter Kern, University of Ulm, Ulm, Germany, for reviewing the section on Alveolar echinococcosis and to Prof Hugo Garcia, Universidad Peruana Cayetano Heredia, Lima, Peru, for providing the CT and MRI images of neurocysticercosis.

REFERENCES

1. Thompson RC. The taxonomy, phylogeny and transmission of Echinococcus. Exp Parasitol 2008;119(4):439–46.
2. Macpherson CN, Bartholomot B, Frider B. Application of ultrasound in diagnosis, treatment, epidemiology, public health and control of *Echinococcus granulosus* and *E. multilocularis*. Parasitology 2003;127(Suppl):S21–35.
3. WHO, IWGE. International classification of ultrasound images in cystic echinococcosis for application in clinical and field epidemiological settings. Acta Trop 2003;85(2):253–61.
4. Brunetti E, Junghanss T. Update on cystic hydatid disease. Curr Opin Infect Dis 2009;22(5):497–502.
5. Hosch W, Junghanss T, Stojkovic M, et al. Metabolic viability assessment of cystic echinococcosis using high-field (1)H MRS of cyst contents. NMR Biomed 2008; 21(7):734–54.
6. Hosch W, Stojkovic M, Janisch T, et al. MR imaging for diagnosing cysto-biliary fistulas in cystic echinococcosis. Eur J Radiol 2008;66(2):262–7.
7. Brunetti E, Kern P, Vuitton DA. Expert consensus for the diagnosis and treatment of cystic and alveolar echinococcosis in humans. Acta Trop 2010;114(1):1–16.
8. Menezes da Silva A. Hydatid cyst of the liver-criteria for the selection of appropriate treatment. Acta Trop 2003;85(2):237–42.
9. Dziri C, Haouet K, Fingerhut A, et al. Management of cystic echinococcosis complications and dissemination: where is the evidence? World J Surg 2009; 33(6):1266–73.
10. Bygott JM, Chiodini PL. Praziquantel: neglected drug? Ineffective treatment? Or therapeutic choice in cystic hydatid disease? Acta Trop 2009;111(2):95–101.
11. Neumayr A, Troia G, de Bernardis C, et al. Justified concern or exaggerated fear: the risk of anaphylaxis in percutaneous treatment of cystic echinococcosis-a systematic literature review. PLoS Negl Trop Dis 2011;5(6):e1154.
12. Kabaalioglu A, Ceken K, Alimoglu E, et al. Percutaneous imaging-guided treatment of hydatid liver cysts: do long-term results make it a first choice? Eur J Radiol 2006;59(1):65–73.
13. Golemanov B, Grigorov N, Mitova R, et al. Efficacy and safety of PAIR for cystic echinococcosis: experience on a large series of patients from Bulgaria. Am J Trop Med Hyg 2011;84(1):48–51.
14. Stojkovic M, Zwahlen M, Teggi A, et al. Treatment response of cystic echinococcosis to benzimidazoles: a systematic review. PLoS Negl Trop Dis 2009;3(9):e524.
15. Brunetti E, Garcia HH, Junghanss T. Cystic echinococcosis: chronic, complex, and still neglected. PLoS Negl Trop Dis 2011;5(7):e1146.
16. Torgerson PR, Keller K, Magnotta M, et al. The global burden of alveolar echinococcosis. PLoS Negl Trop Dis 2010;4(6):e722.
17. Romig T. *Echinococcus multilocularis* in Europe-state of the art. Vet Res Commun 2009;33(Suppl 1):31–4.
18. Eckert J, Deplazes P. Biological, epidemiological, and clinical aspects of echinococcosis, a zoonosis of increasing concern. Clin Microbiol Rev 2004;17(1):107–35.

19. Torgerson PR, Schweiger A, Deplazes P, et al. Alveolar echinococcosis: from a deadly disease to a well-controlled infection. Relative survival and economic analysis in Switzerland over the last 35 years. J Hepatol 2008;49(1):72–7.

20. Bresson-Hadni S, Blagosklonov O, Knapp J, et al. Should possible recurrence of disease contraindicate liver transplantation in patients with end-stage alveolar echinococcosis? A 20-year follow-up study. Liver Transpl 2011;17(7):855–65.

21. Ndimubanzi PC, Carabin H, Budke CM, et al. A systematic review of the frequency of neurocyticercosis with a focus on people with epilepsy. PLoS Negl Trop Dis 2010;4(11):e870.

22. Goel D, Dhanai JS, Agarwal A, et al. Neurocysticercosis and its impact on crude prevalence rate of epilepsy in an Indian community. Neurol India 2011;59(1):37–40.

23. Raghava MV, Prabhakaran V, Jayaraman T, et al. Detecting spatial clusters of Taenia solium infections in a rural block in South India. Trans R Soc Trop Med Hyg 2010;104(9):601–12.

24. Villaran MV, Montano SM, Gonzalvez G, et al. Epilepsy and neurocysticercosis: an incidence study in a Peruvian rural population. Neuroepidemiology 2009;33(1):25–31.

25. Montano SM, Villaran MV, Ylquimicho L, et al. Neurocysticercosis: association between seizures, serology, and brain CT in rural Peru. Neurology 2005;65(2):229–33.

26. Medina MT, Duron RM, Martinez L, et al. Prevalence, incidence, and etiology of epilepsies in rural Honduras: the Salamástudy. Epilepsia 2005;46(1):124–31.

27. Blocher J, Schmutzhard E, Wilkins PP, et al. A cross-sectional study of people with epilepsy and neurocysticercosis in Tanzania: clinical characteristics and diagnostic approaches. PLoS Negl Trop Dis 2011;5(6):e1185.

28. Foyaca-Sibat H, Cowan LD, Carabin H, et al. Accuracy of serological testing for the diagnosis of prevalent neurocysticercosis in outpatients with epilepsy, Eastern Cape Province, South Africa. PLoS Negl Trop Dis 2009;3(12):e562.

29. Praet N, Speybroeck N, Manzanedo R, et al. The disease burden of Taenia solium cysticercosis in Cameroon. PLoS Negl Trop Dis 2009;3(3):e406.

30. del la Garza Y, Graviss EA, Daver NG, et al. Epidemiology of neurocysticercosis in Houston, Texas. Am J Trop Med Hyg 2005;73(4):766–70.

31. Serpa JA, Graviss EA, Kass JS, et al. Neurocysticercosis in Houston, Texas: an update. Medicine (Baltimore) 2011;90(1):81–6.

32. Nash TE, Pretell EJ, Lescano AG, et al. Perilesional brain oedema and seizure activity in patients with calcified neurocysticercosis: a prospective cohort and nested case-control study. Lancet Neurol 2008;7(12):1099–105.

33. Nash TE, Del Brutto OH, Butman JA, et al. Calcific neurocysticercosis and epileptogenesis. Neurology 2004;62(11):1934–8.

34. Nash TE, Garcia HH. Diagnosis and treatment of neurocysticercosis. Nat Rev Neurol 2011;7(10):584–94.

35. Tsang VC, Brand JA, Boyer AE. An enzyme-linked immunoelectrotransfer blot assay and glycoprotein antigens for diagnosing human cysticercosis (Taenia solium). J Infect Dis 1989;159(1):50–9.

36. Wilson M, Bryan RT, Fried JA, et al. Clinical evaluation of the cysticercosis enzyme-linked immunoelectrotransfer blot in patients with neurocysticercosis. J Infect Dis 1991;164(5):1007–9.

37. Rodriguez S, Dorny P, Tsang VC, et al. Detection of Taenia solium antigens and anti-T. solium antibodies in paired serum and cerebrospinal fluid samples from

patients with intraparenchymal or extraparenchymal neurocysticercosis. J Infect Dis 2009;199(9):1345–52.

38. White AC Jr. New developments in the management of neurocysticercosis. J Infect Dis 2009;199(9):1261–2.

39. Nash TE, Singh G, White AC, et al. Treatment of neurocysticercosis: current status and future research needs. Neurology 2006;67(7):1120–7.

40. Rangel-Castilla L, Serpa JA, Gopinath SP, et al. Contemporary neurosurgical approaches to neurocysticercosis. Am J Trop Med Hyg 2009;80(3):373–8.

41. Proano JV, Madrazo I, Avelar F, et al. Medical treatment for neurocysticercosis characterized by giant subarachnoid cysts. N Engl J Med 2001;345(12):879–85.

42. Garcia HH, Pretell EJ, Gilman RH, et al. A trial of antiparasitic treatment to reduce the rate of seizures due to cerebral cysticercosis. N Engl J Med 2004;350(3): 249–58.

43. Del Brutto OH, Roos KL, Coffey CS, et al. Meta-analysis: cysticidal drugs for neurocysticercosis: albendazole and praziquantel. Ann Intern Med 2006;145(1): 43–51.

44. Carpio A, Kelvin EA, Bagiella E, et al. Effects of albendazole treatment on neurocysticercosis: a randomised controlled trial. J Neurol Neurosurg Psychiatry 2008; 79(9):1050–5.

45. Abba K, Ramaratnam S, Ranganathan LN. Anthelmintics for people with neurocysticercosis. Cochrane Database Syst Rev 2010;1:CD000215.

46. Garcia HH, Lescano AG, Lanchote VL, et al. Pharmacokinetics of combined treatment with praziquantel and albendazole in neurocysticercosis. Br J Clin Pharmacol 2011;72(1):77–84.

47. Kaur S, Singhi P, Singhi S, et al. Combination therapy with albendazole and praziquantel versus albendazole alone in children with seizures and single lesion neurocysticercosis: a randomized, placebo-controlled double blind trial. Pediatr Infect Dis J 2009;28(5):403–6.

48. Li MW, Song HQ, Li C, et al. Sparganosis in mainland China. Int J Infect Dis 2011; 15(3):e154–6.

49. Ing MB, Schantz PM, Turner JA. Human coenurosis in North America: case reports and review. Clin Infect Dis 1998;27(3):519–23.

Tropical Bacterial Gastrointestinal Infections

Sadia Shakoor, MBBS, FCPS[a], Anita K.M. Zaidi, MD, SM[b],
Rumina Hasan, MBBS, PhD, FRCPath[a],*

KEYWORDS

- Tropical infections • Diarrhea • Enteric fever • Cholera • *Salmonella* • *Shigella*
- Antimicrobial resistance • Enteric vaccines

KEY POINTS

- Bacterial gastrointestinal infections are prevalent in tropical regions. Recent literature shows a rise in incidence of cholera, which is further augmented by natural disasters.
- Epidemiological trends suggest increasing rates of enteric fever in several endemic regions. In such areas vaccination of high risk populations with *S Typhi* vaccines is recommended.
- Invasive non-typhoidal Salmonellae infections are associated with high HIV incidence in Africa.
- The most common etiology for traveler's diarrhea is Enterotoxigenic strain of *E coli* (ETEC), reflecting the excessive burden of ETEC diarrheal disease in tropical regions.
- Antimicrobial resistance amongst enteric pathogens varies both geographically and temporally. Current resistance information is needed to develop updated antibiotic policies and guidelines.

BURDEN OF GASTROINTESTINAL DISEASES

Climatic and socioeconomic conditions in tropical and subtropical regions predispose to high gastrointestinal infection and diarrheal disease rates. Data from travel clinics and GeoSentinel are a testament to tropical countries being the highest-risk perpetrators of travel-related gastrointestinal infections (**Fig. 1**).[1] The true extent and burden of tropical gastrointestinal disease is, however, difficult to determine. Limited access to health care together with paucity of registries and published reports means that calculated disease rates from these regions are usually based on estimates. Gastrointestinal

The authors have nothing to disclose.
There is no conflict of interest.
[a] Department of Pathology and Microbiology, Aga Khan University, Stadium Road, Karachi 74800, Pakistan; [b] Department of Paediatrics and Child Health, Aga Khan University, Stadium Road, Karachi 74800, Pakistan
* Corresponding author.
E-mail address: rumina.hasan@aku.edu

Infect Dis Clin N Am 26 (2012) 437–453
doi:10.1016/j.idc.2012.02.002
0891-5520/12/$ – see front matter © 2012 Elsevier Inc. All rights reserved.

id.theclinics.com

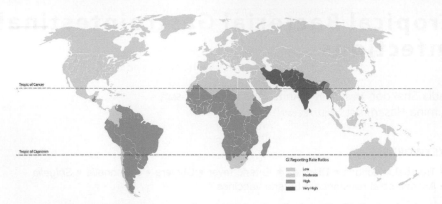

Fig. 1. A profile map of relative rates of acquisition of gastrointestinal infection by destination. Global distribution of reporting rate ratios for all gastrointestinal infections in travelers presenting to 30 GeoSentinel clinics on 6 continents. Twenty-eight countries with available country-specific data are outlined. Where country-specific data are lacking, a country assumes the characteristics of its region. (*Adapted from* Greenwood Z, Black J, Weld L, et al. Gastrointestinal infection among international travelers globally. J Travel Med 2008;15:221; with permission.)

diseases are recognized to exact considerable morbidity and mortality, particularly in children in whom long-term consequences on growth and development are well documented.[2–4] Epidemiology of common tropical bacterial gastrointestinal infections (**Table 1**) indicates that a considerable burden of these infections is due to cholera, salmonellosis, shigellosis, campylobacteriosis, and diarrheagenic *Escherichia coli* (DEC).[31] This review therefore focuses on these high-burden bacterial gastrointestinal infections.

In 2007, 177,963 cases of cholera were reported to the World Health Organization (WHO) from 53 countries, although the actual number of cases is estimated to be much higher.[32] Pandemics of cholera have plagued tropical and subtropical regions involving complex transmission events. The ongoing seventh cholera pandemic caused by *Vibrio cholerae* serotype O1, biotype El Tor originated in the Bay of Bengal (**Fig. 2**).[33,34] In addition, a new strain of *V cholerae*, serotype O139, which also emerged in the Bay of Bengal in 1992, continues to cause epidemics in the South Asia.[33] Several tropical countries have become endemic for cholera.[33] Recent literature shows an increase in incidence further augmented by an increase in natural disasters in tropical regions.[5–13]

Enteric fever is a systemic illness caused by *Salmonella enterica* serotypes Typhi and Paratyphi A, and less commonly by serotypes Paratyphi B and Paratyphi C. Humans are the only natural hosts and reservoirs. More than 21 million cases of typhoid and more than 5 million cases of paratyphoid fever are estimated to have occurred in the year 2000.[35] While enteric fever is a global health concern, the major brunt of morbidity and mortality are borne by tropical regions, especially South Asia.[36,37] Although attempts to measure true incidence of disease are hampered by limited availability of accurate diagnostic tests,[37] recent epidemiologic trends show an increase in rates of enteric fever in endemic regions including Indonesia, India, and Pakistan.[38] In Latin America, however, rates of enteric fever have declined in line with economic development and improved hygiene.[36]

Nontyphoidal Salmonellae (NTS), responsible for sporadic cases and outbreaks of foodborne diarrhea, are zoonotic in etiology. Globally, NTS are estimated to cause

93,757,000 cases of gastroenteritis annually, resulting in 155,000 deaths.[21] Although most disease is self-limiting, invasive infections are a prominent feature of NTS infection in the immunocompromised. The greatest impact of invasive NTS disease is seen in Africa, associated with a high incidence of human immunodeficiency virus in the region.[22] The incidence of invasive salmonellosis appears to be much lower in Asia.[23]

Bacillary dysentery caused by *Shigella* spp is another serious gastrointestinal infection. Four species (*dysenteriae, flexneri, boydii,* and *sonnei*) and 48 serotypes are prevalent.[39] Global burden estimates of shigellosis put the incidence at 80 to 165 million episodes annually, with 99% of these occurring in the developing world.[39] As much as 60% of bacterial dysentery cases in the tropics are caused by *Shigella flexneri.*[39] However, regional differences exist, for example in Thailand, where *Shigella sonnei* is the commonest isolated species.[39] A recent review estimates that approximately 125 million cases of shigellosis occur annually in Asia, of which some 14,000 are fatal.[40]

Another cause of significant morbidity in the tropics is campylobacteriosis, both intestinal and extraintestinal. The epidemiology of *Campylobacter* infections is similar to that of NTS.[41] Whereas *Campylobacter* spp are the commonest cause of bacterial gastroenteritis in the developed world,[42] in the tropics most cases occur in children younger than 5 years.[43]

The most common cause of traveler's diarrhea is the enterotoxigenic strain of *E coli* (ETEC), reflecting the excessive burden of ETEC diarrheal disease in tropical regions.[24] Other serotypes of diarrheagenic *E coli* (DEC) also occur in the tropics along with enteropathogenic *E coli* (EPEC), enteroaggregative *E coli* (EAEC), and diffusely adherent *E coli* (DAEC), causing outbreaks of infantile diarrhea.[24] Enteroinvasive *E coli* (EIEC) causes an illness similar to shigellosis.[24] Enterohemorrhagic *E coli* (EHEC) is associated with serious invasive and noninvasive disease. Toxic dysentery syndromes, however, are relatively uncommon in the tropics apart from a few areas that report high incidence.[24] The low incidence in this case may be attributable to limited access to diagnostic facilities preventing adequate and timely diagnosis of these pathogens.

THE DIAGNOSIS OF BACTERIAL GASTROINTESTINAL INFECTIONS: ARE TROPICS ANY DIFFERENT?

Diagnosis of gastrointestinal infections may be syndromic or etiologic. Common clinical features associated with these infections are shown in **Box 1**.

Most diarrheal syndromes are self-limiting, and culture-based testing is therefore not necessary for therapeutic purposes. The need for diagnostic evaluation arises in the following situations: severe disease or immunocompromised status, illness lasting more than 1 week, or illness associated with systemic symptoms.[44,45] From a public health perspective, however, diagnostic testing is required whenever an outbreak is suspected.[46]

DIAGNOSTIC TESTS
Stool Culture

Despite the turnaround time of 3 to 5 days, stool culture and sensitivity testing remain a gold standard for the diagnosis of bacterial diarrhea. Selective media are used to inhibit normal flora and detect Salmonellae, Shigellae, Vibrionaceae, *Campylobacter*, and toxigenic *E coli*. Culture-based diagnosis of gastroenteritis provides guidance for antimicrobial usage, and generates important microbial surveillance and resistance data.[46]

Table 1
Common tropical bacterial gastrointestinal pathogens

			Pathogens Associated with Recently Reported Outbreaks (Last 5 Years)		
Pathogens	Prevalent Species/Serotype	Region	Countries Reporting Outbreaks	Year(s)	Reported Risk Factors for Outbreaks
Vibrio cholerae	O1 biotype El Tor (serotypes I = Inaba, O = Ogawa)	Africa, Asia, South and Central America	Papua New Guinea[5]	2009–2010	Seasonal (El Nino)
			Central Africa[6]	2010	Seasonal factors
			Haiti[7]	2010	Earthquake
			Pakistan[8]	2010	Floods and IDPs
			Zimbabwe (O, I)[9]	2008–2009	Influx of refugees
			Iraq (I)[10]	2007	Probable sewage contamination of drinking water
			Vietnam[11]	2007–2C08	
			India[12]	2009	Cyclone AILA
	O139	Asia	China (Sichuan province)[13]	2009	Consumption of soft-shelled turtles
Typhoidal Salmonellae (Salmonella enterica serotypes)	Typhi	Asia Africa South and Latin America	India (West Bengal)[14]	2007	Foodborne with a waterborne secondary wave
			Pakistan[15]	2009	Drinking water contamination
Shigella spp	S flexneri S sonnei S dysenteriae S boydii	Asia Africa Latin America	Brazil[16]	2007–2008	Multiple foodborne outbreaks
			Iran[17]	2007	Prison outbreak through contaminated raw vegetables
			Taiwan[18,19]	2007	Groundwater contamination
				2008	Psychiatric ward cross-transmission
Campylobacter spp		Africa Asia South America	Korea[20]	2009	Undercooked chicken

Pathogens endemic in tropics but not reported in recent outbreaks

		Associated factors
Nontyphoidal Salmonellae		Africa, South America, Asia[21–23] — Common as etiology of self-limiting diarrhea, no recently reported outbreaks
Diarrheagenic E coli (DEC)	ETEC EPEC EIEC EHEC EAEC	Asia, South America, Africa[24] — Cause traveler's diarrhea, and outbreaks in infants; no recently reported well-characterized outbreaks
Mycobacterium tuberculosis		Asia, West Africa, Caribbean[25,26] — Gastrointestinal presentation increasingly reported. Likely to coexist with pulmonary tuberculosis, which tends to cluster and is highly infectious
Helicobacter pylori		Asia, Africa, South Amercia[27,28] — Upper gastrointestinal infection and symptoms of gastritis. Rates are higher in developing nations and in tropics
Tropical intestinal diarrhea syndromes with bacterial etiology		
Tropical sprue		Latin America, Southeast Asia, Caribbean[29] — Intestinal malabsorption of putative bacterial etiology (aerobic enteric gram-negative bacteria). Improvement with tetracyclines and folate supplementation. Probably similar to postinfectious irritable bowel syndrome
Whipple disease (Tropheryma whipplei)		Sub-Saharan Africa[30] — Chronic multisystemic infection with diarrhea in approximately 76% of patients. Disease uncommon in tropics but this may be due to underdiagnosis

Abbreviations: EAEC, enteroaggregative E coli; EHEC, enterohemorrhagic E coli; EIEC, enteroinvasive E coli; EPEC, enteropathogenic E coli; ETEC, enterotoxigenic E coli.

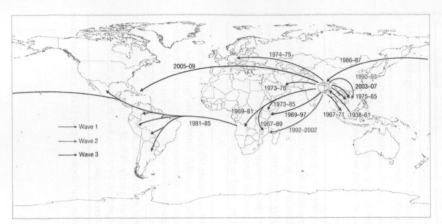

Fig. 2. Transmission events for the seventh *Vibrio cholerae* biotype El Tor pandemic. The information presented is inferred from phylogenetic reconstruction using single nucleotide polymorphisms (SNPs). Data generated by evolutionary parameter estimations in the Bayesian phylogenetic analysis software BEAST suggests the strains spread in 3 independent waves originating in the Bay of Bengal. (*Reproduced from* Mutreja A, Kim DW, Thomson NR, et al. Evidence for several waves of global transmission in the seventh cholera pandemic. Nature 2011;477(7365):464; with permission.)

The limitation for tropical regions in terms of culture, however, is availability, cost-effectiveness, and maintenance of laboratories with culture facilities and procedures.[47] Although National Reference Laboratories (NRLs) exist in WHO regions (tiered laboratory networks), their inaccessibility prevents timely diagnosis of bacterial infections.

Box 1	
Clinical features in specific tropical bacterial gastrointestinal infections	
Infection	**Clinical Features**
Diarrheal illnesses	
Cholera	Acute watery diarrhea ("rice-water"). High risk for rapid development of dehydration and death
Shigellosis	Severe diarrhea ± fever; often dysenteric. High risk of person to person transmission
Nontyphoidal salmonelloses	Acute self-limiting watery diarrhea; only occasionally with fever and dysentery. Zoonotic, foodborne (poultry, eggs, milk products)
Campylobacteriosis	Acute watery diarrhea, severe abdominal pain; often with fever and dysentery. Zoonotic, foodborne (poultry)
ETEC infection	Acute watery traveler's diarrhea; often self-limiting
EPEC/DAEC/EAEC infection	Acute watery diarrhea in infants and toddlers
Enteric fever	
Salmonella Typhi (commonest), followed by *Salmonella* Paratyphi A	Systemic illness; high-grade fever with diarrhea in children and constipation in adults as a rule
Salmonella Paratyphi B and *Salmonella* Paratyphi C are uncommon	High rate of life-threatening complications such as ileal perforations and chronic illness if untreated or inadequately treated

Because the yield of stool cultures for bacterial pathogens remains low,[46] screening tests may be useful in identifying specimens likely to give positive culture results. A summary of screening tests, their principle, sensitivity, and specificity are provided in **Table 2**. Algorithms using both screening and specific testing such as stool culture have been suggested. However, such combination is likely to incur additional costs for outreach health care systems in resource-poor tropical regions. It may therefore be more economical to skip screening tests in favor of specific prevalence-directed pathogen testing in endemic areas.

The unmet need for laboratory capacity building has affected prevalence statistics and availability of surveillance data. Once regional prevalence of pathogens is established, condensed diagnostic algorithms for targeted testing can be introduced in endemic areas, including dipstick testing for *S flexneri* 2a and *V cholerae*.[49,50] Individualized region-specific tiered laboratory systems may be developed whereby first-line testing can be performed using point-of-care (POC) dipstick tests, with confirmatory including culture-based testing being performed in the NRLs.[51]

Nucleic Acid Amplification Tests

Nucleic acid amplification tests (NAAT) have emerged as a sensitive, albeit relatively nonspecific alternative to stool cultures for rapid detection of pathogens from diarrheal stools.[52] Furthermore, microfluidic (dipstick) technologies integrated with NAAT, such as in laboratory chips or in laboratory-on-card systems, are in development; these methods will prove invaluable as low-cost, POC diagnostics of enteric infections in resource-poor tropical regions.[53]

Blood Cultures and Serology

Where invasive infections are suspected, a blood sample must be collected.[54] Blood and bone marrow cultures are the gold standards for detection of systemic salmonellosis. However, blood-culture sensitivity is affected by the number of organisms in the blood (being highest in the first week of illness) and by the volume of blood taken. Prior

Table 2
Summary of screening tests for acute infectious diarrhea

Test	Principle	Sensitivity	Specificity	Comments
Microscopy for fecal leukocytes	Identification of polymorphonuclear cells in stool (iodine, methylene blue stains)	73%	84%	Support diagnosis of inflammatory diarrhea.[45] Absent in noninflammatory enteritides such as cholera
Fecal lactoferrin	Iron-binding glycoprotein found in polymorphonuclear leukocytes	95%	29%	Support diagnosis of inflammatory diarrhea.[45,48] May miss noninflammatory and invasive etiology including *Vibrio cholerae* and ETEC
Fecal calprotectin	Protein released by leukocytes and macrophages in response to intestinal inflammation	—	—	Investigational; Initially developed as a test for inflammatory bowel disease. Potential marker for infectious diarrhea[2]

antibiotic therapy and type of culture media used also affect blood-culture sensitivity.[55] Serologic techniques may prove helpful in blood-culture–negative cases.[56] **Box 2** presents a list of some of the serologic tests based on antibody detection commonly available for diagnosis of enteric fever in the tropics.[37,55,57]

Sensitivity of serologic tests improve when paired sera are tested and with increasing duration of illness. Although in comparison to resource-intensive blood cultures serologic tests are more suitable as POC tests, further development using novel target antigens is warranted to increase their sensitivity.[58] To summarize, a broad range of diagnostic tests are available that need to be directed to imminent needs of tropical regions in relation to the prevalent pathogens.

PATHOPHYSIOLOGY AND PATHOGENESIS

Diarrhea is primarily a consequence of changes in electrolyte and fluid transport during passage through small and/or large intestines.[2] Pathogenesis of acute diarrhea is related to production of bacterial enterotoxins, and invasive and systemic pathogens adopt complicated mechanisms to induce disease.[2] **Table 3** lists pathogenic mechanisms of acute infectious diarrheagenic pathogens. Invasive *E coli*, Shigellae, and Salmonellae elaborate complicated molecular systems to attack enterocytes.[2]

Pathogenesis of enteric fever and molecular apparatus involved has only recently been elucidated. An excellent review by Andrews-Polymenis and colleagues[62] describes how current research has laid down basic mechanisms of disease in enteric

Box 2 Serologic tests for enteric fever			
Test	Sensitivity (%)	Specificity (%)	Comments
Widal: Measures agglutinating antibodies against *Salmonella* Typhi lipopolysaccharide (LPS;O) and flagellar (H) antigens	64	76	Optimally requires testing of paired sera. Widal does not detect *Salmonella* Paratyphi A or Paratyphi B. Cross-reactivity with nontyphoidal Salmonellae and other Enterobacteriaceae is reported
Typhidot: Immunoblot method for specific immunoglobulin (Ig)M and IgG to 50-kDa *Salmonella* Typhi outer membrane protein	67–98	89–100	A qualitative assay. Its modified version; Typhidot M, detects immunoglobulin M as a more specific marker of acute infection Typhidot does not detect *Salmonella* Paratyphi A or Paratyphi B
TUBEX: Detects IgM to *Salmonella* Typhi O9 LPS through its ability to inhibit reaction between 2 colored antigen/antibody coated reagents	56–100	58–100	A 10-min semiquantitative assay that produces a visual readout. Newer versions of the test also detects *Salmonella* Paratyphi A[57]
Typhidot (Malaysian Biodiagnostics Research SDN BHD, Kuala Lumpur, Malaysia). TUBEX (IDL Biotech, Sollentuna, Sweden).			

Table 3
Pathogenic mechanisms associated with diarrheagenic pathogens

Pathogen	Location of Pathology	Incubation	Infectious Dose	Toxin	Mechanism of Action
Vibrio cholerae	Proximal small bowel	12–72 h	10^2–10^6 organisms	Cholera toxin (CT)	Increased levels of cAMP[59]
Shigella spp	Colon	12 h	10^2–10^3 organisms	Shiga toxin (*Shigella dysenteriae* Type 1)	Single-site depurination of 28S ribosomal RNA causes inhibition of protein synthesis and cell death[60]
				Shigella enterotoxin 1 & 2 (ShET 1 & 2) in *Shigella flexneri* 2a	Induces fluid accumulation in rabbit ileal loops[60]
NTS	Colon	6–72 h	200–10^6 organisms	*Salmonella* enterotoxin (Stn); putative role	Immunologic relatedness to CT; cAMP-mediated secretory response in rabbit ileal loops[60]
					Salmonella Pathogenicity Island (SPI)-encoded other factors, eg, T3SS[60]
E coli	—	2–4 d	—	—	—
EHEC	Colon		—	Shiga-like toxin	Similar to Shiga toxin[60,61]
EIEC	Colon		10^6 cells	—	Invasion of enterocytes through invasion-facilitating outer membrane proteins[60,61]
ETEC	Proximal small bowel		10^8 cells	Stable toxin (ST) Labile toxin (LT)	Increased levels of cGMP Similar to cholera toxin[60,61]
EPEC	Small bowel		10^6 cells	Putative new enterotoxin; EspB (EaeB)	3-Step model (adherence, signaling, and intimate adherence)[60,61]
EAEC	Small bowel		—	EAEC heat-stable enterotoxin (EAST 1), several others	Aggregative adhesive fimbriae, formation of biofilm on enteric epithelium[60,61]
Campylobacter	Colon	1–7 d	500–10^4 organisms	LT-like toxin	Increase in cAMP Microtubule-dependent invasion, disruption of cells[60]

Abbreviations: cAMP, cyclic adenosine monophosphate; cGMP, cyclic guanosine monophosphate; EAEC, enteroaggregative *E coli*; EHEC, enterohemorrhagic *E coli*; EIEC, enteroinvasive *E coli*; EPEC, enteropathogenic *E coli*; ETEC, enterotoxigenic *E coli*; NTS, Nontyphoidal salmonellae; T3SS, Type 3 secretion system.

fever. Although *Salmonella* Typhi shares basic pathogenic mechanisms with *Salmonella typhimurium*, a prolonged incubation period (average of 12 days), systemic infection, and gradual development of an inflammatory response in *Salmonella* Typhi infections suggests evasion of host immune defenses to a more sophisticated level. A likely responsible factor is the presence of genes encoding the Vi capsular polysaccharide; however, because this is absent in agents of paratyphoid fever, additional, as yet undiscovered, mechanisms may also exist.

MANAGEMENT
Management of Infectious Diarrhea

The cornerstone of management of acute infectious diarrhea is fluid replacement.[45] Oral rehydration and nutritional therapy (ORNT) regimens proposed by the WHO[63] are commonly used in the tropics. Although refractory vomiting and inability to take fluids orally may prompt parenteral fluid replacement, ORNT is more cost-effective, less invasive, and prevents against overhydration.[46]

The WHO recommends 20 mg of zinc daily for 14 days as a nonantimicrobial adjuvant to ORNT.[63] Zinc blocks basolateral potassium channels and inhibits chloride secretion.[2] Supplementation reduces severity and duration of illness in children.

Antibiotics are recommended for shigellosis and cholera, but not for other forms of acute watery diarrhea.[63] A recent survey of physicians advising travelers with diarrhea in the tropics found a high rate of polypharmacy, and empiric antibiotic usage (61%–95%).[64] While empiric antibiotic usage may be justified in areas with high prevalence of shigellosis and cholera, these areas also have a high rate of self-limiting salmonellosis and campylobacteriosis. Using antibiotics in such situations risks increasing antimicrobial resistance, antibiotic-associated diarrhea, and prolongs pathogen excretion in feces.[46]

Knowledge of current patterns of antimicrobial resistance is useful in establishing antibiotic policies and guidelines. Recent antimicrobial resistance trends of enteric pathogens in the tropics are presented in **Table 4**. However, generalizations regarding prevalence of antimicrobial resistance are difficult because resistance rates vary greatly geographically as well as temporally. NTS and typhoidal Salmonellae, for example, may regress to drug-sensitive phenotypes. Between the periods 1990-1999 and 2000-2004, sensitivity to ampicillin and cotrimoxazole increased in *Salmonella enteritidis* strains from Kenya.[70] Similarly, in India, susceptibility to first-line drugs ampicillin, cotrimoxazole, and chloramphenicol is reemerging in *Salmonella* Typhi strains.[79]

The resistance problem in turn begs the question of whether organism-based diagnostic including antimicrobial sensitivity testing is performed routinely. Indeed, if rapid POC microfluidic tests are widely available in underserved tropical regions, empiric antimicrobials will no longer be administered; hence the cavernous relationship of diagnostic tests to management and, unsurprisingly, to preventive measures.

Management of Enteric Fever: The Fluoroquinolone Resistance Perspective

Enteric fever was routinely treated in the 1960s with chloramphenicol, ampicillin, or cotrimoxazole. Emergence of multidrug-resistant (MDR) strains of typhoidal Salmonellae led to increasing usage of fluoroquinolones. Rapid emergence of fluoroquinolone nonsusceptible strains was soon reported.[79] Nowadays in most areas including the Indian subcontinent, ceftriaxone and cefixime remain the only reliable antimicrobial choices.[36] A summary of empiric treatment of bacterial gastrointestinal infections is given in **Box 3**.

Table 4
Antimicrobial resistance trends of enteric pathogens in the tropics

Pathogen	Tropical Regions	Recent Antibiotic Resistance Rates (%) and Trends
Vibrio cholerae	Africa	Kenya (1999): multiple drug resistance to C, SXT, TE[65]
		Angola (2006): multiple resistance to AMP, C, SXT, TE[66]
	Asia	Iraq: resistant to SXT[10]
		India (2010): multiple resistance to AMP, NA, SXT, C, TE (>70%)[12]
	Latin America	Brazil (1999): AMP, SXT, furazolidone (70%–80%)[67]
Shigella spp	Africa	Tanzania (1999): AMP, C, SXT, TE (>70%)[68]
		Kenya: SXT, TE, AMP (95%–100%)[69]
	Asia	Iran: AMP, SXT, TE (100%)[17]
		Taiwan: NA, SXT (100%)[18]
	Latin America	Brazil: AMP, SXT (>80%). Variable resistance to TE, C[16]
NTS	Africa	*S enteritidis*; AMP, SXT (>90%) in 1999, decreasing trend (2004) *S typhimurium*; AMP, SXT (>90%) (1999–2004)[70]
	Asia	India (2002): AMP (60%), NA (66%), FQ (18%), SXT (34%), C (37%), 3GC (48%)[71]
	Latin America	Mexico: multidrug resistance in *S typhimurium* increased from 0% to 75% (2000–2005)[72]
DEC	Africa	Kenya: resistance rates; AMP (65%), SXT (68%), TE:70%[73]
	Asia	India (2006): AMP (85%), SXT (64%), NA (85%), FQ (79%)[74]
	Latin America	Brazil (2007): SXT (35%), multidrug resistance (3%–5%)[75]
Campylobacter	Africa	Uganda (2005): AMP (20%), FQ (5%), 100% susceptible to E[76]
	Asia	Indonesia (2001): AMP (65%), SXT (70%), TE (65%), FQ (45%), 100% susceptible to E[77]
Typhoidal Salmonellae (TS)	Africa	2002–2008: MDRTS (29%–70%) geographic prevalence variation[78]
	Asia	1992–2005: MDRTS (1.3%–80%) geographic prevalence variation[78]

Abbreviations: AMP, ampicillin; 3GC, third-generation cephalosporins; C, chloramphenicol; DEC, diarrheagenic *E coli*; E, erythromycin; FQ, fluoroquinolones; MDRTS (multidrug-resistant TS), resistant to AMP, SXT, C; NA, nalidixic acid; SXT, cotrimoxazole; TE, tetracycline.

PREVENTION

Most authorities recommend exercising care in selecting food and beverages to prevent diarrhea. In resource-limited tropical regions, however, inculcating this tenet is a challenge. Additional measures on a public scale are required: improving sanitation and sewage disposal and drainage, provision of safe drinking water, and widespread vaccination to generate herd immunity where applicable.[46]

Enteric Vaccines

The WHO prioritizes vaccination against agents causing high morbidity and mortality, especially among children in underdeveloped nations.[2] A summary of the available vaccines for bacterial gastrointestinal infections is given in **Box 4**.

Box 3
Recommended agents for treatment of bacterial gastrointestinal infections

Pathogen	Recommended Agents
Vibrio cholerae	Antibiotics not essential. Oral doxycycline (300 mg single dose in nonpregnant adults), oral azithromycin (1 gram single dose in pregnant females; 20 mg/kg in children as a single dose) decreases symptomatic illness and fecal shedding
Shigella spp	Quinolones (ciprofloxacin 500 mg orally twice daily in adults or 10 mg/kg twice daily in children) or cotrimoxazole (160/800 mg twice daily in adults and 5/25 mg/kg twice daily in children) for 3–5 days
Salmonella enteritidis and other NTS	Antibiotics not indicated in otherwise healthy individuals, as may prolong illness and fecal shedding. Immunocompromised and debilitated patients may be treated according to susceptibility results.
Campylobacter spp	Quinolones (500 mg ciprofloxacin twice daily) or erythromycin (500 mg 4 times daily) for 5 days, although usually self limiting. For children, erythromycin is preferable to quinolones (dosage for erythromycin: 10 mg/kg orally 4 times daily for 5 days)
Diarrheagenic *E coli*	Quinolones (ciprofloxacin 500 mg orally twice daily) or cotrimoxazole (160/800 mg twice daily) for 2–5 days for ETEC, EPEC, EIEC, and DAEC. Dosages for children for severe EPEC and EIEC, or DAEC disease are cotrimoxazole at 5 mg trimethoprim/kg body weight for 3 days. Quinolones should be avoided in children. Caution is required in EHEC-induced postinfectious hemolytic uremic syndrome for which antibiotics are contraindicated
Enteric fever *Salmonella* Typhi, *Salmonella* Paratyphi A (*Salmonella* Paratyphi B and *S* Paratyphi C uncommon)	Treatment of uncomplicated cases with oral cefixime 30 mg/kg/d divided 12-hourly or azithromycin 10 mg/kg/d for 7 days (both children and adults); complicated cases require initial parenteral ceftriaxone 60–80 mg/kg/d divided 12-hourly or cefotaxime 100–150 mg/kg/d divided 8-hourly (both children and adults) followed by oral antibiotics to complete 10–14 days

Vaccines available for cholera include Dukoral, Shanchol, and mORCVAX. The current WHO position is to use these vaccines in areas at risk of outbreaks, and in high-risk populations in endemic areas.[80] Because of the lack of data it is difficult to comment on coverage of these vaccines in target populations.

Commercially available *Salmonella* Typhi vaccines include Ty21a and Vi polysaccharide vaccine. Ty21a provides a 53% to 78% 3- to 7-year protection after 3 doses, whereas Vi polysaccharide vaccine provides 70% protection after 1 dose for 3 years.[81] The WHO recommends routine programmatic vaccination of high-risk populations in endemic countries.[81] Recent field trials of programmatic vaccination in India, Egypt, and Chile have demonstrated good results.[82]

Vaccines against *Shigella* spp and ETEC are less forthcoming, owing to a multitude of serotypes causing infections.[2] A new generation of unlicensed vaccines against these pathogens is currently undergoing clinical trials.[2]

Box 4
Licensed vaccines for bacterial gastrointestinal infections

Vibrio cholerae vaccines

    Inactivated whole cell (serogroup 01) + cholera toxin B-subunit vaccine (Dukoral): oral vaccine for children and adults; 2 doses

    Inactivated Bivalent (O1 and O139) oral cholera vaccines (Shanchol and mORCVAX): recommended for children older than 1 year and adults; 2 doses 2 weeks apart

Salmonella Typhi vaccines

    Ty21a: oral vaccine for children older than 2 years and adults; 3 doses 48 hours apart

    Vi polysaccharide: parenteral vaccine for children older than 2 years and adults; single dose

---

SUMMARY

The tropics are endemic for several bacterial gastrointestinal infections. Globalization and widespread travel have led to geographic boundaries becoming increasingly indistinct as markers of disease occurrence. One must, therefore, consider the occurrence of tropical diseases outside of the tropics. Within the latitudinal limits of the tropics, recent surveillance data is essential to inform diagnostic measures, management, and preventive strategies. Financial and human resource constraints continue to hinder effective implementation of such surveillance measures. However, recent initiatives by nongovernmental funding resources toward generating such data[31] are a welcome change, and may lead to individualized guidelines for gastrointestinal illness in the tropics.

REFERENCES

1. Greenwood Z, Black J, Weld L, et al. Gastrointestinal infection among international travelers globally. J Travel Med 2008;15:221.
2. Petri WA Jr, Miller M, Binder HJ, et al. Enteric infections, diarrhea, and their impact on function and development. J Clin Invest 2008;118:1277.
3. Boschi-Pinto C, Velebit L, Shibuya K. Estimating child mortality due to diarrhoea in developing countries. Bull World Health Organ 2008;86:710.
4. Guerrant RL, Kosek M, Moore S, et al. Magnitude and impact of diarrheal diseases. Arch Med Res 2002;33:351.
5. Rosewell A, Dagina R, Murhekar M, et al. *Vibrio cholerae* O1 in 2 coastal villages, Papua New Guinea. Emerg Infect Dis 2011;17:154.
6. WHO. Global Alert And Response (GAR). Cholera in Central Africa. Available at: http://www.who.int/csr/don/2010_10_08/en/index.html. Accessed March 26, 2012.
7. WHO. Global Alert and Response (GAR). Cholera in Haiti Update 4. Available at: http://www.who.int/csr/don/2010_11_24/en/index.html. Accessed March 26, 2012.
8. WHO. Global Alert and Response (GAR). Cholera in Pakistan. Available at: http://www.who.int/csr/don/2010_10_25/en/index.html. Accessed March 26, 2012.
9. Mason PR. Zimbabwe experiences the worst epidemic of cholera in Africa. J Infect Dev Ctries 2009;3:148.
10. Khwaif JM, Hayyawi AH, Yousif TI. Cholera outbreak in Baghdad in 2007: an epidemiological study. East Mediterr Health J 2010;16:584.

11. Nguyen BM, Lee JH, Cuong NT, et al. Cholera outbreaks caused by an altered *Vibrio cholerae* O1 El Tor biotype strain producing classical cholera toxin B in Vietnam in 2007 to 2008. J Clin Microbiol 2009;47:1568.

12. Panda S, Pati KK, Bhattacharya MK, et al. Rapid situation & response assessment of diarrhoea outbreak in a coastal district following tropical cyclone AILA in India. Indian J Med Res 2011;133:395.

13. Tang XF, Liu LG, Ma HL, et al. Outbreak of cholera associated with consumption of soft-shelled turtles, Sichuan province, China, 2009. Zhonghua Liu Xing Bing Xue Za Zhi 2010;31:1050 [in Chinese].

14. Bhunia R, Hutin Y, Ramakrishnan R, et al. A typhoid fever outbreak in a slum of South Dumdum municipality, West Bengal, India, 2007: evidence for foodborne and waterborne transmission. BMC Public Health 2009;9:115.

15. Farooqui A, Khan A, Kazmi SU. Investigation of a community outbreak of typhoid fever associated with drinking water. BMC Public Health 2009;9:476.

16. Paula CM, Geimba MP, Amaral PH, et al. Antimicrobial resistance and PCR-ribotyping of *Shigella* responsible for foodborne outbreaks occurred in Southern Brazil. Braz J Microbiol 2010;41:966.

17. Ranjbar R, Hosseini MJ, Kaffashian AR, et al. An outbreak of shigellosis due to *Shigella floxnori* serotype 3a in a prison in Iran. Arch Iran Med 2010;13:413.

18. Chao YN, Huang AS, Chiou CS, et al. A waterborne shigellosis outbreak in a primary school, Tai-Chung City, November 2007. Taiwan Epidemiology Bulletin 2008;24:740.

19. Liao YS, Wang YW, Liao CH, et al. A shigellosis outbreak caused by *S. flexneri* X Variant at a psychiatric hospital in Miaoli County. Taiwan Epidemiology Bulletin 2008;25:773.

20. Yu JH, Kim NY, Cho NG, et al. Epidemiology of *Campylobacter jejuni* outbreak in a middle school in Incheon, Korea. J Korean Med Sci 2010;25:1595.

21. Majowicz SE, Musto J, Scallan E, et al. The global burden of nontyphoidal *Salmonella* gastroenteritis. Clin Infect Dis 2010;50:882.

22. Morpeth SC, Ramadhani HO, Crump JA. Invasive non-Typhi *Salmonella* disease in Africa. Clin Infect Dis 2009;49:606.

23. Khan MI, Ochiai RL, von Seidlein L, et al. Non-typhoidal *Salmonella* rates in febrile children at sites in 5 Asian countries. Trop Med Int Health 2010;15:960.

24. O'Ryan M, Prado V, Pickering LK. A millennium update on pediatric diarrheal illness in the developing world. Semin Pediatr Infect Dis 2005;16:125.

25. Donoghue HD, Holton J. Intestinal tuberculosis. Curr Opin Infect Dis 2009;22:490.

26. Gonzalez E, Risco GE, Borroto S, et al. Tuberculosis mortality trends in Cuba, 1998 to 2007. MEDICC Rev 2009;11:42.

27. Fock KM, Ang TL. Epidemiology of *Helicobacter pylori* infection and gastric cancer in Asia. J Gastroenterol Hepatol 2010;25:479.

28. Tanih NF, Dube C, Green E, et al. An African perspective on *Helicobacter pylori*: prevalence of human infection, drug resistance, and alternative approaches to treatment. Ann Trop Med Parasitol 2009;103:189.

29. Batheja MJ, Leighton J, Azueta A, et al. The face of tropical sprue in 2010. Case Rep Gastroenterol 2010;4:168.

30. Fenollar F, Trape JF, Bassene H, et al. *Tropheryma whipplei* in fecal samples from children, Senegal. Emerg Infect Dis 2009;15:922.

31. Money NN, Maves RC, Sebeny P, et al. Enteric disease surveillance under the AFHSC-GEIS: current efforts, landscape analysis and vision forward. BMC Public Health 2011;11(Suppl 2):S7.

32. WHO. Cholera, 2007. Wkly Epidemiol Rec 2008;31:269.

33. Zuckerman JN, Rombo L, Fisch A. The true burden and risk of cholera: implications for prevention and control. Lancet Infect Dis 2007;7:521.
34. Mutreja A, Kim DW, Thomson NR, et al. Evidence for several waves of global transmission in the seventh cholera pandemic. Nature 2011;477(7365): 462–5.
35. Crump JA, Luby SP, Mintz ED. The global burden of typhoid fever. Bull World Health Organ 2004;82:346.
36. Crump JA, Mintz ED. Global trends in typhoid and paratyphoid fever. Clin Infect Dis 2010;50:241.
37. Crump JA, Ram PK, Gupta SK, et al. Part I. Analysis of data gaps pertaining to *Salmonella enterica* serotype Typhi infections in low and medium human development index countries, 1984-2005. Epidemiol Infect 2008;136:436.
38. Ochiai RL, Acosta CJ, Danovaro-Holliday MC, et al. A study of typhoid fever in five Asian countries: disease burden and implications for controls. Bull World Health Organ 2008;86:260.
39. Ram PK, Crump JA, Gupta SK, et al. Part II. Analysis of data gaps pertaining to *Shigella* infections in low and medium human development index countries, 1984-2005. Epidemiol Infect 2008;136:577.
40. Bardhan P, Faruque AS, Naheed A, et al. Decrease in shigellosis-related deaths without *Shigella* spp.-specific interventions, Asia. Emerg Infect Dis 2010;16: 1718.
41. Musher DM, Musher BL. Contagious acute gastrointestinal infections. N Engl J Med 2004;351:2417.
42. Skirrow MB. Epidemiology of *Campylobacter enteritis*. Int J Food Microbiol 1991; 12:9.
43. Calva JJ, Ruiz-Palacios GM, Lopez-Vidal AB, et al. Cohort study of intestinal infection with *Campylobacter* in Mexican children. Lancet 1988;1:503.
44. Baldi F, Bianco MA, Nardone G, et al. Focus on acute diarrhoeal disease. World J Gastroenterol 2009;15:3341.
45. Thielman NM, Guerrant RL. Clinical practice. Acute infectious diarrhea. N Engl J Med 2004;350:38.
46. Guerrant RL, Van Gilder T, Steiner TS, et al. Practice guidelines for the management of infectious diarrhea. Clin Infect Dis 2001;32:331.
47. Wertheim HF, Puthavathana P, Nghiem NM, et al. Laboratory capacity building in Asia for infectious disease research: experiences from the South East Asia Infectious Disease Clinical Research Network (SEAICRN). PLoS Med 2010;7:e1000231.
48. Gill CJ, Lau J, Gorbach SL, et al. Diagnostic accuracy of stool assays for inflammatory bacterial gastroenteritis in developed and resource-poor countries. Clin Infect Dis 2003;37:365.
49. Nato F, Phalipon A, Nguyen TL, et al. Dipstick for rapid diagnosis of *Shigella flexneri* 2a in stool. PLoS One 2007;2:e361.
50. Mukherjee P, Ghosh S, Ramamurthy T, et al. Evaluation of a rapid immunochromatographic dipstick kit for diagnosis of cholera emphasizes its outbreak utility. Jpn J Infect Dis 2010;63:234.
51. Janda JM, Abbott SL. Revisiting bacterial gastroenteritis, part I: issues, possible approaches, and an ever-expanding list of etiologic agents. Clin Microbiol Newslett 2011;33:71.
52. Bennett WE Jr, Tarr PI. Enteric infections and diagnostic testing. Curr Opin Gastroenterol 2009;25:1.
53. Yager P, Edwards T, Fu E, et al. Microfluidic diagnostic technologies for global public health. Nature 2006;442:412.

54. Guarino A, Giannattasio A. New molecular approaches in the diagnosis of acute diarrhea: advantages for clinicians and researchers. Curr Opin Gastroenterol 2011;27:24.

55. Parry CM, Wijedoru L, Arjyal A, et al. The utility of diagnostic tests for enteric fever in endemic locations. Expert Rev Anti Infect Ther 2011;9:711.

56. Baker S, Favorov M, Dougan G. Searching for the elusive typhoid diagnostic. BMC Infect Dis 2010;10:45.

57. Yan M, Tam FC, Kan B, et al. Combined rapid (TUBEX) test for typhoid-paratyphoid A fever based on strong anti-O12 response: design and critical assessment of sensitivity. PLoS One 2011;6(9):e24743.

58. Chart H, Cheasty T, de Pinna E, et al. Serodiagnosis of *Salmonella enterica* serovar Typhi and *S. enterica* serovars Paratyphi A, B and C human infections. J Med Microbiol 2007;56:1161.

59. Ramamurthy T, Nair GB. Foodborne pathogenic vibrios. In: Simjee S, editor. Infectious disease: foodborne diseases. 1st edition. Totowa (NJ): Humana Press Inc; 2007. p. 132–6.

60. Sears CL, Kaper JB. Enteric bacterial toxins: mechanisms of action and linkage to intestinal secretion. Microbiol Rev 1996;60:167. p. 2–16.

61. Meng J, Schroeder CM. Escherichia coli. In: Simjee S, editor. Infectious disease: foodborne diseases. 1st edition. Totowa (NJ): Humana Press Inc; 2007.

62. Andrews-Polymenis HL, Baumler AJ, McCormick BA, et al. Taming the elephant: salmonella biology, pathogenesis, and prevention. Infect Immun 2010;78:2356.

63. The treatment of diarrhoea. A manual for physicians and other senior health workers, 4th Revision. Geneva (Switzerland): WHO Press; 2005.

64. Wyss MN, Steffen R, Dhupdale NY, et al. Management of travelers' diarrhea by local physicians in tropical and subtropical countries—a questionnaire survey. J Travel Med 2009;16:186.

65. Scrascia M, Forcillo M, Maimone F, et al. Susceptibility to rifaximin of *Vibrio cholerae* strains from different geographical areas. J Antimicrob Chemother 2003;52:303.

66. Ceccarelli D, Bani S, Cappuccinelli P, et al. Prevalence of aadA1 and dfrA15 class 1 integron cassettes and SXT circulation in *Vibrio cholerae* O1 isolates from Africa. J Antimicrob Chemother 2006;58:1095.

67. Campos LC, Zahner V, Avelar KE, et al. Genetic diversity and antibiotic resistance of clinical and environmental *Vibrio cholerae* suggests that many serogroups are reservoirs of resistance. Epidemiol Infect 2004;132:985.

68. Navia MM, Capitano L, Ruiz J, et al. Typing and characterization of mechanisms of resistance of *Shigella* spp. isolated from feces of children under 5 years of age from Ifakara, Tanzania. J Clin Microbiol 1999;37:3113.

69. Brooks JT, Ochieng JB, Kumar L, et al. Surveillance for bacterial diarrhea and antimicrobial resistance in rural western Kenya, 1997-2003. Clin Infect Dis 2006;43:393.

70. Gordon MA, Graham SM, Walsh AL, et al. Epidemics of invasive *Salmonella enterica* serovar enteritidis and *S. enterica* serovar Typhimurium infection associated with multidrug resistance among adults and children in Malawi. Clin Infect Dis 2008;46:963.

71. Taneja N, Mohan B, Khurana S, et al. Antimicrobial resistance in selected bacterial enteropathogens in north India. Indian J Med Res 2004;120:39.

72. Zaidi MB, Leon V, Canche C, et al. Rapid and widespread dissemination of multidrug-resistant blaCMY-2 *Salmonella typhimurium* in Mexico. J Antimicrob Chemother 2007;60:398.

73. Bii CC, Taguchi H, Ouko TT, et al. Detection of virulence-related genes by multi-plex PCR in multidrug-resistant diarrhoeagenic *Escherichia coli* isolates from Kenya and Japan. Epidemiol Infect 2005;133:627.

74. Samal SK, Khuntia HK, Nanda PK, et al. Incidence of bacterial enteropathogens among hospitalized diarrhea patients from Orissa, India. Jpn J Infect Dis 2008;61:350.

75. Souza TB, Morais MB, Tahan S, et al. High prevalence of antimicrobial drug-resistant diarrheagenic *Escherichia coli* in asymptomatic children living in an urban slum. J Infect 2009;59:247.

76. Mshana SE, Joloba M, Kakooza A, et al. *Campylobacter* spp among children with acute diarrhea attending Mulago hospital in Kampala, Uganda. Afr Health Sci 2009;9:201.

77. Tjaniadi P, Lesmana M, Subekti D, et al. Antimicrobial resistance of bacterial pathogens associated with diarrheal patients in Indonesia. Am J Trop Med Hyg 2003;68:666.

78. Zaki SA, Karande S. Multidrug-resistant typhoid fever: a review. J Infect Dev Ctries 2011;5:324.

79. Kumar Y, Sharma A, Mani KR. Re-emergence of susceptibility to conventionally used drugs among strains of *Salmonella* Typhi in central west India. J Infect Dev Ctries 2011;5:227.

80. WHO. Cholera vaccines: WHO position paper. Wkly Epidemiol Rec 2010;13:117.

81. WHO. Typhoid vaccines: WHO position paper. Wkly Epidemiol Rec 2008;6:49.

82. Desai SN, Sahastrabuddhe S, Ochiai RL, et al. Enteric vaccines for resource-limited countries: current status and future prospects. Pediatr Ann 2011;40:351.

Vector-Borne Rickettsioses in North Africa

Tahar Kernif, VetD[a,b], Cristina Socolovschi, MD, PhD[a],
Idir Bitam, PhD[b], Didier Raoult, MD, PhD[a], Philippe Parola, MD, PhD[a],*

KEYWORD

- Fleas • Ticks • Lice • Rickettsioses • North Africa

KEY POINTS

- Rickettsioses are an important causes of fever in North Africa and in travellers returned from this area.
- Fever, rash and eschar are typical signs for rickettsioses. When typical signs are lacking, rickettsioses can be misdiagnosed with many other infectious diseases.
- An history of exposure to ticks, lice, or fleas has to be investigate in patients with fever, including the returned travelers.
- Prevention of rickettsioses is based on appropriate mesure to avoid tick, flea, and lice bites.
- Doxycycline remains the treatment of choice for rickettsioses.

INTRODUCTION

Rickettsiae are obligate intracellular bacteria within the family *Rickettsiaceae* of the order *Rickettsiales*. They are associated with both vertebrate and invertebrate hosts, but rickettsial species differ in terms of their associations with arthropods, behavior of the vector to infection, pathophysiology, and outcome of the disease. The rickettsial field has undergone a significant evolution due to technological advances in molecular genetics and genomics. The taxonomy of rickettsiae has been reorganized and continues to be modified as new data become available.[1] Currently, 25 species are recognized in the *Rickettsia* genus, which is divided into 2 main groups: the spotted fever group (SFG) and the typhus group (TG) rickettsia.[2]

Rickettsioses represent some of the oldest known vector-borne diseases, which cause mild to fatal diseases in people. In North Africa, which the United Nations defines

[a] URMITE, UMR CNRS-IRD 6236, World Health Organization Collaborative Centre for Rickettsial Diseases and Other Arthropod-borne Bacterial Diseases, Aix Marseille University, 27 Boulevard Jean Moulin, 13005 Marseille, France; [b] Service d'Ecologie et des Systèmes Vectoriels, Institut Pasteur d'Algérie, Annexe Ruisseau, Algiers, Algeria
* World Health Organization Collaborative Centre for Rickettsioses and other Arthropod Borne Bacterial diseases, Marseille, France.
E-mail address: philippe.parola@univ-amu.fr

Infect Dis Clin N Am 26 (2012) 455–478
doi:10.1016/j.idc.2012.03.007
0891-5520/12/$ – see front matter © 2012 Elsevier Inc. All rights reserved.

as the northernmost region of the African continent, including 8 countries or territories: Algeria, Egypt, Libya, Morocco, South Sudan, Sudan, Tunisia, and western Sahara (http://millenniumindicators.un.org/unsd/methods/m49/m49regi), SFG and TG rickettsiosis have been described since the beginning of the 20th century.[3] The first clinical cases of Mediterranean spotted fever (MSF), which were caused by *Rickettsia conorii*, were described in 1910 by Conor and Brush of the Pasteur Institute in Tunis, Tunisia.[3] Subsequently, Conor and Hayat described the clinical features (an abrupt onset, high fever, headache, chills, arthromyalgias, and conjunctivitis) of another 4 clinical cases in Tunisia.[4] The exanthema was papular rather than macular, which they termed bouton, often turned red–purple in color, and involved the palms and soles. The duration of the illness was 12 to 15 days with no fatal cases.[4] In 1928, Burnet and Olmer conducted the first experimental infection of a chimpanzee in Tunisia. After 10 days with a fever, the chimpanzee died.[5] After the discovery of tache noire, an eschar at the point of inoculation of the infectious agent in Marseille, France, all researchers believed in the existence of the disease's vector. At that time, Olmer believed that the vector of the disease was the brown dog tick. In 1930, in Tunisia, this hypothesis was confirmed by Durand and Conseil, who inoculated patients with crushed infected *Rhipicephalus sanguineus* ticks and noted that the patients subsequently contracted MSF.[6] These results were confirmed later by Blanc and Caminopetros in Greece.[7]

The first observations of the role of lice in epidemic typhus transmission (caused by *Rickettsia prowazekii*) were observed in Tunisia by Nicolle,[8] a discovery for which he received the Nobel Prize in 1928. In 1903, Tunis was heavily populated by typhus patients, and Charles Nicolle, director of the Pasteur Institute in Tunis, observed that patients could infect others out on the street and that their clothing was also infectious. After the patients had a hot bath and were dressed in hospital clothing, they ceased to be infectious. Later, he fed uninfected lice to experimentally infected bonnet monkeys (*Macacus sinicus*) and then transferred the lice to uninfected monkeys that later developed typhus.[8] Moreover, Plazy, Marcandier, and Pirot observed the first Mediterranean cases of murine typhus, which was caused by *Rickettsia typhi*, in sailors on warships from Toulon, France. From 1926 to 1932, 135 cases of murine typhus were observed on warships from Toulon. Observations were even made by Lépine in Greece and Liban, by Blanc in Morocco, and by Nicolle in Tunis that indicated the presence of the microorganism in the brains of rats.[9]

After the 1930s, there was an absence of rickettsiosis investigations in North Africa for about 60 years. However, in the early 1970s, *R prowazekii* itself was isolated from the blood of Egyptian donkeys.[10] In contrast, other investigators had previously failed to isolate *R prowazekii* from many species of wild animals and ticks in Egypt and Sudan.[11] Since 1990, there have been a few fragmentary reports on the ecology and epidemiology of rickettsioses in North Africa, including a sero-survey of MSF infections, indicating that the seroprevalence of *R conorii* antibodies among blood donors was 1% in Egypt[12] and 5% to 9% in Tunisia, Algeria, and Morocco.[13,14] Subsequently, an important increase in the number of MSF cases was recorded in northern African countries.[15–17] Moreover, murine typhus is often unrecognized in Africa. However, 43 patient cases from southern Sudan were linked to *R typhi* in 1988 by a sero-survey,[18] and in northern Africa (ie, Tunisia and Algeria), several sporadic cases of typhus were reported in the last decade.[19] Furthermore, *R typhi* antibodies were present in healthy individuals and in patients with acute fevers of an undetermined origin in Tunisia.[16,20]

Several SFG rickettsiae have been detected in arthropods, and among these rickettsiae, some are recognized as emerging pathogens or as potential pathogens. The use of polymerase chain reaction (PCR) and sequencing methods for the identification of SFG and TG rickettsiae in ticks and fleas has led to new questions regarding the geographic distribution of rickettsiae in North Africa and the arthropod–rickettsia association. Here, the authors present an overview of the various flea-, tick-, and louse-borne rickettsioses described to date in North Africa. They also discuss some epidemiologic circumstances that have contributed to the emergence or re-emergence of these rickettsioses in this area.

EXPOSURE

Rickettsiae are small obligate intracellular bacteria that are strongly associated with eukaryotic cells. They are often found in arthropods (ticks, mites, and other insects, including lice, fleas, beetles, and homopterans), amoebae, and leeches. Only blood-sucking arthropods are able to transmit the disease to people, and transmission occurs via transdermal inoculation with the arthropod's saliva. Rickettsiae from the SFG are transmitted by ticks, fleas, and mites, and rickettsiae from the TG are transmitted by fleas and lice. The arthropods can act as vectors and sometimes as the principal reservoirs of the rickettsiae.[2] Thus, exposure to the disease is closely linked to exposure to the arthropod vectors. Most of the vectors favor specific optimal environmental conditions, biotopes, and hosts. These factors determine the geographic repartition of the vector and, consequently, the risk area for the diseases.[1]

DISEASES
Tick-Borne Rickettsioses

In many cases, tick-borne rickettsiae infect and colonize the organs of ticks, particularly the salivary glands and ovaries of adult females. This infection pattern enables some species of ticks to transmit rickettsiae to vertebrate hosts during feedings and from 1 tick generation to the next.[1] In North Africa, 8 rickettsial species, all human pathogens, have been detected from ticks or human cases, including *R conorii* subspecies *conorii*, *R conorii* subspecies *israelensis*, *R aeschlimannii*, *R sibirica mongolitimonae*, *R massiliae*, *R slovaca*, *R raoultii*, and *R monacensis* (**Fig. 1**, **Table 1**).[21–27]

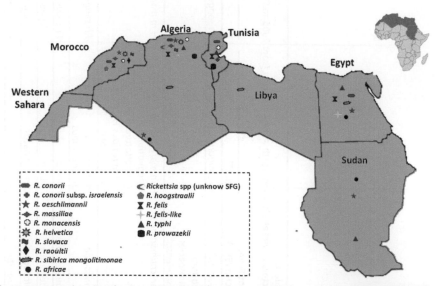

Fig. 1. Geographic distribution of Spotted fever group (SFG) and typhus group (TG) *rickettsiae* (isolated in vectors and/or in human) in North Africa.

Table 1
Vectors of rickettsioses in North Africa reported from 2005 to 2011

Spot Fever Group (SFG)	Algeria		Morocco		Tunisia		Egypt		Sudan	
	Tick (T)	Fleas (F)	T	F	T	F	T	F	T	F
R conorii[a]	Rh sanguineus	—	Rh sanguineus	—	—	—	—	—	—	—
R conorii subspecies israelensis[b]	—	—	—	—	—	—	—	—	—	—
R aeschlimannii[a]	H m marginatum H aegyptium H impeltatum H m rufipes H dromedarii	—	H m marginatum	—	H impeltatum H.dromedarii	—	H aegyptium H dromedarii H impeltatum	—	H dromedarii H truncatum	—
R massiliae	Rh turanicus Rh sanguineus	—	Rh sanguineus	—	—	—	—	—	—	—
R monacensis	I ricinus	—	I ricinus	—	I ricinus	—	—	—	—	—
R helvetica	I ricinus	—	I ricinus	—	I ricinus	—	—	—	—	—
R slovaca	D marginatus	—	D marginatus	—	—	—	—	—	—	—
R raoultii	—	—	D marginatus	—	—	—	—	—	—	—

Agent						
R sibirica mongolitimonae[b]	—	—	—	—	—	—
R africae	H dromedarii	—	—	—	—	Am lepidum, Am variegatum
R felis[a]	C felis, C canis, Ar erinacei, X cheopis	—	C felis	—	—	C felis, E gallinacea
R hoogstraalii	—	Hae sulcata	—	—	—	—
Rickettsia species	Rh sarguineus, Hae erinacei	—	—	—	—	—
Typhus Group (TG)	**Lice (L)**	F	L	F	L	F
R typhi[a]	X cheopis	F	—	—	—	X cheopis, L segnis
R prowazekii[a]	—	—	P h corporis[c]	—	—	—

Abbreviations: Am, Amblyomma; Ar, Archeopsylla; C, Ctenocephalides; D, Dermacentor; d, detritum; E, Echidnophaga; H, Hyalomma; Hae, Haemaphysalis; I, Ixodes; L, Leptopsylla; m, marginatum; Rh, Rhipicephalus; X, Xenopsylla.
[a] Rickettsia in people and vectors.
[b] Rickettsia in people.
[c] Pediculus humanus corporis by Nicolle in Tunis 1909.

Mediterranean spotted fever

MSF, also known as boutonneuse fever, is caused by *R conorii* subspecies *conorii* and is endemic in the Mediterranean countries. *Rh sanguineus*, the brown dog tick, is the main vector, and it may also act as the reservoir of the disease (**Fig. 2**).[1] MSF is the most abundant human tick-borne rickettsiosis known to occur in North Africa.[17] After an incubation period of around 6 days, the onset of MSF is abrupt. Typical patients have a high fever, influenza-like symptoms, a local necrotic inflammation with a black crust known as an eschar (the tache noire) at the tick bite site, and a generalized maculopapular rash.[1,28] Occasionally, the eschar is not found, but it is also rarely observed at multiples sites, as a consequence of multiple bites by infected ticks.[28] Severe forms, including major neurologic manifestations and multiple organ involvement, may occur in 5% to 6% of cases.[1]

Several case series of MSF have been published in recent years from North Africa. In particular, cases have been increasingly reported in Algeria.[17] In a prospective study conducted in 2004 in Oran, 93 MSF cases were confirmed using serologic tools. The clinical signs of these patients were as follows: the presence of an underlying disease (44%), sudden onset (78%), fever (100%), loss of weight (63%), conjunctivitis (43%), and the presence of eschar (70%). The existence of severe and malignant forms was reported in 6.4% of MSF cases, as characterized by the occurrence of complications and death (3.2%).[29] The clinical signs of MSF for 34 children hospitalized in Oran hospital were moderate fever, splenomegaly (38.2%), and digestive signs such as vomiting (10%), diarrhea (12%), and hepatomegaly (9%).[30] An eschar was present in 91% of the cases and typically at the cephalic level (retro-auricular, the lobule of the ear, scalp), but sometimes within the trunk region. Neurologic signs included headaches (29.4%), meningism (17.6%), convulsions (5%), meningitis (6%), coughing (6%), and arthralgia, particularly in the knees (5.7%). The analysis of the epidemiologic and clinical aspects of MSF in Algeria was extended to the following years. As in a study conducted in 2005,[17] uncommon aspects were found, such as an increased incidence and the presence of multiple inoculation eschars in 12% of the patients. Also, 49% of the patients were hospitalized with a severe form of MSF, and the global death rate was 3.6%. Furthermore, the MSF incidence was 54.5% in patients hospitalized with major neurologic manifestations and multiple organ involvement.[17] In the last study in Algeria on 39 patients, underlying conditions were present in 13 patients (33%): diabetes (10.2%), hypertension (5%), chronic renal failure (2.5%), cervical cancer (2.5%), bronchial

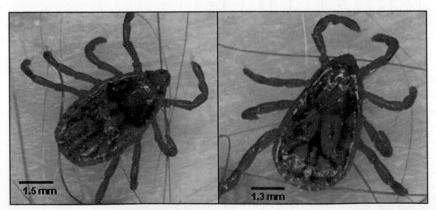

Fig. 2. Adult, female (nonengorged) and male stage of *Rhipicephalus sanguineus,* the brown dog tick, implicated in the transmission of *Rickettsia conorii* in the North Africa.

cancer (2.5%), and tobacco consumption (15%).[31] Moreover, lymphadenopathy was found near the eschar of 8 (20.5%) patients. A parallel study on the epidemiologic and clinical aspects of MSF was conducted in eastern Algeria in Batna.[32] In this study, only 4.6% of the 108 included patients with eruptive fever were confirmed by an MSF diagnosis using molecular and serologic tools.

MSF has been described in Algeria's neighboring countries, such as Tunisia and Morocco. In 2007, 45 MSF patients were diagnosed in Morocco; 75% had inoculation eschars (25% of them presented several inoculation eschars). The rate of case fatalities of MSF was reported to be 5% in these patients.[15] One prospective study was conducted at the ophthalmology unit at Monastir (Tunisia), and 30 patients with confirmed MSF underwent a complete ophthalmic examination. Unilateral or bilateral posterior segment involvement was described in 83% of patients. White retinal lesions were frequent, but only 30% of the patients had ocular complaints. Most of these abnormalities were resolved after 3 to 10 weeks, and final visual acuity was restored in 93% of the affected eyes.[33] In that same hospital in Monastir, 200 patients were diagnosed with MSF during the period from January 1987 to December 2006. Clinically, fever was the most common symptom (100%), followed by rashes (98.5%), headaches (76.5%), arthromyalgias (64.5%), eschar (63%), conjunctival hyperemia (23%), local lymphadenopathy (18%), coughing (10.5%), and meningitis (1%).[34] In Sousse, central Tunisia, the diagnosis of MSF was confirmed in 62 cases among 269 patients with acute unknown fevers. Severe forms were reported in 3.5% of the patients, with favorable outcomes.[16]

In North Africa, most MSF cases are diagnosed during July and October, similar to what is reported in southern Europe.[1,16,17] This is probably linked to the increased aggressiveness and propensity of Rh sanguineus to bite hosts during warmer conditions.[35] Direct contact with dogs or domestic animals has been reported in 76.5% to 95.2% of the cases, and a history of a tick bite has been given in 38% to 50.3% of the cases.[15–17,30,34,36,37] The tick was still attached to 10.2% of the patients at the time of the consultation in the largest recent series Algeria.[17] Recently, it was experimentally demonstrated that Rh sanguineus readily bites people when exposed to higher temperatures.[35]

Israeli spotted fever

R conorii subspecies israelensis was first isolated by Goldwasser in 1974 in Israel, where Israeli spotted fever (ISF) disease is endemic.[38] Later, the disease appeared to be more widely spread in the Mediterranean countries than first believed, because cases from Italy and Portugal were reported. Previously, R conorii subspecies israelensis was detected in a Rh sanguineus tick in Sicily.[1] The clinical manifestations of ISF are similar to those of other spotted fever group infections, but an inoculation eschar is rarely observed. Additionally, a history of tick exposure is not always present.[38] In Sfax (southern Tunisia), 2 cases of ISF, which were confirmed by the detection of rickettsial DNA in skin biopsies, have been described. One patient had a fever of 38°C, chills, a headache, and arthromyalgia without hemodynamic abnormalities. A second patient was admitted with a fever of 41°C, conjunctivitis, and cardiovascular collapse and treated in an intensive care unit for 1 day. This patient worked in the livestock importation industry, and his illness developed 5 days after his return from a 2-week trip to Libya.[26]

R aeschlimannii infections

R aeschlimannii was first isolated from Hyalomma marginatum marginatum ticks collected from Morocco in 1992.[1] The first human infection caused by R aeschlimannii was in a French patient who became ill after returning from a trip to Morocco. The patient exhibited symptoms similar to those of MSF, including an eschar on his ankle, a high fever, and a generalized maculopapular rash. The definitive diagnosis was made by PCR amplification of rickettsial DNA in the patient's early serum.[39] Recently, 2 new cases were reported in Algeria.[40] One patient, an 80-year-old man, reported contact with dogs parasitized by ticks. He had a 7-day history of a high fever, a headache, myalgia, and vomiting. Upon physical examination, a generalized maculopapular rash, 2 eschars (right shoulder and knee), and bilateral hemorrhagic signs on the retina were observed. A second patient, a 36-year-old man, reported a 15-day history of fever with a headache. He presented with a maculopapular rash and purpuric lesions on his arms.[40]

R aeschlimannii was detected by molecular tools in *H marginatum marginatum* from Algeria[41] and Morocco.[24] *H marginatum marginatum* is known as the Mediterranean *Hyalomma* and may represent, for example, up to 42% of the ticks found on cattle in Morocco. This rickettsia has also been detected in *H aegyptium* ticks collected from Algerian tortoises, in *H dromedarii, H impeltatum, H marginatum rufipes,* and *H truncatum* collected from camels or cows from Egypt, Sudan, Algeria, and Tunisia.[21,42–45]

R sibirica mongolitimonae infections

R sibirica mongolitimonae causes lymphangitis-associated rickettsiosis (LAR). This rickettsia, formerly known as *R sibirica* HA-91, was first isolated from *H asiaticum* ticks collected in the Alashian region of Inner Mongolia.[46] In 1996, the first human infection was diagnosed in southern France in a woman who had a febrile rash and a single inoculation eschar on her groin.[47] A *R sibirica mongolitimonae* infection was also diagnosed in 2 French travelers.[27,46] A 62-year-old woman returned from a trip to southern Algeria, without history of tick-bites and camel contact, presented fever, myalgias, and headache. She developed 2 inoculation eschars on the left foot and hypochondrium associated with a generalized maculopapular rash involving the palms and soles but not the face. In September 2009, a previously healthy 52-year-old man living in France was admitted with a 10-day history of fever, asthenia, headache, and arthromyalgia. Three days earlier, he had returned from a 2-week trip to Egypt. He had a fever (38°C), painful axillary lymphadenopathies, and an inoculation eschar surrounded by an inflammatory halo on the left scapular area (**Fig. 3**), without rash. The diagnosis of the both cases was made on the basis of serology, molecular tools, and a positive culture.[27,46] Although *R sibirica mongolitimonae* is apparently associated with *Hyalomma* subspecies ticks in North Africa, more experimental data are needed to determine the tick vectors and reservoirs of this rickettsia.

Other tick-borne rickettsiae

R slovaca was isolated in 1968 from *Dermacentor marginatus* ticks in Czechoslovakia, and in 1997, it was first described as a human pathogen and the agent of tick-borne lymphadenopathy (TIBOLA), which is also known as *Dermacentor*-borne necrotic erythema and lymphadenopathy (DEBONEL).[48] As other bacterial agents have been reported to cause the same symptoms, the term SENLAT (scalp eschars and neck lymphadenopathy following tick bites) has been proposed for this clinical entity.[49] This bacterium has been found in *D marginatus* and *D reticulatus* ticks in a great majority of European countries,[1,48] and only in *D marginatus* ticks collected in vegetation from Morocco[24] and the mountains of Chréa, Algeria.[23] These mountains are increasingly visited by tourists, and there is a risk of being bitten by *D marginatus* ticks carrying *R slovaca* in this area.[23] Moreover, several rickettsial isolates from *Dermacentor* subspecies ticks collected in Russia and France in 2008 have been characterized using multigene sequencing and classified as new and unique *Rickettsia* species now

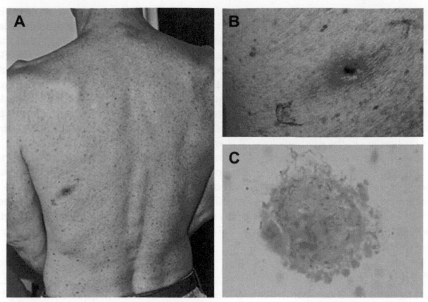

Fig. 3. (*A*) Eschar on the scapular area of a patient infected with *Rickettsia sibirica mongoliti-monae*. (*B*) Close-up view of eschar. (*C*) *R sibirica mongolitimonae* growing in L929 cells, stained in red by Gimenez staining. ([*C*] *From* Socolovschi C, Barbarot S, Lefebvre M, et al. Rickettsia sibirica mongolitimonae in traveler from Egypt. Emerg Infect Dis 2010;16(9):1495–6.)

known as *R raoultii*.[50] In 2002, *R raoultii* was detected by PCR in a *D marginatus* tick taken from the scalp of a patient in France who had developed a typical clinical picture of TIBOLA. In a French study on SENLAT, 8% of patients had *R raoultii* infections.[48] *R raoultii* has been detected in *D marginatus* ticks in Morocco.[24] This tick is found in the cooler and more humid areas of the Mediterranean region, which are associated with the Atlas Mountains, and the tick is restricted to small areas of Morocco and Tunisia.[23,24]

In 1992, a novel rickettsial agent was isolated from *Rh sanguineus* ticks collected near Marseille (France). It was characterized as a distinct species within the SFG group of rickettsiae and named *R massiliae*.[51] *R massiliae* is an emerging pathogen, with only 3 cases of human infections described in Italy, southern France, and Argentina.[52] This phenomenon is in stark contrast with the high infection rate found in *Rhipicephalus* ticks, which have a worldwide distribution that spans America, Africa, and Europe.[1,52] The few reported cases might be because of the low pathogenicity of these bacteria or misdiagnoses. In North Africa, this rickettsia has been detected in 4.7% of *Rh sanguineus* and 26.7% of *Rh bursa* from Morocco,[24,53] in 4 *Rh turanicus* (2 collected on cattle, 1 collected on a goat, 1 collected on a hedgehog), and 4 specimens of *Rh sanguineus* (collected on a hedgehog) from Algeria.[41]

The presence of *Rickettsia helvetica* and *R monacensis* has been described in *Ixodes ricinus* ticks in Algeria, Tunisia and Morocco.[22–25] *R helvetica* is a member of the SFGR and presumptively associated with human illnesses. In 2 patients from Spain, *R monacensis* was detected in blood samples using molecular tools, and 1 rickettsial strain was isolated by shell vial culture. One patient was an 84-year-old man from La Rioja (Spain) who had a fever and maculopapular rash without an inoculation eschar. The second patient was a 59-year-old woman from the Basque region of

Spain. She had a history of a tick bite, fever, and a rash at the tick bite site.[54] With these results, *R monacensis* joins the list of autochthonous *Rickettsia* subspecies confirmed as human pathogens in North Africa.

To date, *Rickettsia africae*, the agent responsible for African tick bite fever (ATBF) and mainly associated with *Amblyomma* ticks, is considered the most common rickettsioses in sub-Saharan Africa (**Fig. 4**).[55] However, it has been detected in northern Africa too. In Sudan, *R africae* has been detected in *Amblyomma lepidum* and *A variegatum*.[45] In addition, *R africae* has been detected in *H dromedarii* collected on camels (*Camelus dromedarius*) in Algeria and in *H dromedarii* in Egypt.[56,57] The role of *H dromedarii* in the epidemiology of *R africae* requires further investigation.

Finally, *Rickettsia* endosymbiont of *Haemaphysalis sulcata* was detected in *Haemaphysalis* subspecies ticks from Morocco in 2008.[24] Recently, this rickettsia was isolated from soft tick *Carios capensis* in Georgia, United States and from *H sulcata* in Croatia and named *Rickettsia hoogstraalii*.[58] Moreover, another *Rickettsia* species from SFGR was detected in 11.25% of *Rh sanguineus* and in 77% of *H erinacei* ticks collected in hedgehogs from Algeria.[59] The *Rickettsia* species is phylogenetically close to *Rickettsia heilongjiangensis*.

Flea-Borne Rickettsioses

To date, there are 2 flea-borne rickettsioses. The first is *Rickettsia felis,* an emerging pathogen that belongs to the SFG, and the second is *R typhi* from the TG. Besides flea-borne pathogens such as *Yersinia pestis,* the plague agent that is transmitted by the rat flea *Xenopsylla cheopis,* fleas, and human flea-borne infections has been scarcely studied in North Africa. These 2 flea-borne rickettsioses have worldwide distributions, and in recent years, several scientific reports related to the presence of these rickettsiae in North African countries have been authored.

Flea-borne spotted fever

R felis was probably first detected in the cat flea *Ctenocephalides felis* (**Fig. 5**) in 1918 by Sikora. This work was overlooked until 1990, when an ELB agent was found in *C felis* fleas using electron microscopy.[60] This agent was demonstrated to be a *Rickettsia*-like organism. The first evidence of the pathogenicity of *R felis* was noted in 1994 when this agent was detected in blood samples obtained from a patient in Texas,

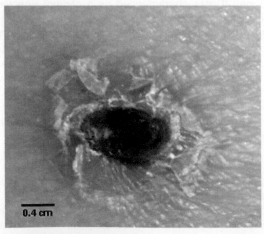

Fig. 4. Tick bite fever eschar.

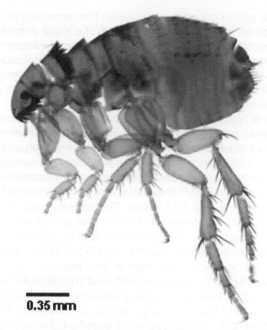

0.35 mm

Fig. 5. Femelle *Ctenocephalides felis felis* fleas, main vector of *Rickettsia felis*.

United States.[61] Within the last 20 years, growing numbers of reports have been published that implicate *R felis* as a human pathogen, which parallels the fast-growing number of reports on the worldwide detection of *R felis* in arthropods other than fleas, such as ticks, mites, mosquitoes, and booklice.[62] In a rickettsial study in Tunisia from 1998 to 2003, 8 patients with *R felis* infections were confirmed using serologic tools. Most of the patients lived in urban areas, and 1 patient came from Libya. All 8 patients had fevers and a maculopapular rash. Two patients had peripheral adenopathy on admission: cervical and inguinal in the first patient and axillary and inguinal in the second patient. Also, 1 patient with *R felis* infection had pulmonary involvement. Although none had an eschar or a history of a flea bite, 3 patients had contact with animals.[63] In addition, flea spotted fever has been reported in 2 patients from Batna, eastern Algeria, and in another patient from Sousse, central Tunisia.[16,32]

Initially, *R felis* was detected in *C canis* fleas collected from rodents in the Oran district of Algeria.[64] In that same study, *R felis*-like organisms were detected in *Archeopsylla erinacei* from hedgehogs, which was similar to the *Rickettsia RF2125* detected in fleas from Thailand. Subsequently, in Algeria, a high prevalence (95.5%) of *R felis* was reported in fleas collected from hedgehogs,[59] and a new flea species, *Xenopsylla cheopis*, was described as a potential vector of this bacterium.[65] In Morocco, *R felis* DNA was detected in 29% of *C felis* fleas collected from cats and dogs, as well as from a herd of sheep from the same location.[66] Moreover, *R felis* was detected in 100% of *Echidnophaga gallinacea* fleas collected from 5 *Rattus rattus* (black rats) trapped in Mansoura and Zagazig (Egypt). Two additional spotted fever groups of *Rickettsia* subspecies. were identified in 2 *X cheopis,* from a black rat in Suez and a Norwegian rat in Alexandria, but definitive species identifications were not possible.[67]

Flea-borne typhus
The ubiquitous murine typhus is caused by *R typhi*, and its main vector is the rat flea (*X cheopis*). Most persons become infected when flea feces containing *R typhi*

contaminate broken skin or are inhaled; however, infections may also result from flea bites. Clinically, after an incubation period of 7 to 14 days, the most common symptoms include a fever, which can last 3 to 7 days, headache, rash, and arthralgia. The rash associated with murine typhus is described as being nonpruritic, macular, or maculopapular and starts on the trunk and then spreads peripherally, sparing the palms and soles. The mortality rate for murine typhus is low (1%) with the use of appropriate antibiotics.[68]

Since 1993, murine typhus has been re-emerging in Tunisia, both among the indigenous population and travelers.[69] In 2005, 7 cases were documented in Tunisia. Clinical features were as follows: a sudden onset of a fever, maculopapular rash (5 cases), prostration (4 cases), meningism (3 cases) and pneumonia (4 cases). Several complications of the murine typhus were described, including neuropsychiatric abnormalities, meningitis, and renal failure.[69] In the last study on murine typhus in Tunisia on 43 patients, the mean age was 43.1 years. The patients were from rural areas in 58.1% of the cases, and the cases were more prevalent during the summer and autumn. The most frequent clinical presentation was an isolated fever (67.5%), but a cutaneous rash and headache were noted in 44.1% and 60.5% of the cases, respectively. No patients reported exposure to rats or their fleas.

In 2008, 2 cases of *R typhi* infection were confirmed in patients in Oran, Algeria.[19] One patient, a 42-year-old male pharmacist who reported contact with cats and dogs, consulted for a 10-day history of a high fever, sweating, headache, arthralgia, myalgia, cough, and 6-kg weight loss. No rash, eschar, or specific signs were found. The second patient, a 25-year-old farmer, was hospitalized for a 5-day history of fever, headache, diarrhea, and lack of response to a treatment with amoxicillin. He reported contact with cats and cattle, and a discrete macular rash and pharyngitis were observed.[19] In Batna (eastern Algeria), murine typhus was responsible for 3.7% (4 of 108 cases) of the cases of febrile exanthemas.[32]

Murine typhus is mainly transmitted by the fleas of rodents and is associated with cities and ports where urban rats are abundant. The rat reservoir not only serves as a host for the flea vector but also makes rickettsiae available in the blood for fleas, which transmit rickettsiae back to a rat host during subsequent feedings.[68] Although murine typhus often goes unrecognized in Africa, in 1967, 32% of the serum specimens from *Acomys* (spiny mice) near the Red Sea (Egypt) tested positive for TG agglutinins.[70] In addition, the prevalence of the *R typhi* antibody in dog sera was only 0.4%, while 25% of *Rattus norvegicus* and 11% of *Rattus rattus* rodents had measurable antibodies.[71] Anti-*R typhi* antibodies were reported in 1 louse and in mice in Algeria.[72] Subsequently, *R typhi* was detected in *X cheopis* and *Leptopsylla segnis* from rats from 9 cities in Egypt and in 4 *X cheopis* fleas in 2 regions of western Algeria.[65,67]

Body Louse-Borne Rickettsioses

Transmission of *R prowazekii*, the etiologic agent of epidemic typhus, from lice to people occurs by contamination of the bite site with feces containing rickettsiae or by contamination of conjunctivae or mucous membranes with the crushed bodies or feces of infected lice.[73,74] Clinically, the incubation period of epidemic typhus is usually 10 to 14 days. Patients usually have 1 to 3 days of malaise before the abrupt onset of severe headaches and fever. In a study in Burundi,[75] a crouching attitude caused by myalgia was reported, and abdominal pain was also common.[74] Other symptoms vary and include severe myalgias, arthralgias, rashes, and nonspecific constitutional symptoms (ie, malaise, anorexia, chills), and central nervous system (CNS) manifestations (eg, delirium, coma, and seizures) occur in up to 80% of the cases.[74,75] Recently, a case of epidemic typhus in a 64-year-old woman with generalized febrile exanthema was reported in the Batna region of Algeria.[76] She was a native Algerian who had always lived in the Batna area, a mountainous town in eastern Algeria at an elevation of 1038 m. Her symptoms started 8 days before hospitalization with a fever, asthenia, arthralgia, and a headache. Four days after the onset of symptoms, she developed a generalized maculopapular skin rash. On admission, she had a temperature of 40.2°C and a maculopapulous rash involving her whole body, except for the face, palms, and soles. She complained of severe asthenia, headache, and arthralgia. No inoculation eschar was found, and no body lice were found on her clothing. The clinical examination was otherwise normal.[76] More recently, another case of epidemic typhus was diagnosed in the same region of Algeria.[32]

Finally, the eradication of epidemic typhus is not simple. If a person with a *R prowazekii* infection is simultaneously infested with lice (**Fig. 6**), an epidemic focus of epidemic typhus can re-emerge. In addition, *R prowazekii* infections can be acquired through reservoirs other than people, such as flying squirrels in the United States.[74]

RICKETTSIOSES IN TRAVELERS FROM NORTH AFRICA

The increase in international traffic for various reasons, such as tourism, professional interests, and family matters, results in greater vulnerability of travelers throughout the world to the transmission of old, new, and re-emerging infectious diseases. During their trip, travelers are exposed to unusual infectious diseases, and the main symptom that is frequently present in those who return ill is fever.[77] Several rickettsiosis have been described in European travelers from North Africa. The Geosentinel network investigated the epidemiology of rickettsial diseases among 99,355 ill returned travelers between 1996 and 2008. Three of 231 SFGRs were reported among international travelers from North African countries.[55] Recently, 4 cases of MSF were reported in Belgian travelers returning from Morocco after a visit to friends and relatives in their country of origin. One patient presented a clinical picture of meningoencephalitis with serious neurologic impairment; the second patient presented with a lung embolism. The third patient presented with septic shock and multiple organ failure, and the fourth patient presented fever and a markedly swollen inguinal lymph node.[78,79] A fatal case of ISF after a Mediterranean cruise has been reported in Switzerland in patient without animal contact and history of tick bite.[80] This patient visited several archeological sites in Libya (Cyrene, Apollonia, Ptolemais, Leptis Magna, Sabratha). At 6 days after symptom onset, the patient was confused and exhibited bilateral dysdiadochokinesis in association with a maculopapular rash involving the trunk, limbs, palms, and soles and petechial lesions on the right arm.

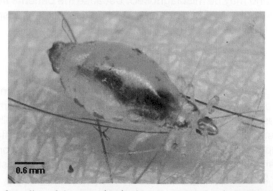

Fig. 6. The adult femelle of human body louse, *Pediculus humanus humanus* (or *P h corporis*).

Interestingly, the first human infection caused by R aeschlimannii was reported in 2002 in a patient returning from Morocco to France.[39] In addition, 2 cases from 16 reported in the English literature about R sibirica mongolitimonae infection were described in travelers from Algeria and from Egypt.[27,46]

Besides tick-borne rickettsiosis, several murine typhus cases have been reported after travels in Tunisia, Morocco, and Egypt.[77,81] Of the 32 murine typhus cases that were diagnosed from 2008 to 2010 at the World Health Organization (WHO) Collaborative Center for Rickettsial diseases (Marseille, France), 40.6% (n = 13/32) were acquired in African countries. All cases were observed during the late summer and early autumn, and the patients suffered from a persistent fever.[77] Most patients were travelers from Tunisia. Additionally, 1 case of epidemic typhus was imported into France from Algeria. In October 1998, a 65-year-old man was evaluated in Marseille for fever, nausea, vomiting, myalgias, and diarrhea. He was a native Algerian who lived in France but had visited Msila, a small town in east central Algeria, for 3 months. The patient recalled pruritis and scratching during his stay in Algeria. However, no lice were found on his clothing. He had a temperature of 40°C, mild confusion, a discrete rash, and splenomegaly. This diagnosis was confirmed by serologic testing and the isolation of R prowazekii in his blood.[82] A supplementary element of the complexity in the epidemiology of R prowazekii infection is Brill-Zinsser disease. Under stress conditions or a waning immune system, R prowazekii infection can be reactivated in people years or decades after the primary infection. Two cases of Brill-Zinsser disease have been reported in travelers.[83,84] Using serologic tools (high immunoglobulin [Ig] G and the absence of IgM titers to R prowazekii), Brill-Zinsser disease was diagnosed in 1999 in a 65-year-old man who had epidemic typhus in 1960 during the Algerian civil war. At admission to a hospital, he presented a fever, rash, and severe asthenia.[83] In 2011, the second case of Brill-Zinsser disease was reported in a French patient born in Morocco who had no history of epidemic typhus. After 2 days of a high-grade fever associated with a headache, myalgia, fatigue, and mild cough, a 69-year-old man living in France sought care from his general practitioner on March 7, 2011. Amoxicillin was prescribed for the putative diagnosis of an acute respiratory infection. The patient was raised in Morocco, and, at 19 years of age, he immigrated to France, where he lived in an urban area. He subsequently traveled every 3 years to urban areas in Morocco for 1-month summer holidays. He denied any history of hospitalization for severe febrile illnesses and any exposure to louse bites. In the weeks before disease onset, he had not taken any new drug and had no immunoglobulin deficiency.[84] In conclusion, rickettsioses have emerged in the field of travel medicine and may be misdiagnosed, because the patients frequently present with nonspecific symptoms. These diseases should be highly suspected in febrile patients returning from the North Africa.

DIAGNOSTIC

The diagnosis of rickettsial infections is often difficult. The clinical signs and symptoms (eg, fever, headache, nausea, vomiting, and muscle aches) resemble many other infectious diseases during early stages when antibiotic treatment is most effective. A history of exposure to the appropriate vector (eg, tick, louse, or flea) is helpful but cannot be relied upon. To date, an immunofluorescence assay (IFA) on serum samples is used as a reference technique in most laboratories for the diagnosis of human rickettsioses (Table 2).[1] Sensitivity and specificity vary depending on the species involved, and cut-off levels are determined by each laboratory. In the WHO collaborative center for rickettsial diseases in Marseille, titers of ≥1/128 for IgG and ≥1/32 for

Table 2			
New approaches to rickettsiosis diagnosis			
Tools	Samples	Test	Note
Serology	Serum samples	Immunofluorescence assay	• The reference method • Cut-off at the WHO collaborative Center in Marseille: titers of ≥1/128 for IgG and ≥1/32 for IgM in acute phase serum specimens and/or evidence of seroconversion with a fourfold increase in IgG titer
Western Blot study	Serum samples	Western Blot study with cross-adsorption	• Make a distinction between several rickettsial species from SFG or TG, in some cases, also with other intracellular bacteria • Available only in few reference centers
Molecular assay	EDTA anticoagulated whole blood, skin biopsies, swab, cerebral spinal fluid, paraffin-embedded specimens, detached arthropods.	• Real-time PCR • Regular PCR	• Screening test: real-time PCR for SFG and TG rickettsiae • Confirmation test: rickettsia-specific real-time PCR (epidemiology) or regular PCR targeting rickettsial-specific genes: gltA, ompA, ompB, 16S RNA, sca4 genes
Histology and immunohistochemistry (IH)	Formalin-fixed, paraffin-embedded tissue specimens	Giemsa or Gimenez stains	• Immunohistochemical methods provide superior visualization of SFG rickettsiae
Culture	Heparin anticoagulated whole blood, skin biopsies, or arthropods	Cell culture (Vero, L929, HEL, XTC-2, or MRC5 cells), shell vial	• Reference laboratories with a P3 safety level • Presence of team capable of maintaining living host cells

Abbreviations: SFG, spotted fever group; TG, typhus group.

IgM in acute-phase serum specimens and/or evidence of seroconversion with a four-fold increase in IgG titer are considered evidence of a recent infection with a *Rickettsia* species. The main issue with IFA is a cross-reactivity between species and, in some cases, with other intracellular bacteria. An early and late (separated by 2–3 weeks) serum sample should be tested. If antibody titers remain negative in these 2 samples, a second later sample (4–6 weeks) must be obtained, because, for some rickettsioses, seroconversion is only observed after 2 to 3 weeks.

In recent years, great collaborations between North African countries and France have been undertaken in the field of rickettsial diseases. Thus, the sera of patients with clinical suspicion of rickettsiosis have been sent to WHO Collaborative Center for Rickettsial Diseases and Other Arthropod-borne Bacterial Diseases, Aix Marseille University, Marseille.[15–17,20,29,30,34,36,37] When cross-reactions have been noted between several rickettsial antigens, western blotting and cross-adsorption studies have been employed to determine the rickettsial species in the Marseille laboratory.[29,85] However, this technique is very expensive and cannot be completely performed in the laboratory. Cell culture is still the ultimate means to identify and characterize rickettsiae and to confirm a clinical diagnosis of rickettsial disease. It is not, however, as sensitive as immunoassays in confirming clinical diagnoses, or molecular assays in detecting rickettsiae in acute samples.[1,85,86]

Molecular methods, including standard PCR and quantitative real-time PCR (qPCR), which target specific rickettsial genes, are actually used to detect *Rickettsia* speceis in human samples, such as EDTA blood, skin biopsies, swabs of skin lesions, cerebral spinal fluid, and paraffin-embedded specimens, and in detached arthropods. Recently, the advantages of skin swab samples for the diagnosis of rickettsial diseases have been evaluated in Algeria.[31] A first molecular screening is systematically performed with a set of primers and a probe targeting SFG *Rickettsia*. If clinically and epidemiologically suspected, a screening is then performed to target TG *Rickettsia*. When a diagnosis at the species level cannot be obtained using specific qPCR, conventional PCR followed by the sequencing of the *gltA*, *ompA*, and/or *ompB* genes is performed.[86] With the maturation of gene and genome sequencing, the molecular characterization of rickettsiae is now more frequently used than any other means of description or typing. Thus, 99 years after the description of MSF by Conor, the first molecular identification of the agent (*R conorii* subspecies *conorii*) of the disease in an inoculation eschar was performed in Tunisia.[87]

TREATMENT

Before confirmation of a diagnosis, early empiric antibiotic therapies should be prescribed in any suspected tick-transmitted rickettsiosis. Doxycycline (200 mg/d) remains the treatment of choice for tick- and flea-transmitted SFG rickettsioses, including in children. In cases of an allergy to tetracyclines, chloramphenicol or josamycin (a macrolide) may be administered, and fluoroquinolones and newer macrolides may also be used (**Table 3**).[1] However, the administration of fluoroquinolone only is associated with an increased MSF severity. Therefore, researchers do not recommend the use of this regimen for the treatment of the spotted fever group of rickettsioses.[88] In pregnant women, josamycin or newer macrolides can be used. In patients with severe diseases, doxycycline should be administered intravenously up to 24 hours after apyrexia.[1]

In North Africa, doxycycline has remained the treatment of choice and is prescribed for most rickettsioses.[15–17,19,20,30] In Tunisia, tetracycline and doxycycline are prescribed to 50% to 85% of rickettsial patients. The mean duration of treatment has been 5 to 7 days, and apyrexia has been noted 3 days after the beginning of

Table 3
Antibiotic treatments for rickettsiosis

Rickettsiosis	Patient Cohort	Selected Antibiotic Regimens	References
Mediterranean spotted fever[e,f] (R conorii conorii)	Adults	• Doxycycline, 2 oral 200-mg doses separated by a 12-h interval • Doxycycline, 200 mg single dose or 100 mg twice a day for 2 to 5 days[a,b] • Josamycin, 2 oral doses of 1 g every 8 h for 5 days[c]	1
	Children	• Doxycycline, 2.2 mg/kg every 12 h for children weighing (<45 kg) or adult dosage for other, for 5 to 10 days[a,b,d] • Clarythromycin, 15/mg/kg/d in 2 divided doses for 7 days • Azithromycin, 10 mg/kg/d in 1 dose for 3 days • Josamycin, 50 mg/kg every 12 h for 5 days	1
	Pregnant women	• Josamycin, 50 mg/kg every 12 h for 5 days[b,c]	1
Epidemic typhus[e,f] (R prowazekii)	Adults and children	• Doxycycline, 200 mg single dose or 100 mg twice a day for 5 days, or 2–4 days after defervescence[a,b] • Doxycycline, 200 mg single dose in outbreak situations	74
Endemic typhus[e,f] (R typhi)	Adults	• Doxycycline, 100 mg twice a day for 3 days after symptoms have resolved • Doxycycline, 200 mg single dose in outbreak situations	69
	Children	• Doxycycline, 0.9 mg/kg every 12 h (<45 kg) (maximum 100 mg per dose)[d]	

[a] Oral or intravenous. Intravenous formulation was generally used for patients with vomiting or severe disease. Longer courses of doxycycline treatment may be warranted for patients with severe disease.

[b] Chloramphenicol could be an alternative if it is the sole available drug for empiric treatment of severe cases, as may be the situation in developing countries.

[c] Josamycin is not available in the United States. Based on the results in children and in vitro studies, azythromycin or clarythromycin could represent alternatives.

[d] The risk of dental staining by doxycycline is negligible when a short course of therapy is given (5–10 days).

[e] Fluroquinolone treatment should be avoided.

[f] Tetracycline antibiotics are contraindicated during pregnancy because of the risks associated with interference in the development of teeth and long bones in the fetus.

Table 4
Protective measures for rickettsial infections

Arthropods	Main Measures	Alternative Measures	References
Tick	• Inspection after travel in tick-endemic area • Removal of attached ticks with tweezers or forceps close to the skin • Routine disinfection of the bite wound to avoid contamination of the bite site with skin bacteria	• Permethrin-treated clothing significantly reduces tick bites and tick-borne pathogen transmission • Repellents on the skin • Antibiotic prophylactic therapy after a tick bite is not recommended • Monitoring of persons who have undergone tick removal up to 30 days for signs and symptoms	89
Flea	• Flea control measures on pets, especially domesticated cats	• Foliage in the yard should be trimmed so that it does not provide harborage for rodents, opossums, and stray or feral cats • Screens should be placed on windows and crawl spaces to prevent entry of animals into the house • Food sources, such as open trash cans, fallen food, and pet food that could encourage wild animals to take up residence around the home should be eliminated	69
Louse	• Bathing the patient and changing and boiling infested clothes Or • Remove and leave infested clothing unworn for a week	• Eradication of lice with an insecticide (10% DDT, 1% malathion, or 1% permethrin)	74

antibiotic treatment. However, no side effects have been noted.[20] In Algeria, most MSF patients (80.8%) have been treated with doxycycline (200 mg/d for 3–8 days), while other patients have been treated with a macrolide antibiotic (josamycin; 15.6%, including children and pregnant women), chloramphenicol (1.8%), and fluoroquinolones (1.8%). The outcome has been favorable for 96.4% of the patients. A discrete skin desquamation has been observed in 59.3% of the patients, and apyrexia appeared after a mean of 2.6 days (a range of 1–7 days). Asthenia and myalgia have persisted in 72% of the patients from anywhere to a few weeks to 6 months.[17] In Morocco, 70% of MSF patients have been treated with doxycycline, 16% with fluoroquinolones, 10% with thiamphenicol, and 2% with josamycine.[15] Moreover, MSF is still often misdiagnosed in children, as are other eruptive febrile diseases. The consequences of these misdiagnoses include delays in appropriate therapies, a risk of the development of a more severe form, and even a fatal outcome.[37]

SUMMARY

The incidence of vector-borne rickettsioses in North Africa is generally unfamiliar to physicians and health authorities. In past decades, several pathogens or suspected pathogens of SFG rickettsiae have been identified: *R massiliae, R conorii* subspecies *israelensis, R slovaca, R helvetica, R monacensis, R raoultii, R africae, R sibirica mongolitimonae*, and *R felis*, and the presence of *R conorii* and 2 TG rickettsial infections have been confirmed. In addition, the curiosity of clinicians and their specific interests in rickettsioses are probably not the sole explanations for the increase in the number of reported cases in Algeria, Tunisia, and Morocco since 1993. In contrast, infections due to these pathogens are likely underestimated and misdiagnosed in other North African countries and should be considered in differential diagnoses of unknown fevers. However, an increased aggressiveness of ticks to bite people, which might be linked to climatic changes, can be hypothesized. Moreover, 3 rickettsial species, including 1 endosymbiont species and 2 other noncharacterized *Rickettsia* species, have been reported in North Africa and await further identification and description of their pathogenesis. However, the *Rickettsia* endosymbiont of *H sulctata* has been recognized as a novel species and recently named *Rickettsia hoogstraalii*.

These results are due to several works of center reference countries such as Algeria, Tunisia, and Morocco in collaboration with the French National Reference Center. The authors' results should strongly encourage other North African countries to investigate the medical aspects of rickettsioses in people and to use appropriate diagnostic tests to confirm this etiology. It may be interesting to add molecular tools (such as qPCR) as a point-of-care strategy in this area. However, entomologic and climatic studies would help to test the hypothesis that a modification of the tick vector life cycle or behavior explains the increased incidence of cases, as suggested by several authors, and may provide a link between the behavior or life cycle changes and the increased number of severe forms that have been observed by clinicians in recent years. SFG and TG rickettsioses can be effectively prevented through tick, flea, and lice control measures (**Table 4**). Finally, entomologic surveys will allow for a better understanding of arthropod-borne rickettsioses and will help to highlight the epidemiologic aspects of SFG and TG rickettsioses in North Africa.

REFERENCES

1. Parola P, Paddock CD, Raoult D. Tick-borne rickettsioses around the world: emerging diseases challenging old concepts. Clin Microbiol Rev 2005;18(4): 719–56.

2. Merhej V, Raoult D. Rickettsial evolution in the light of comparative genomics. Biol Rev Camb Philos Soc 2011;86(2):379–405.

3. Conor A, Bruch A. Une fièvre éruptive observée en Tunisie. Bull Soc Pathol Exot Filiales 1910;8:492–6.

4. Conor A, Hayat A. Nouveaux faits concernant la Fièvre Boutonneuse de Tunisie. Bull Soc Pathol Exot Filial 1910;10:759–64.

5. Olmer D, Olmer J. La fièvre boutonneuse, fièvre exanthémique du littoral méditerranéen. Paris: Masson et Cie; 1933.

6. Durand P, Conseil E. Transmission expérimentale de la fièvre boutonneuse par *Rhipicephalus sanguineus*. C R Acad Sci [D] (Paris) 1930;190:1244.

7. Blanc G, Caminopetros J. Epidemiological and experimental studies on Boutonneuse fever done at the Pasteur Institute in Athens. Arch Inst Pasteur Tunis 1932;20:394.

8. Nicolle C, Comte C, Conseil E. Transmission expérimentale du typhus exanthématique par le pou de corps. C R Acad Sci 1909;149:486–9.

9. Bertozzi I. Le typhus murin dans le bassin méditerranéen. Marseille (France): Dissertation; 1935.

10. Ormsbee RA. The hypothesis of extrahuman reservoirs of *Rickettsia prowazekii*. In: International symposium on the control of lice and louse-borne diseases. Seminal publication edition. Washington, DC: PAHO-WHO; 1972. p. 104–8.

11. Ormsbee RA, Hoogstraal H, Yousser LB, et al. Evidence for extra-human epidemic typhus in the wild animals of Egypt. J Hyg Epidemiol Microbiol Immunol 1968;12(1):1–6.

12. Botros BA, Soliman AK, Darwish M, et al. Seroprevalence of murine typhus and fievre boutonneuse in certain human populations in Egypt. J Trop Med Hyg 1989;92(6):373–8.

13. Meskini M, Beati L, Benslimane A, et al. Seroepidemiology of rickettsial infections in Morocco. Eur J Epidemiol 1995;11(6):655–60.

14. Letaief AO, Yacoub S, Dupont HT, et al. Seroepidemiological survey of rickettsial infections among blood donors in central Tunisia. Trans R Soc Trop Med Hyg 1995;89(3):266–8.

15. Boudebouch N, Sarih M, Socolovschi C, et al. Spotted fever group rickettsioses documented in Morocco. Clin Microbiol Infect 2009;15(Suppl 2):257–8.

16. Kaabia N, Bellazreg F, Hachfi W, et al. Rickettsial infection in hospitalised patients in central Tunisia: report of 119 cases. Clin Microbiol Infect 2009;15(Suppl 2): 216–7.

17. Mouffok N, Parola P, Lepidi H, et al. Mediterranean spotted fever in Algeria—new trends. Int J Infect Dis 2009;13(2):227–35.

18. Woodruff PW, Morrill JC, Burans JP, et al. A study of viral and rickettsial exposure and causes of fever in Juba, southern Sudan. Trans R Soc Trop Med Hyg 1988; 82(5):761–6.

19. Mouffok N, Parola P, Raoult D. Murine typhus, Algeria. Emerg Infect Dis 2008; 14(4):676–8.

20. Kaabia N, Letaief A. Characterization of rickettsial diseases in a hospital-based population in central Tunisia. Ann N Y Acad Sci 2009;1166:167–71.

21. Bitam I, Kernif T, Harrat Z, et al. First detection of *Rickettsia aeschlimannii* in *Hyalomma aegyptium* from Algeria. Clin Microbiol Infect 2009;15(Suppl 2):253–4.

22. Dib L, Bitam I, Bensouilah M, et al. First description of *Rickettsia monacensis* in *Ixodes ricinus* in Algeria. Clin Microbiol Infect 2009;15(Suppl 2):261–2.

23. Kernif T, Messaoudene D, Ouahioune S, et al. Spotted fever group rickettsiae identified in *Dermacentor maginatus* and *Ixodes ricinus* ticks in Algeria. Ticks Tick Borne Dis 2012. [Epub ahead of print].

24. Sarih M, Socolovschi C, Boudebouch N, et al. Spotted fever group rickettsiae in ticks, Morocco. Emerg Infect Dis 2008;14(7):1067–73.
25. Sfar N, M'ghirbi Y, Letaief A, et al. First report of *Rickettsia monacensis* and *Rickettsia helvetica* from Tunisia. Ann Trop Med Parasitol 2008;102(6):561–4.
26. Znazen A, Hammami B, Lahiani D, et al. Israeli spotted fever, Tunisia. Emerg Infect Dis 2011;17(7):1328–30.
27. Socolovschi C, Barbarot S, Lefebvre M, et al. *Rickettsia sibirica mongolitimonae* in traveler from Egypt. Emerg Infect Dis 2010;16(9):1495–6.
28. Rovery C, Raoult D. Mediterranean spotted fever. Infect Dis Clin North Am 2008; 22(3):515–30.
29. Mouffok N, Benabdellah A, Richet H, et al. Reemergence of rickettsiosis in Oran, Algeria. Ann N Y Acad Sci 2006;1078:180–4.
30. Benabdellah A, Mouffok N, Bensaad M, et al. Mediterranean spotted fever: clinical and laboratory characteristics of 34 children in Oran (Algeria). Pathol Biol (Paris) 2007;55(10):539–42.
31. Mouffok N, Socolovschi C, Benabdellah A, et al. Diagnosis of rickettsioses from eschar swab samples, Algeria. Emerg Infect Dis 2011;17(10):1968–9.
32. Mokrani K, Tebbal S, Raoult D, et al. Spotted fever rickettsioses Batna, eastern Algeria. Ticks Tick Borne Dis 2012. [Epub ahead of print].
33. Khairallah M, Ladjimi A, Chakroun M, et al. Posterior segment manifestations of *Rickettsia conorii* infection. Ophthalmology 2004;111(3):529–34.
34. Romdhane FB, Loussaief C, Toumi A, et al. Mediterranean spotted fever: a report of 200 cases in Tunisia. Clin Microbiol Infect 2009;15(Suppl 2):209–10.
35. Parola P, Socolovschi C, Jeanjean L, et al. Warmer weather linked to tick attack and emergence of severe rickettsioses. PLoS Negl Trop Dis 2008;2(11):e338.
36. Letaief A, Souissi J, Trabelsi H, et al. Evaluation of clinical diagnosis scores for Boutonneuse fever. Ann N Y Acad Sci 2003;990:327–30.
37. Mouffok N, Parola P, Abdennour D, et al. Mediterranean spotted fever in Algerian children. Clin Microbiol Infect 2009;15(Suppl 2):290–1.
38. Mumcuoglu KY, Keysary A, Gilead L. Mediterranean spotted fever in Israel: a tick-borne disease. Isr Med Assoc J 2002;4(1):44–9.
39. Raoult D, Fournier PE, Abboud P, et al. First documented human *Rickettsia aeschlimannii* infection. Emerg Infect Dis 2002;8(7):748–9.
40. Mokrani N, Parola P, Tebbal S, et al. *Rickettsia aeschlimannii* infection, Algeria. Emerg Infect Dis 2008;14(11):1814–5.
41. Bitam I, Parola P, Matsumoto K, et al. First molecular detection of *R. conorii, R. aeschlimannii,* and *R. massiliae* in ticks from Algeria. Ann N Y Acad Sci 2006; 1078:368–72.
42. Demoncheaux JP, Socolovschi C, Davoust B, et al. Detection of *Rickettsia aeschlimannii* in *Hyalomma dromedarii* ticks collected from dromedary (*Camelus dromedarius*) in Tunisia. Ticks Tick Borne Dis 2012. [Epub ahead of print].
43. Djerbouh A, Kernif T, Beneldjouzi A, et al. The first molecular detection of *Rickettsia aeschlimannii* in the ticks of camels from southern Algeria. Ticks Tick Borne Dis 2012. [Epub ahead of print].
44. Loftis AD, Reeves WK, Szumlas DE, et al. Rickettsial agents in Egyptian ticks collected from domestic animals. Exp Appl Acarol 2006;40(1):67–81.
45. Morita C, El Hussein AR, Matsuda E, et al. Spotted fever group rickettsiae from ticks captured in Sudan. Jpn J Infect Dis 2004;57(3):107–9.
46. Fournier PE, Gouriet F, Brouqui P, et al. Lymphangitis-associated rickettsiosis, a new rickettsiosis caused by *Rickettsia sibirica mongolotimonae*: seven new cases and review of the literature. Clin Infect Dis 2005;40(10):1435–44.

47. Raoult D, Brouqui P, Roux V. A new spotted-fever-group rickettsiosis. Lancet 1996;348(9024):412.
48. Parola P, Rovery C, Rolain JM, et al. *Rickettsia slovaca* and *R. raoultii* in tick-borne rickettsioses. Emerg Infect Dis 2009;15(7):1105–8.
49. Angelakis E, Pulcini C, Waton J, et al. Scalp eschar and neck lymphadenopathy caused by *Bartonella henselae* after tick bite. Clin Infect Dis 2010;50(4): 549–51.
50. Mediannikov O, Matsumoto K, Samoylenko I, et al. *Rickettsia raoultii* sp. nov., a spotted fever group rickettsia associated with *Dermacentor* ticks in Europe and Russia. Int J Syst Evol Microbiol 2008;58(Pt 7):1635–9.
51. Beati L, Raoult D. *Rickettsia massiliae* sp. nov., a new spotted fever group rickettsia. Int J Syst Bacteriol 1993;43(4):839–40.
52. Garcia-Garcia JC, Portillo A, Nunez MJ, et al. A patient from Argentina infected with *Rickettsia massiliae*. Am J Trop Med Hyg 2010;82(4):691–2.
53. Boudebouch N, Sarih M, Socolovschi C, et al. Molecular survey for spotted fever group rickettsiae in ticks from Morocco. Clin Microbiol Infect 2009;15(Suppl 2): 259–60.
54. Jado I, Oteo JA, Aldamiz M, et al. *Rickettsia monacensis* and human disease, Spain. Emerg Infect Dis 2007;13(9):1405–7.
55. Jensenius M, Davis X, von SF, et al. Multicenter GeoSentinel analysis of rickettsial diseases in international travelers, 1996-2008. Emerg Infect Dis 2009;15(11):1791–8.
56. Kernif T, Djerbouh A, Mediannikov O, et al. Rickettsia africae in *Hyalomma dromedarii* ticks (Acari-Ixodidae) from Sub-Saharan Algeria. Ticks Tick Borne Dis 2012. [Epub ahead of print].
57. Abdel-Shafy S, Allam NA, Mediannikov O, et al. Molecular detection of spotted fever group rickettsiae associated with ixodid ticks in Egypt. Vector Borne Zoonotic Dis 2012. DOI:10.1089/vbz.2010.0241.
58. Duh D, Punda-Polic V, Avsic-Zupanc T, et al. *Rickettsia hoogstraalii* sp. nov., isolated from hard- and soft-bodied ticks. Int J Syst Evol Microbiol 2010;60(Pt 4): 977–84.
59. Khaldi M, Socolovschi C, Benyettou M, et al. Rickettsiae in arthropods collected from the North African Hedgehog (*Atelerix algirus*) and the desert hedgehog (*Paraechinus aethiopicus*) in Algeria. Comp Immunol Microbiol Infect Dis 2012; 35(2):117–22.
60. Adams JR, Schmidtmann ET, Azad AF. Infection of colonized cat fleas, *Ctenocephalides felis* (Bouche), with a rickettsia-like microorganism. Am J Trop Med Hyg 1990;43(4):400–9.
61. Schriefer ME, Sacci JB Jr, Dumler JS, et al. Identification of a novel rickettsial infection in a patient diagnosed with murine typhus. J Clin Microbiol 1994; 32(4):949–54.
62. Parola P. *Rickettsia felis*: from a rare disease in the USA to a common cause of fever in sub-Saharan Africa. Clin Microbiol Infect 2011;17(7):996–1000.
63. Znazen A, Rolain JM, Hammami A, et al. *Rickettsia felis* infection, Tunisia. Emerg Infect Dis 2006;12(1):138–40.
64. Bitam I, Parola P, De La Cruz KD, et al. First molecular detection of *Rickettsia felis* in fleas from Algeria. Am J Trop Med Hyg 2006;74(4):532–5.
65. Bitam I, Baziz B, Kernif T, et al. Molecular detection of *Rickettsia typhi* and *Rickettsia felis* in fleas from Algeria. Clin Microbiol Infect 2009;15(Suppl 2):255–6.
66. Boudebouch N, Sarih M, Beaucournu JC, et al. *Bartonella clarridgeiae, B henselae* and *Rickettsia felis* in fleas from Morocco. Ann Trop Med Parasitol 2011; 105(7):493–8.

67. Loftis AD, Reeves WK, Szumlas DE, et al. Surveillance of Egyptian fleas for agents of public health significance: *Anaplasma, Bartonella, Coxiella, Ehrlichia, Rickettsia,* and *Yersinia pestis.* Am J Trop Med Hyg 2006;75(1):41–8.

68. Civen R, Ngo V. Murine typhus: an unrecognized suburban vectorborne disease. Clin Infect Dis 2008;46(6):913–8.

69. Letaief AO, Kaabia N, Chakroun M, et al. Clinical and laboratory features of murine typhus in central Tunisia: a report of seven cases. Int J Infect Dis 2005; 9(6):331–4.

70. Hoogstraal H, Kaiser MN, Ormsbee RA, et al. *Hyalomma (Hyalommina) rhipicephaloides Neumann* (Ixodoidea: Ixodidae): its identity, hosts, and ecology, and *Rickettsia conori, R. prowazeki,* and *Coxiella burneti* infections in rodent hosts in Egypt. J Med Entomol 1967;4(4):391–400.

71. Soliman AK, Botros BA, Ksiazek TG, et al. Seroprevalence of *Rickettsia typhi* and *Rickettsia conorii* infection among rodents and dogs in Egypt. J Trop Med Hyg 1989;92(5):345–9.

72. Dumas N. Rickettsiosis and chlamydiosis in Hoggar (Republic of Algeria): epidemiological sampling. Bull Soc Pathol Exot Filiales 1984;77(3):278–83.

73. Bechah Y, Capo C, Raoult D, et al. Infection of endothelial cells with virulent *Rickettsia prowazekii* increases the transmigration of leukocytes. J Infect Dis 2008; 197(1):142–7.

74. Bechah Y, Capo C, Mege JL, et al. Epidemic typhus. Lancet Infect Dis 2008;8(7): 417–26.

75. Raoult D, Ndihokubwayo JB, Tissot-Dupont H, et al. Outbreak of epidemic typhus associated with trench fever in Burundi. Lancet 1998;352(9125):353–8.

76. Mokrani K, Fournier PE, Dalichaouche M, et al. Reemerging threat of epidemic typhus in Algeria. J Clin Microbiol 2004;42(8):3898–900.

77. Walter G, Botelho-Nevers E, Socolovschi C, et al. Murine typhus in returned travelers: a report of thirty-two cases. Am J Trop Med Hyg 2012. [Epub ahead of print].

78. Demeester R, Claus M, Hildebrand M, et al. Diversity of life-threatening complications due to Mediterranean spotted fever in returning travelers. J Travel Med 2010;17(2):100–4.

79. Laurent M, Voet A, Libeer C, et al. Mediterranean spotted fever, a diagnostic challenge in travellers. Acta Clin Belg 2009;64(6):513–6.

80. Boillat N, Genton B, D'Acremont V, et al. Fatal case of Israeli spotted fever after Mediterranean cruise. Emerg Infect Dis 2008;14(12):1944–6.

81. Rozsypal H, Aster V, Skokanová V. Murine typhus - rare cause of fever return from Egypt. Klin Mikrobiol Infekc Lek 2006;12(6):244–6 [in Czech].

82. Niang M, Brouqui P, Raoult D. Epidemic typhus imported from Algeria. Emerg Infect Dis 1999;5(5):716–8.

83. Stein A, Purgus R, Olmer M, et al. Brill-Zinsser disease in France. Lancet 1999; 353(9168):1936.

84. Faucher J-F, Socolovschi C, Aubry C, et al. Brill-Zinsser Disease in Moroccan Man, France, 2011. Emerg Infect Dis 2012;18(1):171–2.

85. La Scola B, Raoult D. Laboratory diagnosis of rickettsioses: current approaches to diagnosis of old and new rickettsial diseases. J Clin Microbiol 1997;35(11): 2715–27.

86. Renvoise A, Rolain JM, Socolovschi C, et al. Widespread use of real-time PCR for rickettsial diagnosis. FEMS Immunol Med Microbiol 2012;64(1):126–9.

87. Sfar N, Kaabia N, Letaief A, et al. First molecular detection of *R. conorii* subsp. *conorii* 99 years after the Conor description of Mediterranean spotted fever, in Tunisia. Clin Microbiol Infect 2009;15(Suppl 2):309–10.

88. Botelho-Nevers E, Rovery C, Richet H, et al. Analysis of risk factors for malignant Mediterranean spotted fever indicates that fluoroquinolone treatment has a deleterious effect. J Antimicrob Chemother 2011;66(8):1821–30.
89. Socolovschi C, Mediannikov O, Raoult D, et al. Update on tick-borne bacterial diseases in Europe. Parasite 2009;16(4):259–73.

Arboviruses and Viral Hemorrhagic Fevers (VHF)

Eyal Meltzer, MD, DTM&H[a,b,*]

KEYWORDS

- Arbovirus • Viral hemorrhagic fever • Flavivirus • Filovirus • Arenavirus • Alphavirus
- Bunyavirus

KEY POINTS

- Arboviruses are transmitted through the bite of hematophagous arthropods. In addition to humans, many arboviruses infect Avifauna. Through highly mobile reservoirs, rapid and dramatic changes in epidemiology can easily occur.
- Viral hemorrhagic fever (VHF) is typified by a combination of endothelial dysfunction causing a capillary leak syndrome and a bleeding diathesis, caused by thrombocytopenia and diffuse intravascular coagulation.
- In addition to arboviruses, the VHF syndrome may be caused by several rodent and bat viruses (Ebola and Lassa viruses respectively).
- In addition to VHF, arboviruses may cause a variety of organ specific syndromes, including encephalitis, pneumonitis, nephritis and arthritis.
- Several arboviral infections (mainly Flaviviruses) are vaccine preventable. By and large, treatment is supportive, with the exception of Arenaviruses, where ribavirin is the drug of choice.

PREFACE

In 1780, Philadelphia was visited by a massive epidemic of an unusual febrile disease, with fatalities associated with severe hemorrhage.[1] The disease, then described by Dr Benjamin Rush, is now recognized as dengue fever. A century later, a febrile tugboat captain disembarked in Memphis, Tennessee and died within 24 hours. In the following weeks, 1500 Memphians succumbed to yellow fever, the town half depopulated by the ensuing panic.[2] Yet a century later, a Zairian English teacher returned

The author has nothing to disclose.

[a] Department of Medicine C, Sheba Medical Center, Center for Geographic Medicine, Tel Hashomer 52621, Israel; [b] Department of Internal Medicine, Sackler School of Medicine, Tel Aviv University, Tel Aviv 69978, Israel

* Department of Medicine C, Sheba Medical Center, Center for Geographic Medicine, Tel Hashomer 52621, Israel.

E-mail address: emeltzer@post.tau.ac.il

Infect Dis Clin N Am 26 (2012) 479–496
doi:10.1016/j.idc.2012.02.003
0891-5520/12/$ – see front matter © 2012 Elsevier Inc. All rights reserved.

id.theclinics.com

home from a field trip with fever and diarrhea; he died of profuse bleeding and shock after 13 days. In the ensuing weeks, most of his family and hospital attendants also died of a similar disease: the first recognized Ebola outbreak.[3]

These outbreaks, although centuries apart, illustrate the dramatic nature of viral hemorrhagic fever (VHF) outbreaks. These agents naturally remain at the focus of medical attention.

Many of the agents causing VHF are arthropod borne, or arboviruses. In addition to the VHF syndrome, arboviruses cause other clinical syndromes, including encephalitis and arthritis. Also, several viruses that are not arthropod borne can cause VHF.

The aim of this review is to describe the epidemiology and clinical features of salient agents of VHF, arboviral and nonarboviral, and of other arboviruses.

ARBOVIRUSES: TAXONOMY AND EPIDEMIOLOGY

Arboviruses are mostly small RNA viruses that belong to 4 families: *Flaviviridae, Bunyaviridae, Reoviridae,* and *Togaviridae* (**Fig. 1**). They are grouped together because of their similar mode of transmission: through the bite of hematophagous arthropods (mosquitoes, ticks, midges, and sandflies). Arboviruses plague all continents and climate zones. By and large, these agents are maintained in a variety of animal reservoirs, especially avian and mammalian, with man being an accidental host. A notable exception is dengue virus, which is anthroponotic. The implications are that with the sole exception of dengue, arboviral diseases are noneradicable. Also, that via highly mobile reservoir hosts (birds and even human travelers), rapid and dramatic changes in arboviral epidemiology can easily occur. This idea was amply illustrated by the 1999 introduction of West Nile virus (WNV) to the Western Hemisphere.[4]

It should also be kept in mind that human arboviral pathogens are only a fraction of all arboviruses and that the potential for emerging infection is real.

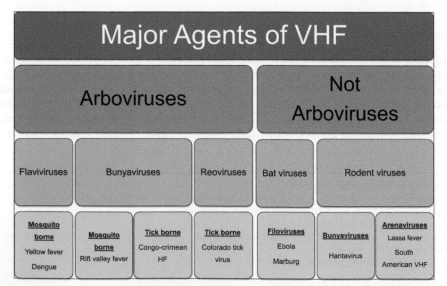

Fig. 1. Agents of viral hemorrhagic fever. Togaviruses, a large family of Arboviruses, are not included because they do not cause the VHF syndrome.

FLAVIVIRUSES

Of the 70 flavivirus species only a few are major human pathogens, including yellow fever, dengue, WNV, St Louis encephalitis (SLEV), Japanese encephalitis (JEV), Murray Valley encephalitis, and tick-borne encephalitis (TBE). As illustrated in **Fig. 2**, most of the world's population is at risk of flaviviral infections. A brief epidemiology of the major flaviviruses follows.

Dengue Virus

Dengue is by far the most prevalent human arboviral infection, with some 50 million infections yearly, and probably 500,000 fatalities.[5] Although a sylvatic cycle among Asian simians may exist,[6] dengue is largely an anthroponosis and may, therefore, be a target for eradication. Although well described since the eighteenth century,[1] the second half of the twentieth century had seen a spectacular growth in the burden of dengue. *Aedes aegypti,* the main vector of dengue virus, is extremely well adapted for survival in urban settings. The rapid urbanization of much of the tropics and subtropics has created ideal conditions for the vector, which, coupled with the dense human population and the long duration of viremia, underlies the burden of dengue. In fact, in many tropical locales in Southeast Asia, most of the adult population will have antibodies against all circulating dengue serovars.

Human activity (eg, car tire shipments) can lead to infected aedes mosquitoes being transported thousands of miles, resulting in the introduction of dengue to new areas. Thus, a massive outbreak of the dengue 2 virus (DEN-2) in Cuba in 1981 was in fact an introduction of the Southeast Asian virulent strain of DEN-2.[7]

Dengue is often perceived as a tropical disease. However, aedes mosquitoes range throughout the eastern seaboard of the United States. Autochthonous cases of dengue have been documented in Texas,[8] raising the threat of major urban outbreaks in the future. In Eurasia, *Aedes albopictus*, another dengue vector, is currently increasing its range throughout the Levant and Europe. Autochthonous cases of dengue have recently been documented in Croatia[9] and France.[10] In the twenty-first century, dengue is set to become everybody's problem rather than a third world disease.

Yellow Fever

Yellow fever is also a mosquito-borne flavivirus, transmitted by *A aegypti* from primate reservoirs. It occurs in sub-Saharan Africa, from Mauritania and Ethiopia in the north to

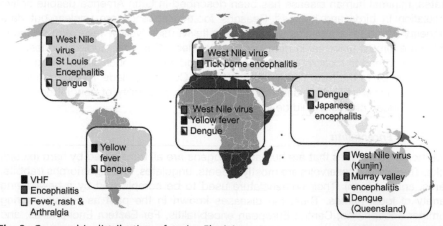

Fig. 2. Geographic distribution of major Flaviviruses.

Angola and Kenya in the south, and in most of tropical South America. However, its epidemiology is different in the two continents. In South America, sylvatic transmission is the rule and most cases occur in people traveling to the Jungle. In Africa, in addition to sylvatic transmission, urban transmission occurs, leading to occasional large-scale urban outbreaks. Most world cases are currently reported from Africa. In fact, in several West African countries, yellow fever is actually a reemerging disease, where the discontinuation of mass vaccination approximately 30 years ago has created a large, susceptible population.[11]

Japanese Encephalitis

The JEV serologic group of flaviviruses includes 8 virus species, including JEV, WNV, SLEV, Murray Valley encephalitis virus, and other minor species (see **Fig. 2**). Most of these viruses have avian hosts and are transmitted by culicine mosquitoes. For JEV, pigs may serve an important role as additional amplifying hosts. The range of JEV extends throughout East and Southeast Asia, from the Russian Far East in the north to the Torres Strait region in Northern Australia. Its range has been increasing in the latter half of the twentieth century. Within this vast range, several epidemiologic patterns exist: from marked seasonal outbreaks in temperate and monsoon dependent regions to holoendemic regions with year-round transmission. The actual burden of human disease differs greatly between regions, probably reflecting varying degrees of anthropophilia of local *Culex* species.[12]

SLEV and Murray Valley encephalitis virus are closely related to JEV and cause a similar neuroinvasive disease in the Americas and Australia respectively. SLEV was the leading diagnosed cause of viral encephalitis in the United States until it was eclipsed by WNV.[13]

West Nile Virus

WNV was initially described and recognized in Africa and the Levant. It is transmitted by mosquitoes from avian reservoirs and in many areas (eg, the Balkans and Israel) occurs seasonally, in time with the annual migration of birds from Eurasia to Africa. For reasons that are unclear, occasional years are epidemic. Thus, in 2000 and 2010, the incidence in Israel was markedly high.[14] In 1999, WNV was first detected in the Western Hemisphere. By 2005, it had spread throughout Latin America down to Argentina. However, although several large epidemics have occurred in the United States, minimal human disease has been described in Latin America despite active circulation in birds and horses.[4] Reasons for this absence are unclear but data suggests a role for antibodies against other flaviviruses (yellow fever and dengue), which are almost universal in many tropical locales.[4] Genomic studies suggest that WNV had spread to most regions (eg, Australia and India) through single introductory events, similar to the New York event in 1999.[15] Currently, clade 1 WNV dominates throughout most of Eurasia and the Americas. The possibility of new introductions of other African clades should be kept in mind.

Tick-Borne Encephalitis

Tick-borne flaviviruses that are human pathogens are all transmitted by hard (ixodid) ticks. Their natural reservoirs are mostly rodents, ungulates, and lagomorphs (rabbits, hares, and so forth). Their nomenclature used to be complicated by a bewildering variety of local names. Thus, the diseases known in the past as Russian spring summer encephalitis, Central European encephalitis, Far Eastern Encephalitis, and others are all in fact varieties of TBE.

Most tick-borne flaviviruses tend to be restricted to small endemic foci with human disease occurring in small numbers. Thus, Kyasanur Forest virus, its varieties of Alkhurma and Nanjianyin viruses, and the Omsk virus (all of whom cause a VHF syndrome) are restricted to southern India, Saudi Arabia, Western China, and Siberia respectively. TBE, however, is widely distributed in a great arc across Eurasia, from the Russian Far East to central Europe and Scandinavia.[16] Within this range, there are foci of hyperendemic disease, whereby most of the population tests seropositive. It is likely that the actual range of TBE is in fact larger (serosurveys suggest its existence in Italy and Anatolia for example);[17,18] however, cross-reacting antibodies to animal tick-borne flaviviruses hampers the interpretation of serosurveys if neutralizing antibody tests are not used. TBE can occasionally be acquired by the ingestion of milk from infected animals or by handling animal carcasses.

BUNYAVIRUSES

Bunyaviruses are a large family of RNA viruses that affect animals and plants. Of the 5 Bunyavirus genera, 4 include human pathogens: *Orthobunyavirus, Nairovirus, Phlebovirus*, and *Hantavirus* (**Fig. 3**). All but the Hantaviruses are Arboviruses and their epidemiology are discussed here.

Orthobunyavirus: Oropouche, Tahyna, La Crosse, and Related California Encephalitis Viruses

These phleboviruses are mosquito borne, with small mammals serving as reservoirs.

La Crosse virus is the most prevalent of the California virus group of Bunyaviruses (which also include California encephalitis virus and Jamestown Canyon virus. Its main hosts are squirrels and chipmunks. Most cases occur in the Mississippi and Ohio River basins during the summer months and are often associated with recreational activities in wooded areas.

Tahyna virus is another member of the California virus group. It is reported as a cause of a mild, nonspecific febrile disease from Central Europe to Russia and China and also in Africa.[19,20] It can occasionally be a cause of meningoencephalitis.

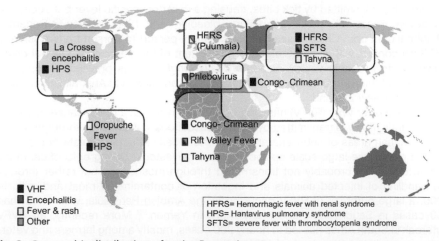

Fig. 3. Geographic distribution of major Bunyaviruses.

Oropouche is another Orthobunyavirus that is prevalent throughout much of South America and some Caribbean islands. It is unique in having a midge vector (*Culicoides paraensis*), which enables urban transmission. Large outbreaks have been described, especially in the Brazilian Amazon basin, where Oropouche is second only to dengue as a cause of arboviral fever.[21] In a recent study evaluating acute febrile patients in South America, Orthobunyaviruses were the third diagnosed group after dengue and the Alphaviruses. In this study, Oropouche was second to group C Orthobunyaviruses, a varied group of viruses that are clinically indistinguishable from the Oropouche virus.[22]

Nairoviruses: Congo-Crimean Hemorrhagic Fever

Congo-Crimean hemorrhagic fever (CCHF) is endemic in all of Africa, the Balkans, the Middle East, and Central and Southern Asia. *Hyalomma*, its principal tick vector, is found south of the 50°N, which serves as the northern geographic limit of the disease. Within this vast area, some countries report cases/outbreaks yearly, in others human cases have not been recorded despite evidence of viral circulation, and in some countries CCHF has not been recorded at all (eg, Israel, Jordan, and Lebanon). The largest number of cases is reported from Turkey, Iran, southern Russia, and Uzbekistan.[23]

Phleboviruses: Toscana and Related Viruses, Severe Fever With Thrombocytopenia Syndrome, and Rift Valley Fever

Phleboviruses differ markedly in their epidemiology, vectors, and clinical features.

Toscana, Sicily, Naples, and some other Phleboviruses are transmitted by Phlebotomine sandflies. Their natural reservoir host has not been definitely determined. They are prevalent in the Mediterranean region, where they cause sandfly fever (also known as papataci fever), a nonspecific febrile disease often with rash and myalgias. However, they also cause meningitis and encephalitis. In fact, in some countries, such as Italy, Toscana virus has been found to be a major cause of aseptic meningitis during the summer months.[24]

Severe fever with thrombocytopenia syndrome (SFTS) is a newly described phleboviral disease that has caused several outbreaks in China. Although details are sparse, it is probably transmitted by tick bites, causing a mild nonspecific fever but occasionally severe illness with multiorgan failure, bleeding, and 12% fatalities.[25] Recently, additional data from China raises the possibility of person-to-person transmission of SFTS via contact with infected blood.[26] The extent of this infection is still not clear. However, its probable vector, *Haemaphysalis longicornis*, is prevalent throughout much of East Asia and Oceania: from China, Korea, and Japan to Australia, the Pacific Islands, and New Zealand.

Rift Valley fever virus (RVFV) has long been recognized as a major cause of severe VHF in Africa. RVFV is transmitted by aedes mosquitoes. It is endemic throughout arid and savannah areas of sub-Saharan Africa and mostly affects ungulate hosts.[27] As such, it can cause large-scale epizootics among livestock. During epizootics, many human cases are probably not transmitted through mosquitoes but rather through the handling of infected animals and ingestion of contaminated meat and milk. In 2000, a large outbreak of RVFV occurred in the Arabian Peninsula, with more than 800 cases in Saudi Arabia and many more in Yemen.[28] More recently, an RVFV outbreak in South Africa has led to nearly 200 cases, mostly among farmers and veterinarians, resulting in the death of 10% of the affected population.[29]

REOVIRUSES

Reoviruses comprise a numerous family of animal and plant viruses, including such human pathogens as rotavirus. Arthropod-borne reoviruses belong to 2 genera: Coltiviruses, which are tick-borne, and Seadornaviruses, which are mosquito-borne (**Fig. 4**).

Coltiviruses: *Colorado tick fever virus* is found in the Rocky Mountain region of the United States and in Canada. The virus's distribution follows that of its vector, *Dermacentor andersoni*.[30] Additional Coltiviruses circulate in this area, including the Salmon River virus and perhaps others. All cause a similar illness: a nonspecific fever that is sometimes accompanied with rash and occasionally with meningoencephalitis. *Eyach virus* is a Coltivirus circulating in Central and Western Europe, which causes a similar disease.[31]

Seadornaviruses: These mosquito-borne viruses have only been associated with human disease in the last 2 decades. *Banna virus* is associated with febrile disease and with meningoencephalitis in China. It can infect a variety of vertebrate hosts. The virus may in fact circulate throughout much of Southeast Asia where cases are commonly mistaken for those of the cocirculating JEV.[32] Additional Seadornaviruses are currently known and are at the frontier of emerging infection research. To date, similar viruses have not been documented outside of Asia.

TOGAVIRUSES: ALPHAVIRUSES

All human Alphaviruses are mosquito borne. As illustrated in **Fig. 5**, they exist on all continents. In addition to encephalitis and fever with rash, Alphaviruses can cause a unique form of viral arthritis that can lead to prolonged morbidity, which will be described later.

Chikungunya Virus

Chikungunya virus (CHIK) emerged in Africa where it is maintained by primate reservoirs and transmitted by aedes mosquitoes. Urbanization, by combining a large concentration of susceptible hosts and allowing explosive proliferation of aedes mosquitoes, has enabled large epidemics of the disease. CHIK was documented in Southeast Asia early in the twentieth century; in fact, when dengue hemorrhagic fever

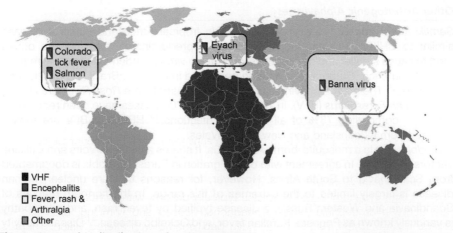

Fig. 4. Geographic distribution of major reoviruses.

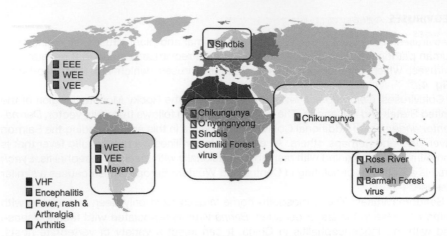

Fig. 5. Geographic distribution of major Alphaviruses. EEE, Eastern equine encephalitis; WEE, Western equine encephalitis; VEE, Venezuelan equine encephalitis.

(DHF) emerged in Thailand in the 1960s, CHIK was initially considered as a possible causative agent.[33] More recently, in 2005, a massive outbreak of CHIK developed in the Mascarenes, involving most of the population in Reunion and Mauritius. From this focus, CHIK involved many Indian Ocean countries, affecting especially India, where 1,400,000 of cases occurred.[34] The reasons for the dramatic Indian Ocean outbreak remain unclear. However, genetic studies have demonstrated viral point mutations causing enhanced viral transmission by aedes albopictus mosquitoes.[35]

Aedes albopictus (commonly referred to as the Asian tiger mosquito) is an emerging vector with increasing presence in many regions. It has become established in the Middle East and in some Southern European countries. In 2006, more than 200 cases of CHIK were diagnosed in the Emilia-Romagna region in Northern Italy. The outbreak was probably initiated by a viremic traveler returning from India in an area where *A albopictus* was well established.[36] In 2010, an autochthonous case of CHIK was diagnosed in Southeast France, again resulting from an Indian strain introduced by travelers.[37] The likelihood of similar importations in the future is high.

Other Arthritogenic Alphaviruses

Semliki forest and *O'nyongnyong* circulate in tropical Africa and cause a disease similar to CHIK.[38] For unclear reasons, CHIK predominates, whereas the others tend to cause smaller and rarer outbreaks. *Mayaro virus* is endemic to tropical regions of South America. Outbreaks have been described in Manaus, Brazil, Venezuela, and elsewhere.[39] The main Alphaviruses occurring in Australia are *Ross River virus* (RRV) and *Barmah Forest virus* (BFV). In 2008, more than 7000 cases have been reported in Australia, composing 78% of all arboviral infections.[40] RRV and BFV are mostly reported from Queensland and New South Wales.

Sindbis virus is a mosquito-borne Alphavirus. It shares avian reservoirs and Culicine vectors with WNV. In agreement with bird migration in Eurasia, Sindbis is documented from Scandinavia to South Africa. However, for reasons that are unclear, human disease is largely limited to the extremes of this range. In the northern reaches of Scandinavia and Western Russia, a disease typified by fever, rash, and arthropathy is variously known as Pogosta, Karelian fever, and Ockelbo disease.[41] Disease activity seems to peak in a 7-year cycle.

Encephalitic Alphaviruses: Eastern, Western, and Venezuelan Equine Encephalitis Viruses

These viruses are restricted to the Americas. Eastern equine encephalitis (EEE) virus is a summertime disease in the Gulf and east coastal areas of the United States, whereas Western equine encephalitis (WEE) virus is mostly diagnosed in states west of the Mississippi River. EEE is maintained in avian hosts, with horses and humans serving as dead end hosts because viremia is usually low. WEE causes higher-level viremia, and horses may, therefore, have a larger role in the virus ecology. Venezuelan equine encephalitis (VEE) virus is maintained in an enzootic cycle among rodents in South America. Intermittently, some strains cause large epizootics among horses, with concomitant epidemics in humans. The largest in recent times has been an epidemic in Venezuela and Colombia, which, in 1995, caused an estimated 100,000 human cases, 3000 of which experienced neurologic complications, with 300 associated deaths.[42] As these numbers suggest, most cases of VEE do not evolve into severe neuroinvasive disease. It is probable that in endemic countries a significant portion of disease currently diagnosed as dengue fever may in fact be attributed to VEE.[43]

NONARBOVIRAL AGENTS OF VHF: FILOVIRUSES, ARENAVIRUSES, AND HANTAVIRUSES

The VHF syndrome is not unique to Arboviruses. In fact, some of the most virulent agents of VHF are not Arboviruses. Arenaviruses and Hantaviruses have rodent reservoirs in common, and infection is usually caused via exposure to rodent excreta (**Fig. 6**). Filoviruses are probably bat viruses. Much regarding their epidemiology is conjectured, but human exposure may result from exposure to bush meat. Infected wild animals, such as apes or ungulates, may have acquired the virus via ingestion of fruit dropped by bats and contaminated by their saliva.[44] Some of these agents are unique among all the VHF agents in their ability for human-to-human infection. This fact underlay the inadvertent creation of hospital-based epidemics of VHF.

Filoviruses: Ebola and Marburg Viruses

The filoviruses derive their name from their elongated, hairlike appearance on electron microscopy. Human pathogenic filoviruses are restricted to Africa (a nonvirulent

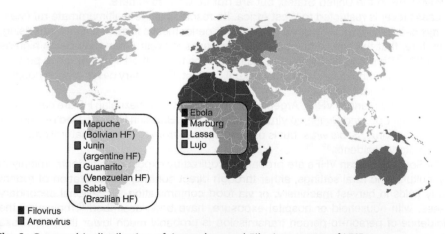

Fig. 6. Geographic distribution of Arenavirus and Filovirus agents of VHF.

filovirus, Ebola Reston, has been detected in the Philippines). Their natural hosts are fruit bats that occur from Gabon to Sudan in the north to Angola in the south.

Ebola epidemics or cases have been recorded in the Democratic Republic of Congo, Sudan, Cote d'Ivoire, and Uganda, with different serotypes in each case. As was seen in the first Ebola outbreak in Yambuku, Zaire,[3] close contact with infected persons was the main risk factor for infection. Hospitals, through the reuse of syringes, and absence of minimal infection-control measures, have served as the most important form of disease dissemination. However, with standard infection-control measures, the likelihood of secondary cases is probably low. This can be inferred from a case of Ebola that was treated in a South African hospital. Despite the fact that the diagnosis was only made after the patient was discharged from hospital, of more than 300 hospital personnel with significant exposure, there was only one secondary case and that was in all likelihood attributed to a needle-stick exposure.[45] Another important epidemiologic feature of Ebola virus VHF is that the testis is often involved in the infection (sometimes with clinical orchitis) and that viral shedding in semen may continue for weeks. Prevention of sexual transmission through barrier control or abstinence until negative viral culture is, therefore, important.

Marburg virus owes its name to the first recorded outbreak, which involved imported West African green monkeys and laboratory personnel in Marburg, Germany. More recently, large epidemics have been documented in Angola. Gold mining has been associated with Marburg outbreaks,[46] with exposure to bat excreta as the probable link. However, here, as with Ebola, hospitals served as outbreak amplifiers, mainly through the absence of barrier nursing and the reuse of injection equipment in vaccine administration.[47]

Arenaviruses: Lassa Fever and South American HF Viruses

Arenaviridae is a large family of viruses, most of whom are not pathogenic to humans. All share rodents as natural reservoir hosts. Humans mostly become infected through ingestion or inhalation of rodent ejecta, directly or through contaminated food. As illustrated in **Fig. 6**, VHF caused by Arenaviruses is restricted to Africa and South America. Other Arenaviruses cause neuroinvasive disease, including the globally distributed *Lymphocytic choriomeningitis virus* and the more recently recognized *Whitewater Arroyo* virus in the United States, but are not be discussed here.

Lassa fever is restricted to West Africa. Its reservoir is the multimammate rat (*Mastomys natalensis*), which is a highly prevalent peridomestic rodent. It is not surprising, therefore, that the annual number of Lassa cases in West Africa may be as high as 300,000.[48] Similar to the Filoviruses, Lassa can be transmitted from person to person, through close contact, and probably sexual contact. Secondary cases among hospital personnel are not rare.

The South American VHFs: Argentinean, Bolivian, and Venezuelan HF are caused by *Junin, Machupo, and Guanarito* viruses respectively. Brazilian HF is caused by another lethal Arenavirus, *Sabia virus*, but is only recognized from one known natural case and 2 laboratory accidents.[49]

All South American VHFs are probably acquired by exposure to rodents, mostly in agricultural and rural settings, either through direct contact, aerosolization of rodent body fluids in harvest machinery, or via food contamination. Occasional secondary cases, with household or hospital exposure, have been described[50]; however, the incidence of person-to-person transmission is probably much lower than for Lassa fever.

Hantaviruses

Hantaviruses are extant in both the Old World and the New (see **Fig. 3**). All are hosted by rodents, and person-to-person transmission is not important for these Bunyaviruses. In Eurasia, Hemorrhagic fever with Renal Syndrome (HFRS) is recognized from Eastern Russia, Korea (where the virus was first recognized), and China to the Balkans (where it is known as Dobrava disease or Balkan nephropathy). The agents of HFRS, *Hantaan virus* and *Dobrava virus,* predominate in Eastern Asia and in Europe respectively and are hosted by field mice; most cases are described in rural areas, with dramatic differences in incidence even within countries. Thus, in China, northeastern provinces account for most cases, with peak incidence in the spring and fall.[51]

Puumala fever is a milder form of HFRS, it is also known as nephropathia epidemica or vole fever. Its reservoir hosts are indeed voles, which inhabit both rural and suburban habitats. Puumala is mostly recognized in Northern Europe, including Scandinavia and Western Russia. The true incidence of Puumala is probably grossly underestimated. Even so, thousands of cases are reported yearly in Europe.[52] An unusual feature of Puumala is a cyclic surge in cases. Vole populations tend to peak every several years, probably in association with abundant mast seasons in European beech forests, which may correlate with increases in human disease.[53]

An additional *Hantavirus,– Seoul virus,* is hosted by the gray rat (*Rattus norvegicus*) and in fact is distributed globally, along with its host. Surprisingly, few cases are recorded worldwide but some have occurred in facilities and personnel involved with animal medical research.[54]

In the Americas, a phylogenetically divergent group of Hantaviruses causes a different disease: Hantavirus pulmonary syndrome (HPS). In addition to *Sin Nombre virus,* the type species isolated during the first recognized outbreak of HPS in 1993, many other species exist from Canada to Argentina, each with its attendant rodent host.[55] There are large differences in the virulence of Hantavirus strains in the Americas. Thus, although HPS has been described only occasionally from Latin American countries, the true incidence of Hantavirus infections is much higher. For example, the seroprevalence of Hantavirus infection in rural communities in Panama ranged from 16.5% to 60.4%; however, all acute cases presented with a nonspecific fever and none with HPS.[56]

CLINICAL FEATURES: MAIN SYNDROMES

It is unfortunately beyond the scope of this article to describe in detail the clinical features of each of the agents previously discussed. However, despite the large number of agents, most cases will fall within a few clinical syndromes. A few illustrative examples are given here. It should be kept in mind that apart from a few agents like Ebola, most cases of most arboviral diseases will not be typical but rather nonspecific febrile illnesses or even clinically unapparent infections.

Fever With Rash and Arthralgia: Classical Dengue Fever

After an incubation period of 4 to 7 days, fever develops abruptly and is often accompanied by severe frontal headache and retro-orbital pain. Severe musculoskeletal and lumbar pain combined with hyperesthesia of the skin may interrupt locomotion. Anorexia, vomiting, and loose stools may occur. After 3 to 4 days, with defervescence, an indistinct macular/scarlatiniform rash develops, sparing the palms and soles; areas of spared skin within the rash are typical and are evocatively described as white islands in a red sea. A second bout of fever and symptoms may ensue (saddleback pattern). Localized clusters of petechiae and minor bleeding (eg, epistaxis) can occur.

As described by Rush,[1] recovery may be followed by a prolonged period of listlessness, easy fatigability, and even depression; the disease was also aptly named break-heart fever.

The VHF Syndrome

The symptoms of VHF result from a combination of endothelial dysfunction that causes a capillary leak syndrome, and a bleeding diathesis caused by thrombocytopenia and diffuse intravascular coagulation. The resultant shock leads to death, although specific organ dysfunction (eg, brain, liver, heart, lungs, and gut) may contribute to the picture.

Typical VHF: Dengue Hemorrhagic Fever/Dengue Shock Syndrome

DHF/Dengue Shock Syndrome (DSS) is mostly described in infants but may occur in all age groups. In a small minority of patients with dengue, defervescence is accompanied with signs of shock manifested by central cyanosis, restlessness, diaphoresis, and cool, clammy skin and extremities. Abdominal pain is a common complaint. A rapid and weak pulse, a narrowing of the pulse pressure to less than 20 mm Hg, and in the most extreme cases, an unobtainable blood pressure are accompanied by diffuse petechiae, ecchymoses, and bleeding from mucosal and venipuncture sites. Noncardiogenic pulmonary edema and myocardial dysfunction may complicate the course. However, capillary leakage usually resolves spontaneously in 48 hours with a rapid resolution of the VHF syndrome.

Most Severe VHF: Ebola Virus

After an incubation period that ranges from 2 to 19 days, fever begins abruptly, accompanied by myalgia and headache. The fever is joined by some combination of nausea and vomiting and especially diarrhea, abdominal, and chest pain. Other common features include photophobia, conjunctival injection, sore throat, and lymphadenopathy. Central nervous system involvement is often manifested by somnolence, delirium, or coma. As the disease progresses, bleeding manifestations, such as petechiae, hemorrhages, ecchymoses around needle puncture sites, and mucous membrane hemorrhages, occur in most patients. Around day 5, most patients develop a maculopapular rash, prominent on the trunk, followed in a few days with either recovery or death from shock and multiorgan dysfunction. Convalescence is protracted and may be accompanied by arthralgia, orchitis, recurrent hepatitis, uveitis, and rarer phenomena.

VHF with prominent liver involvement (yellow fever): The course of yellow fever follows a saddleback, 3-stage pattern. These stages were described since very early times as the early period of infection, indistinguishable from early dengue as described previously, a period of remission whereby after several days the fever resolves for a few hours to several days, and then a period of intoxication whereby a capillary leak leads eventually to multiorgan failure and death. During this period, severe hepatitis causes clinical jaundice (the source of the disease's name) and is accompanied by encephalopathy and by mucosal and other bleeding, especially from the gut (the ominous black vomit). Although jaundice may be profound, should patients survive this period, recovery is usually complete without chronic liver damage.

VHF with prominent kidney involvement (hantavirus HFRS): After an incubation period of typically 2 weeks, fever, headache, myalgias, conjunctival injection, and blurred vision develop, followed by a blanching erythematous rash. After 4 to 7 days, a severe capillary leak syndrome ensues, with shock, oliguria, and bleeding phenomena. This phase, if not fatal, is resolved by a period of polyuria, heralding renal recovery, and protracted asthenia. Milder forms, such as Puumala, although lacking the VHF phase, will still evolve through an oliguric and polyuric phase, usually with hematuria and proteinuria. Although cases of severe HFRS usually resolve completely, the milder forms may lead to chronic renal injury and contribute to hypertension and chronic renal failure in endemic locales.

VHF with prominent pulmonary involvement (hantavirus HPS): HPS presents as a nonspecific fever, similar to early HFRS. However, after usually 4 to 5 days, mild cough and dyspnea rapidly evolve to noncardiogenic pulmonary edema and respiratory failure. This pulmonary capillary leak syndrome is of short duration and should patients survive with supportive care, rapid and complete recovery will occur in a few days.

Arboviral encephalitis: There is little to distinguish arboviral from other causes of encephalitis. However, it is important to recall that apart from a generic encephalitic syndrome of fever, headache, altered consciousness (and possibly seizures), almost any form of acute neurologic syndrome has been described, including meningitis, acute flaccid paralysis mimicking polio, cranial neuropathies, polyradiculopathies, cerebellitis with ataxia, or damage to basal ganglia, with late-onset parkinsonism. A varying proportion of patients remain with long-term sequelae.

Alphavirus arthritis (Chikungunya): Although arboviral encephalitis is similar to other encephalitides, *Alphavirus arthritis* is a unique syndrome. Following an incubation period of up to 12 days, fever ensues, accompanied by headache, photophobia, retro-orbital pain, pharyngitis, and vomiting. An accompanying blanching erythematous or maculopapular rash completes this early denguelike picture. Fever may abate and recrudesce, giving rise to a saddleback pattern. Arthralgia is, however, the leading feature, often polyarticular, involving small joints and sites of previous injuries; joints may swell without significant effusion. These symptoms may last from 1 week to several months and are accompanied by myalgia. Studies following the large Indian Ocean outbreak have demonstrated that a significant proportion of patients will be disabled for 2 years and more.[57] Follow-up of large numbers, with the use of advanced laboratory and imaging methods, has shown persistent arboviral arthritis to be an active inflammatory process, with erosive arthritis.[58] The implications regarding the long-term morbidity burden of Alphavirus outbreaks when millions of cases are infected are clear.

DIAGNOSIS OF VHF

As can be expected from the earlier descriptions, an exhaustive differential diagnosis of VHF-causing agents may include most of the medical conditions affecting humans and is, therefore, beyond the scope of this review. Indeed, milder forms of infections of VHF agents can be mistaken for anything between influenza, gastroenteritis, primary HIV, syphilis, and so forth. However, when considering the manifestations of severe forms of VHF, whether one is practicing in endemic regions or caring for returning travelers, it is important to keep in mind fulminant hepatic failure from viral hepatitis or toxins, severe leptospirosis (Weil disease), malaria, typhoid, rickettsial diseases, and Borrelia with relapsing fever.

The diagnosis of a specific agent can be achieved by either demonstrating seroconversion or by viral isolation. However, viral culture should only be attempted in well-equipped Biosafety level-4 laboratories because most of the VHF agents pose a real risk for laboratory personnel. The viral RNA can be demonstrated by polymerase chain reaction in blood samples during acute illness; however, for some agents, viremia is brief and at a low level, and the negative predictive value of genomic tests is variable and tends to be low. Serum antigen tests exist commercially for a few of these agents (eg, NS-1 protein for dengue). A definitive serologic diagnosis usually requires plaque reduction studies, which may only be available at a national or even international level. A variety of serologic tests are marketed for many of the major arboviral agents. However, these are hampered by cross-reactivity between many Arboviruses. In the case of travelers, interpretation is further complicated by previous *Flavivirus* (yellow fever, JEV, and TBE) vaccination.

TREATMENT AND PREVENTION OF VHF

In the management of the 1873 Memphis yellow fever epidemic, iced champagne was highly recommended (and gratefully received).[2] It is unfortunate that for most of the VHF agents, therapeutics have not greatly improved. Supportive care, with fluid reple-tion, correction of coagulopathy, and specific target organ support (from dialysis to ventilatory support) are the mainstay of treatment. For simpler forms of VHF, such as DHF/DSS, supportive care with intravenous volume repletion leads to a fatality rate that should not be more than 1%.[4]

Exceptions to this rule are Arenavirus infections. Ribavirin, a purine nucleoside, was found to be highly effective in patients with Lassa fever in all stages of the disease. If given before the seventh day of illness, ribavirin reduced the mortality rate from 55% to 5%.[59] Although the evidence base for its use in other Arenavirus infections is less rigorous, ribavirin is also recommended for cases of South American HF viruses.[60] Some evidence suggests that ribavirin may be beneficial in early Hantavirus HFRS[61]; however, its use in HPS has not been shown to be beneficial.[62]

With the absence of effective therapies for most agents, the onus has remained on prevention. Improved housing, rodent proofing, and vector control seem to be straight-forward measures. However, urbanization and perhaps even climate change have actually increased the scope of some vectors, which is manifested by the resurgence of *A aegypti* and the spread of *A albopictus*.

The twentieth century saw the introduction of some arboviral vaccines: the yellow fever vaccine, one of the most successful in history, Japanese encephalitis vaccine, and the TBE vaccine (in Europe). However, for all other arboviruses, there is no vaccine available.

For no arboviral disease is a vaccine more urgently needed as it is for dengue. A plethora of vaccine candidates has been discussed in the literature over decades; at long last a vaccine candidate, Sanofi Pasteur's live, attenuated tetravalent dengue vaccine (based on a yellow fever 17D vaccine strain), is currently undergoing field trials and may enter phase 3 trials soon.[63] That many of these infections are neglected trop-ical diseases has all but abolished the economic incentive of pharmaceutical compa-nies for development of arboviral vaccines.

SUMMARY

As they have in the past, VHFs continue to pose a major threat in most world regions today. VHF agents, especially arboviruses, are at the forefront of emerging infection detection. The absence of specific therapy and vaccine prevention for most of these pathogens poses a grave concern for human health in the developing and developed worlds alike.

REFERENCES

1. Rush B. An account of the bilious remitting fever, as it appeared in Philadelphia in the summer and autumn of the year 1780. In: Rush B, editor. Medical inquiries and

observations. Philadelphia: J. Conrad & Co; 1805. p. 115–34. Available at: http://books.google.com/books?id=y3EFAAAAQAAJ&dq=inauthor%3A%22Benjamin%20Rush%22&hl=iw&pg=PR5#v=onepage&q&f=false. Accessed March 25, 2012.

2. Erskine JH. A report on yellow fever as it appeared in Memphis, Tenn., in 1873. Public Health Pap Rep 1873;1:385–92.

3. WHO investigation commission. Ebola haemorrhagic fever in Zaire, 1976. Bull World Health Organ 1978;56(2):271–93.

4. Petersen LR, Hayes EB. West Nile virus in the Americas. Med Clin North Am 2008;92(6):1307–22.

5. Dengue haemorrhagic fever: diagnosis, treatment, prevention and control. 2nd edition. Geneva (Switzerland): World Health Organization; 2009. Available at: http://whqlibdoc.who.int/publications/2009/9789241547871_eng.pdf. Accessed September 30, 2009.

6. de Silva AM, Dittus WP, Amerasinghe PH, et al. Serologic evidence for an epizootic dengue virus infecting toque macaques (Macaca sinica) at Polonnaruwa, Sri Lanka. Am J Trop Med Hyg 1999;60(2):300–6.

7. Rico-Hesse R, Harrison LM, Salas RA, et al. Origins of dengue type 2 viruses associated with increased pathogenicity in the Americas. Virology 1997;230(2):244–51.

8. Brunkard JM, Robles López JL, Ramirez J, et al. Dengue fever seroprevalence and risk factors, Texas-Mexico border, 2004. Emerg Infect Dis 2007;13(10): 1477–83.

9. Gjenero-Margan I, Aleraj B, Krajcar D, et al. Autochthonous dengue fever in Croatia, August–September 2010. Euro Surveill 2011;16(9):pii–19805. Available at: http://www.eurosurveillance.org/ViewArticle.aspx?ArticleId=19805. Accessed March 25, 2012.

10. La Ruche G, Souarès Y, Armengaud A, et al. First two autochthonous dengue virus infections in metropolitan France, September 2010. Euro Surveill 2010;15(39):19676.

11. Tomori O. Yellow fever in Africa: public health impact and prospects for control in the 21st century. Biomedica 2002;22(2):178–210.

12. Misra UK, Kalita J. Overview: Japanese encephalitis. Prog Neurobiol 2010;91(2): 108–20.

13. Romero JR, Newland JG. Viral meningitis and encephalitis: traditional and emerging viral agents. Semin Pediatr Infect Dis 2003;14(2):72–82.

14. Kopel E, Amitai Z, Bin H, et al. Surveillance of West Nile Virus Disease, Tel Aviv District, Israel, 2005 to 2010. Euro Surveill 2011;16(25):pii–19894. Available at: http://www.eurosurveillance.org/ViewArticle.aspx?ArticleId=19894. Accessed March 25, 2012.

15. May FJ, Davis CT, Tesh RB, et al. Phylogeography of West Nile virus: from the cradle of evolution in Africa to Eurasia, Australia, and the Americas. J Virol 2011;85(6):2964–74.

16. Lasala PR, Holbrook M. Tick-borne flaviviruses. Clin Lab Med 2010;30(1):221–35.

17. Ergunay K, Ozer N, Us D, et al. Seroprevalence of West Nile virus and tick-borne encephalitis virus in Southeastern Turkey: first evidence for tick-borne encephalitis virus infections. Vector Borne Zoonotic Dis 2007;7(2):157–61.

18. Pugliese A, Beltramo T, Torre D. Seroprevalence study of tick-borne encephalitis, Borrelia burgdorferi, dengue and Toscana virus in Turin Province. Cell Biochem Funct 2007;25(2):185–8.

19. Jentes ES, Robinson J, Johnson BW, et al. Acute arboviral infections in Guinea, West Africa, 2006. Am J Trop Med Hyg 2010;83(2):388–94.

20. Lu Z, Lu XJ, Fu SH, et al. Tahyna virus and human infection, China. Emerg Infect Dis 2009;15(2):306–9.
21. Mouráão MP, Bastos MS, Gimaqu JB, et al. Oropouche fever outbreak, Manaus, Brazil, 2007-2008. Emerg Infect Dis 2009;15(12):2063–4.
22. Forshey BM, Guevara C, Laguna-Torres VA, et al, NMRCD Febrile Surveillance Working Group. Arboviral etiologies of acute febrile illnesses in Western South America, 2000-2007. PLoS Negl Trop Dis 2010;4(8):e787.
23. WHO. Crimean-Congo haemorrhagic fever (CCHF) Fact sheet and map. Available at: http://www.who.int/csr/disease/crimean_congoHF/en/on. Accessed September 30, 2011.
24. Cusi MG, Savellini GG, Zanelli G. Toscana virus epidemiology: from Italy to beyond. Open Virol J 2010;4:22–8.
25. Yu XJ, Liang MF, Zhang SY, et al. Fever with thrombocytopenia associated with a novel bunyavirus in China. N Engl J Med 2011;364(16):1523–32.
26. Liu Y, Li Q, Hu W, et al. Person-to-person transmission of severe fever with thrombocytopenia syndrome virus. Vector Borne Zoonotic Dis 2012;12(2):156–60.
27. Clements AC, Pfeiffer DU, Martin V, et al. A Rift Valley fever atlas for Africa. Prev Vet Med 2007;82(1–2):72–82.
28. Madani TA, Al-Mazrou YY, Al-Jeffri MH, et al. Rift Valley fever epidemic in Saudi Arabia: epidemiological, clinical, and laboratory characteristics. Clin Infect Dis 2003;37(8):1084–92.
29. WHO. Rift Valley fever, South Africa - update. Wkly Epidemiol Rec 2010;85(21): 185–6.
30. Attoui H, Mohd Jaafar F, de Micco P, et al. Coltiviruses and Seadornaviruses in North America, Europe, and Asia. Emerg Infect Dis 2005;11(11):1673–9.
31. Charrel RN, Attoui H, Butenko AM, et al. Tick-borne virus diseases of human interest in Europe. Clin Microbiol Infect 2004;10(12):1040–55.
32. Liu H, Li MH, Zhai YG, et al. Banna virus, China, 1987-2007. Emerg Infect Dis 2010;16(3):514–7.
33. Hammon WM, Rudnick A, Sather GE. Viruses associated with epidemic hemorrhagic fevers of the Philippines and Thailand. Science 1960;131:1102–3.
34. Pialoux G, Gaüzère BA, Jauréguiberry S, et al. Chikungunya, an epidemic arbovirosis. Lancet Infect Dis 2007;7(5):319–27.
35. Tsetsarkin KA, Chen R, Leal G, et al. Chikungunya virus emergence is constrained in Asia by lineage-specific adaptive landscapes. Proc Natl Acad Sci U S A 2011;108(19):7872–7.
36. Rezza G, Nicoletti L, Angelini R, et al, CHIKV study group. Infection with chikungunya virus in Italy: an outbreak in a temperate region. Lancet 2007;370(9602): 1840–6.
37. Grandadam M, Caro V, Plumet S, et al. Chikungunya virus, southeastern France. Emerg Infect Dis 2011;17(5):910–3.
38. Mathiot CC, Grimaud G, Garry P, et al. An outbreak of human Semliki Forest virus infections in Central African Republic. Am J Trop Med Hyg 1990;42(4): 386–93.
39. Mourão MP, Bastos MD, de Figueiredo RP, et al. Mayaro fever in the city of Manaus, Brazil, 2007-2008. Vector Borne Zoonotic Dis 2012;12(1):42–6.
40. Australian Government Department of Health and Ageing, the Communicable Diseases Network Australia. Arboviral diseases and malaria in Australia, 2008–09: annual report of the National Arbovirus and Malaria Advisory Committee. Commun Dis Intell 2010;34(3):225–41. Available at: http://www.health.gov.au/internet/main/publishing.nsf/content/cda-cdi3403b.htm. Accessed October 01, 2011.

41. Sane J, Guedes S, Kurkela S, et al. Epidemiological analysis of mosquito-borne Pogosta disease in Finland, 2009. Euro Surveill 2010;15(2):pii–19462. Available at: http://www.eurosurveillance.org/ViewArticle.aspx?ArticleId=19462. Accessed March 25, 2012.

42. Weaver SC, Salas R, Rico-Hesse R, et al. Re-emergence of epidemic Venezuelan equine encephalomyelitis in South America. VEE study group. Lancet 1996; 348(9025):436–40.

43. Aguilar PV, Estrada-Franco JG, Navarro-Lopez R, et al. Endemic Venezuelan equine encephalitis in the Americas: hidden under the dengue umbrella. Future Virol 2011;6(6):721–40.

44. Groseth A, Feldmann H, Strong JE. The ecology of Ebola virus. Trends Microbiol 2007;15(9):408–16.

45. Richards GA, Murphy S, Jobson R, et al. Unexpected Ebola virus in a tertiary setting: clinical and epidemiologic aspects. Crit Care Med 2000;28(1):240–4.

46. Bausch DG, Nichol ST, Muyembe-Tamfum JJ, et al, International Scientific and Technical Committee for Marburg Hemorrhagic Fever Control in the Democratic Republic of the Congo. Marburg hemorrhagic fever associated with multiple genetic lineages of virus. N Engl J Med 2006;355(9):909–19.

47. Jeffs B, Roddy P, Weatherill D, et al. The Medecins Sans Frontieres intervention in the Marburg hemorrhagic fever epidemic, Uige, Angola, 2005. I. Lessons learned in the hospital. J Infect Dis 2007;196(Suppl 2):S154–61.

48. Ogbu O, Ajuluchukwu E, Uneke CJ. Lassa fever in West African sub-region: an overview. J Vector Borne Dis 2007;44(1):1–11.

49. Armstrong LR, Dembry LM, Rainey PM, et al. Management of a Sabiá virus-infected patients in a US hospital. Infect Control Hosp Epidemiol 1999;20(3):176–82.

50. Kilgore PE, Peters CJ, Mills JN, et al. Prospects for the control of Bolivian hemorrhagic fever. Emerg Infect Dis 1995;1(3):97–100.

51. Liu X, Jiang B, Bi P, et al. Prevalence of haemorrhagic fever with renal syndrome in mainland China: analysis of national surveillance data, 2004-2009. Epidemiol Infect 2011;1–7. [Epub ahead of print].

52. Heyman P, Ceianu CS, Christova I, et al. A five-year perspective on the situation of haemorrhagic fever with renal syndrome and status of the hantavirus reservoirs in Europe, 2005-2010. Euro Surveill 2011;16(36):pii–19961. Available at: http://www.eurosurveillance.org/ViewArticle.aspx?ArticleId=19961. Accessed March 25, 2012.

53. Clement J, Maes P, van Ypersele de Strihou C, et al. Beechnuts and outbreaks of nephropathia epidemica (NE): of mast, mice and men. Nephrol Dial Transplant 2010;25(6):1740–6.

54. Zhang YZ, Dong X, Li X, et al. Seoul virus and hantavirus disease, Shenyang, People's Republic of China. Emerg Infect Dis 2009;15(2):200–6.

55. Macneil A, Nichol ST, Spiropoulou CF. Hantavirus pulmonary syndrome. Virus Res 2011;162(1–2):138–47.

56. Armien B, Pascale JM, Munoz C, et al. Incidence rate for hantavirus infections without pulmonary syndrome, Panama. Emerg Infect Dis 2011;17(10):1936–9.

57. Larrieu S, Pouderoux N, Pistone T, et al. Factors associated with persistence of arthralgia among chikungunya virus-infected travellers: report of 42 French cases. J Clin Virol 2010;47(1):85–8.

58. Manimunda SP, Vijayachari P, Uppoor R, et al. Clinical progression of chikungunya fever during acute and chronic arthritic stages and the changes in joint morphology as revealed by imaging. Trans R Soc Trop Med Hyg 2010;104(6):392–9.

59. McCormick JB, King IJ, Webb PA, et al. Lassa fever. Effective therapy with riba-virin. N Engl J Med 1986;314(1):20–6.
60. Kilgore PE, Ksiazek TG, Rollin PE, et al. Treatment of Bolivian hemorrhagic fever with intravenous ribavirin. Clin Infect Dis 1997;24(4):718–22.
61. Rusnak JM, Byrne WR, Chung KN, et al. Experience with intravenous ribavirin in the treatment of hemorrhagic fever with renal syndrome in Korea. Antiviral Res 2009;81(1):68–76.
62. Mertz GJ, Miedzinski L, Goade D, et al, Collaborative Antiviral Study Group. Placebo-controlled, double-blind trial of intravenous ribavirin for the treatment of hantavirus cardiopulmonary syndrome in North America. Clin Infect Dis 2004;39(9):1307–13.
63. Guy B, Barrere B, Malinowski C, et al. From research to phase III: preclinical, industrial and clinical development of the Sanofi Pasteur tetravalent dengue vaccine. Vaccine 2011;29(42):7229–41.

Tropical Fungal Infections

Li Yang Hsu, MBBS, MRCP, MPH[a],*, Limin Wijaya, MBBS, MRCP, DTM&H[b],
Esther Shu-Ting Ng, MBBS, MRCP[a], Eduardo Gotuzzo, MD[c]

KEYWORDS

- Tropical fungal infections • Epidemiology • Returning travelers • Dimorphic fungi
- Antifungal therapy

Fungal infections in humans are more prevalent and diverse in the tropics and subtropics,[1] likely because warm and humid climates are more conducive for the growth and dissemination of fungi. Several of the dimorphic and geographically delimited fungi such as *Lacazia loboi* are found only in the tropical zone, but infections by these organisms may present anywhere in the world owing to the increasing frequency of human migration and travel.[2,3] In global surveys of travel-related diseases, fungal infections are invariably among the most common causes of dermatologic disorders in returning travelers.[4]

One commonly used classification for fungal infections is based on the tissue that is initially colonized.[1,5] Superficial mycoses are restricted to the outermost layer of the epidermis (stratum corneum) and do not cause any inflammation. Cutaneous mycoses involve the integumentary system, including nails and hair, and generally elicit inflammation of the skin. Subcutaneous mycoses describe infection of the deeper layers of tissue, with the fungi usually being directly implanted following minor trauma. Unlike the previously mentioned mycoses, these infections may invade beyond the initial colonized area, involving muscle, deep fascia, and even bone. The respiratory and gastrointestinal tracts are the main portals of entry for systemic mycoses, which can be further classified into primary and opportunistic mycoses based on whether the fungus in question is able to cause an infection in a normal host.[5] Several fungi, such as *Sporothrix schenckii* and certain dematiaceous molds, are able to manifest as either subcutaneous or systemic mycoses depending on the portal of entry and the immune status of the human host.

No specific funding was utilized in the writing of this manuscript.
L.Y.H. has received research funding from Pfizer Inc, and Merck, Sharpe & Dohme as well as paid consultancy from Pfizer Inc.
L.W., E.S.N., and E.G. have no competing interests to declare.

[a] Department of Medicine, National University Health System, 5 Lower Kent Ridge Road, Singapore 119074, Singapore; [b] Department of Infectious Diseases, Singapore General Hospital, Outram Road, Singapore 169608, Singapore; [c] Instituto de Medicina Tropical Alexander von Humboldt, Universidad Peruana Cayetano Heridia, Av. Honorio Delgardo 430-Urb. Ingeniería-SMP-Lima 3, 31 Lima, Peru
* Corresponding author.
E-mail address: liyang_hsu@yahoo.com

Infect Dis Clin N Am 26 (2012) 497–512
doi:10.1016/j.idc.2012.02.004
0891-5520/12/$ – see front matter © 2012 Elsevier Inc. All rights reserved.

id.theclinics.com

In this review, the authors briefly discuss superficial and subcutaneous mycoses that are far more prevalent or restricted to the tropics (**Fig. 1, Table 1**), as well as fungal infections in returning travelers. Systemic mycoses caused by dimorphic fungi have been extensively reviewed recently[6–8] and are not further discussed except in the context of travel-related infections.

SUPERFICIAL AND CUTANEOUS MYCOSES

These very common mycoses affect up to 25% of the global population and occur predominantly in the tropics, although they have a worldwide distribution.[9]

The most common superficial mycoses are pityriasis versicolor, tinea nigra, and the piedras. Pityriasis versicolor is caused by various *Malassezia* spp and is characterized by the presence of asymptomatic (rarely, mild itch) fine hyperchromic or hypochromic macules on the torso, neck, and arms, occasionally extending to face, groin, and thighs.[10] Major risk factors include warm and humid environments, corticosteroids, and tanning lotions. Young adults are more frequently affected, with no gender bias.[10] Differential diagnoses include pityriasis alba and rosea, solar dermatitis, and postlesional melanodermas.[10,11] Laboratory diagnosis is made by finding clusters of round budding yeast cells on microscopy of skin scrapings with 10% potassium hydroxide solution. Woods (ultraviolet) light is useful in the clinic setting, with macules emitting a characteristic yellow-green fluorescence.[12] Treatment comprises topical therapy (imidazoles, allylamines, ciclopirox olamine, 20% sodium hypochlorite, or 50% propileneglycol) for 2 to 4 weeks for limited/initial cases and systemic azoles for extensive/recurrent cases. Avoiding or removing risk factors is helpful in preventing relapse.[10,12]

Tinea nigra presents as chronic, asymptomatic, irregular, scaly, hyperpigmented (tan, brown, or black) patches or spots on the palms, occasionally involving soles, arms, and torso. It is caused by the pigmented yeast *Hortaea werneckii*, occurring predominantly in children and young adults in coastal tropical regions, with the

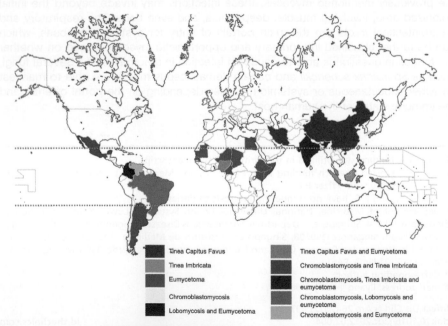

Tinea Capitus Favus	Tinea Capitus Favus and Eumycetoma
Tinea Imbricata	Chromoblastomycosis and Tinea Imbricata
Eumycetoma	Chromoblastomycosis, Tinea Imbricata and eumycetoma
Chromoblastomycosis	Chromoblastomycosis, Lobomycosis and eumycetoma
Lobomycosis and Eumycetoma	Chromoblastomycosis and Eumycetoma

Fig. 1. Geographic distribution of major superficial, cutaneous, and subcutaneous mycoses.

most important predisposing factor being hyperhidrosis of hands and feet.[12,13] Laboratory diagnosis is made by finding dark septate hyphae with clusters of blastoconidia on microscopy, whereas dermatoscopy in the clinic setting, showing hyperchromic fungal growth, may be helpful in differentiating this condition from nevi and melanoma.[12,14] Control of hyperhidrosis is sufficient for treating tinea nigra, although keratolytics and topical antifungals may also be used.[12]

White and black piedra are caused by *Trichosporon* spp and *Piedraia hortae*, respectively, which are chronic asymptomatic infections of the hair shafts (scalp and, less commonly, beard, axilla, and pubic hair) in children and young adults. Predominant risk factors are humidity and poor personal hygiene. Soft white concretions or nodules are seen in white piedra, whereas black hard nodules are seen in black piedra. Laboratory diagnosis is made via observation of masses of septate hyphae and arthroconidia on microscopy of infected hair, and treatment is identical for both conditions, involving clipping of infected hair followed by application of topical antifungals or keratolytics, one effective option being 2% ketoconazole shampoo.[12]

Cutaneous mycoses and onychomycoses are predominantly caused by dermatophytes, with *Candida* spp being the most common nondermatophyte cause. Dermatophytosis is somewhat inappropriately named tinea (ie, ringworm in Latin) followed by the body part affected, whereas onychomycosis is another term for tinea unguium or fungal nail infection.[1] The major pathogenic dermatophyte genera are *Trichophyton*, *Microsporum*, and *Epidermophyton*, with different species being transmitted between humans (anthropophilic), from animals (zoophilic), or from soil (geophilic).[1,5] Ameen[15] has recently described the global epidemiology of the causative species, highlighting the changing epidemiology as a consequence of migration and socioeconomic conditions. In general, the clinical presentation is that of a circumscribed scaly and itchy rash, with interdigital erosive changes in tinea pedis and hair loss in tinea capitis. In tinea unguium, affected nail plates have a thickened, dirty, and granular appearance.[1,5]

As with superficial mycoses, laboratory diagnosis is made via observation of fungal organisms in skin scrapings or hair on microscopy, mounted in 10% potassium hydroxide. Cultures are unnecessary for making a diagnosis. However, it is impossible to distinguish the various dermatophytes by microscopy alone, and cultures are therefore useful for epidemiologic trending.[1,5] Therapy is site specific, with topical antifungals or Whitfield ointment (salicylic acid and benzoic acid in a suitable base) being successful in most cases of tinea corporis, cruris, or pedis, whereas oral antifungals remain the mainstay of therapy for tinea capitis and onychomycosis as well as extensive tinea corporis and tinea pedis.[1,16] A couple of the more unusual tropical dermatophytoses are briefly described.

Tinea capitis favosa or favus is a specific chronic scalp dermatophytosis caused almost primarily by *Trichophyton schoenleinii*, although cases have rarely been attributed to other dermatophytes.[1,17] The fungus, and therefore the disease, is currently geographically restricted to Iran, some parts of Africa, and China, although sporadic cases are seen in various parts of the world.[17] The prevalence of favus is higher in boys and in children aged between 6 and 10 years, and few individuals are infected after puberty. The disease has 3 stages of severity, with the classic lesion being that of a cup-shaped yellow crust on the scalp termed the scutulum.[17] The fungus can be seen on microscopy of affected hair, but culturing on Sabouraud agar is required for definite identification of *T schoenleinii*. Treatment is identical to that of tinea capitis; *T schoenleinii* remains susceptible to griseofulvin unlike other dermatophytes for which resistance may be increasing.[1,16,17]

Tinea imbricata or Tokelau is caused by the strict anthropophilic dermatophyte *Trichophyton concentricum* and is restricted to Polynesian and Melanesian archipelagoes

Table 1
Cutaneous and subcutaneous mycoses that are more prevalent in the tropics

Mycoses	Pathogens	Distribution	Diagnosis	Therapy
Superficial mycoses				
Pityriasis versicolor	*Malassezia* spp	Global (more common in the tropics)	• Woods light (clinic) • Microscopy of skin scrapings	Topical antifungals, systemic antifungals for severe/ recurrent cases
Tinea nigra	*Hortaea werneckii*	Tropical coastal regions	• Dermatoscopy (clinic) • Microscopy of skin scrapings	Control of hyperhidrosis; rarely, keratolytics or topical antifungals
White piedra	*Trichosporon* spp	Global (more common in the tropics)	Microscopy of infected hair	Removal of infected hair, then topical antifungals or keratolytics
Black piedra	*Piedraia hortae*	Global (more common in the tropics)	Microscopy of infected hair	Removal of infected hair, then topical antifungals or keratolytics
Cutaneous mycoses				
Dermatophytosis (including favus and tinea imbricata)	*Trichophyton* spp, *Microsporon* spp, *Epidermophyton* spp	Global (more common in the tropics); *Trichophyton schoenleinii* virtually restricted to Iran, Africa, and China; *Trichophyton concentricum* restricted to Polynesian and Melanesian archipelagos and Central and South America	• Clinical presentation • Microscopy of skin scraping	Site specific with topical antifungals or Whitfield ointment; oral antifungals for extensive disease • Favus: griseofulvin • Tinea imbricata: griseofulvin or terbinafine

Subcutaneous mycoses				
Chromoblastomycosis	Dematiaceous molds, especially *Fonsecaea* spp, *Cladophialophora* spp, and *Phialophora* spp	Global (most common in India, Thailand, Madagascar, Amazonian regions, Dominican Republic)	• Microscopy of skin scrapings • Fungal cultures (slow growth) • Serology and PCR, experimental	• Small lesions: surgical excision or liquid nitrogen, thermotherapy • Extensive lesions: itraconazole, terbinafine, newer azoles
Eumycetoma	Various fungal species (most commonly *Madurella mycetomatis* and *Scedosporium apiospermum*)	Global (more common in India and Africa)	• Clinical presentation • Ultrasonography or magnetic resonance imaging appearance • Fine-needle aspiration cytology (early lesions) • Deep surgical biopsy	• Surgical excision • Systemic antifungals (itraconazole or terbinafine) • Newer azoles may be useful for recurrent disease
Lobomycosis	*L loboi*	Amazon rainforest	• Microscopy of tissue samples	• Surgical excision • Cryosurgery for isolated lesions • Clofazimine
Sporotrichosis	*S schenckii* complex	Global (more common in tropical and subtropical regions)	• Tissue culture • ELISA (limited use) • PCR, experimental	• Itraconazole (terbinafine and potassium iodide for nonresponders)

Abbreviations: ELISA, enzyme-linked immunosorbent assay; PCR, polymerase chain reaction.

of South Pacific, Southeast Asia, and Central and South America, areas with high humidity. Susceptibility to the disease is inherited in either an autosomal recessive manner or an autosomal dominant manner with incomplete penetrance, with the disease most often beginning in childhood. The clinical appearance is characteristic, comprising thick, concentric, scaly plaques covering the skin surface; palms, hair-bearing areas, and nails are rarely affected. Diagnosis is based on clinical appearance, confirmed by direct microscopic examination of skin scrapings showing thin branching filaments with few arthroconidia. However, culturing in Sabouraud media or polymerase chain reaction (PCR) testing is necessary for identifying the fungus. Treatment is with oral griseofulvin or terbinafine, with azoles generally demonstrating poorer response. Nonetheless, recurrence rates are high no matter what agent is prescribed.[18]

SUBCUTANEOUS MYCOSES

There are several distinct clinical syndromes in the mycoses of implantation, some of which may be caused by a variety of different fungi. Because subcutaneous zygomycosis and phaeohyphomycosis are found worldwide, with no significant increased prevalence in the tropics, they are not discussed further.

Chromoblastomycosis

Chromoblastomycosis is a term encompassing a group of chronic subcutaneous mycoses caused by specific species of dematiaceous molds, mainly those belonging to the genera *Fonsecaea*, *Cladophialophora*, and *Phialophora*. Although these fungi are present worldwide, chromoblastomycosis is more common in parts of India, Thailand, Madagascar, Amazonian Latin America (particularly Brazil), and the Dominican Republic.[19–22] The most commonly implicated fungus is *Fonsecaea pedrosoi* in Amazonian and temperate regions of Latin America, whereas *Cladophialophora carrionii* is commonly found in drier climates, including the subtropical parts of India and Thailand.[20–22]

Unlike other subcutaneous infections caused by dematiaceous molds, the lesions of chromoblastomycosis are unique in having thick-walled hyperpigmented multicellular structures called muriform cells or sclerotic bodies.[21,23] Certain dematiaceous molds such as *Exophiala jeanselmei* may separately cause chromoblastomycosis, eumycetoma, and subcutaneous phaeohyphomycosis,[23] but it remains unclear at present whether it is host or pathogen-associated factors that result in the type of subcutaneous mycosis manifested.

Because the fungi are inoculated via puncture wounds, those infected tend to be rural workers, belong to the lower socioeconomic classes, and are barefoot, with the distal limbs being most commonly affected.[19–23] Men are more commonly affected in Latin America and parts of Asia, whereas women are predominantly affected in southern Africa, and children younger than 15 years are rarely affected.[24] Disease progression is very slow and may be asymptomatic at the start, appearing as small skin-colored papules that insidiously enlarge to form verrucose warty growth complexes.[21] More rapid growth of lesions, albeit still in term of months, has been described.[22] Satellite lesions may develop as a result of autoinoculation or lymphatic dissemination, and complications include secondary bacterial infection and lymphedema; keloidal scarring; and, rarely, neoplastic transformation to squamous cell carcinoma. Disease extension to underlying muscle or bone is rare unless there is concomitant immunosuppression.[25]

The diagnosis is readily confirmed by direct microscopy (in 10% potassium hydroxide) of skin scrapings taken from characteristic black dots present on the lesions, showing the typical muriform cells. Fungal cultures are slow because the organisms generally take weeks to grow.[21,25] Serologic and PCR tests are available but are used almost exclusively for research purposes at present.

Treatment of chromoblastomycosis is difficult, complicated by the lack of comparative trials and variable rates of treatment failure, ranging up to 85% in line with the extent of disease.[25] Surgical excision or cryosurgery with liquid nitrogen should be limited to small lesions, with wide surgical margins, as remnant infecting fungus may spread within the scar tissue.[26,27] Thermotherapy using devices such as benzene pocket warmers, either as monotherapy or in combination with antifungals, has been successfully but not systematically assayed in Japan.[26,28] The mainstay of therapy remains high-dose, long-term (minimum 6–12 months) oral antifungals. Itraconazole, terbinafine, and 5-flucytosine in combination have been variously prescribed in the past.[25,26] The new azoles, particularly posaconazole, show great promise for the treatment of extensive and/or refractory chromoblastomycosis[29] but are highly expensive.

Eumycetoma

Eumycetoma is a chronic, granulomatous, suppurative fungal infection of the subcutaneous and deeper tissues, usually of the foot and lower limbs (**Fig. 2**). English physicians first described the condition in Madura, India, in 1842, giving rise to the term Madura foot or maduromycosis.[30] It has a wider distribution than chromoblastomycosis, being endemic in equatorial Africa, India, Mexico, and the Middle East, although sporadic cases have been described from most tropical and temperate countries.[21,23,31] A diverse and large group of fungi cause eumycetomas, with the most common being *Madurella mycetomatis* (black grain eumycetomas in India and Africa), *Magnaporthe grisea*, *Acremonium* spp, and *Scedosporium apiospermum* (white grain eumycetomas in temperate countries, including the United States).[21,31] The predisposing factors are virtually identical to that of chromoblastomycosis.

As with chromoblastomycosis and other subcutaneous mycoses, the fungi are introduced via penetrating trauma and present initially as an asymptomatic subcutaneous mass that gradually progresses, forming multiple sinuses that drain out pus and aggregated fungi (grains).[21,23,31] These aggregated fungi are also known as sclerotia and are a multicellular version of the muriform cells in chromoblastomycosis. They vary in color depending on the fungus and are also found within the lesions in granulomata that are formed as a result of the host neutrophilic inflammatory response.[31] Unlike chromoblastomycosis, the infection frequently involves the muscle and bone if left untreated, although tendons and nerves are spared until the disease is advanced.[23] Enlarged regional lymph nodes are also unusual in this disease.

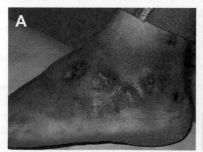 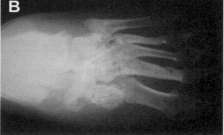

Fig. 2. Eumycetoma. (*A*) Multiple chronic sinuses and skin hyperpigmentation from an underlying eumycetoma. (*B*) Underlying osteomyelitis from eumycetoma.

Diagnosis is traditionally dependent on clinical presentation; the classical triad of subcutaneous mass, sinuses, and fungal grains; and laboratory identification of the infecting fungus, the laboratory identification being vital for treatment success.[31,32] During the early stages, eumycetomas are difficult to distinguish clinically from chromoblastomycosis. Subsequently, other clinical differentials include chronic osteomyelitis, actinomycosis (which forms identical mycetomas), botryomycosis, tuberculosis, and certain skin tumors.[21,23,30,31] Ultrasonography is a noninvasive technique of differentiating the possible diagnoses; fungal grains produce sharp hyperreflective echoes, and numerous thick-walled cavities without acoustic enhancement are seen.[32] Actinomycetomas appear similar, but the smaller and less consistent grains are less distinct.[32] Magnetic resonance imaging shows promise as a useful diagnostic adjunct for those patients who can afford it and is helpful for planning surgery; fungal grains appear as minute hypointense foci within the hyperintense signals given off by the surrounding granulomata (dots-in-circles).[31,33,34] Fine-needle aspiration cytology is useful even in early disease and can distinguish between eumycetomas and actinomycetomas.[35] It is cheap, rapid, and well tolerated. However, deep surgical biopsies tend to have better yield in terms of fungal cultures because these avoid picking up surface bacterial contamination that may interfere with the slower growth of the fungi. Molecular methods of fungal identification show future promise but are currently research based only.[36]

Aggressive surgical excision combined with systemic antifungals is the mainstay of therapy for eumycetoma, with limb amputation for advanced cases.[21,31–33] As with chromoblastomycosis, treatment success is very much dependent on extent and duration of disease, with local and regional lymph node recurrences being frequent.[21,31] Itraconazole and terbinafine are the current drugs of choice for eumycetoma, with the more expensive voriconazole and posaconazole as alternative options.[31] Criteria for cure include complete clinical and radiologic (ultrasound absence of hyperreflective echoes and cavities) resolution of the lesions as well as repeating negative serology tests if this has been performed.[21,37,38] Treatment recommendations are based on case series and noncomparative studies because there has been no randomized controlled trial to date.

Lobomycosis

First described in 1930 by Brazilian dermatologist Jorge Lobo,[39] lobomycosis or lacaziosis is an uncommon chronic subcutaneous mycosis caused by L loboi.[40] Human disease is geographically restricted to natives of and travelers to the Amazon rainforest in South America, although sporadic cases have been reported from Mexico, Central America, the United States, and France.[21] Besides humans, bottlenose dolphins are the only other known animals that are infected in the wild.[41] The incubation period is long, ranging from several months to years, as is evidenced by individuals developing the disease years after their visits to endemic regions.[42] The disease is more common in young men aged between 21 and 40 years who work in the forest.[43] The natural reservoir of the fungus is unknown but is presumed to be in the rural environment in view of disease distribution.[21,43]

The most common clinical presentation is that of chronic keloidal lesions in exposed skin, with occasional regional lymph node involvement but no systemic involvement.[43] The most frequently affected area is the pinna of the ear (**Fig. 3**), followed by the limbs, with new lesions arising locally or via lymphatic dissemination.[21,43] Infiltrative, gummatous, macular, and/or disseminated lesions may also present occasionally, representing the other end of the clinical spectrum.[43] Patients are generally well, with no symptoms other than pruritus and possible restriction of movements at affected sites,

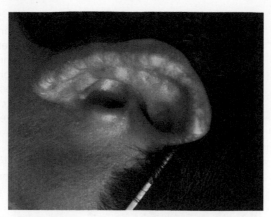

Fig. 3. Lobomycosis of the pinna.

except when rare complications such as secondary bacterial infection or carcinomatous change develop.[43] Clinical differential diagnoses include keloids, xanthomas, and dermatofibrosarcoma protuberans.[21]

Diagnosis is confirmed via direct microscopy of tissue samples in 10% potassium hydroxide, showing abundant chains of round hyaline cells with thick and birefringent cell walls.[21,43] There has been no successful attempts at culturing L loboi in vitro. Serologic testing is complicated by cross-reactions with *Paracoccidioides brasiliensis*, which shares similar geographic endemicity.[44]

Wide surgical excision of the affected area remains the treatment of choice.[21,43] As with other subcutaneous mycoses, relapses are common in extensive disease. Cryosurgery and electrodissection are options for isolated lesions.[21,43] Experience with medical therapy is limited, with success reported for clofazimine (for at least 2 years) and mixed results for itraconazole.[21,43,45,46]

Sporotrichosis

The S schenckii complex, the rapidly growing group of related dimorphic fungi causing sporotrichosis, has a worldwide distribution, although the disease is primarily reported from tropical and warmer temperate regions.[47,48] Unlike other subcutaneous mycoses, large clusters of cases and outbreaks have occurred with regard to sporotrichosis, generally caused by contact with the same contaminated environmental source, that is, wooden pit props in the South Africa Rand gold mines outbreak, sphagnum moss, and even cats, among others.[49]

Most cases of sporotrichosis involve the subcutaneous and cutaneous tissues, with osteoarticular, pulmonary, and meningeal disease occurring rarely and disseminated infection occurring mainly in the setting of immunosuppression.[21,50] Subcutaneous infections are subdivided into 2 categories: fixed cutaneous and lymphocutaneous diseases.[51] The former is less common, with infection confined entirely to the site of inoculation, presenting as a scaly, verrucous, or ulcerative nodule.[51] The latter results from lymphatic spread of infection, with an initial subcutaneous nodule at the site of inoculation that may ulcerate to form a nontender sporotrichotic chancre. Satellite lesions appear along a lymphatic chain, followed by lymphadenopathy **(Fig. 4)**.[21,51,52] The major clinical differentials are leishmaniasis, nontuberculous mycobacterial (especially *Mycobacterium marinum*) infections, nocardiosis, and tuberculoid Hansen disease.[21,53] Spontaneous healing seldom occurs.

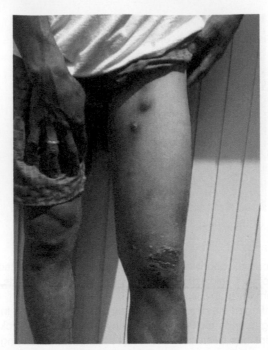

Fig. 4. Sporotrichotic chancre with satellite nodules.

Unlike other subcutaneous mycoses, microscopy of tissue biopsy specimens is not sensitive, although, rarely, finding extracellular asteroid bodies of eosinophilic spicules surrounding a central yeast is diagnostic.[21,54] More commonly, a nonspecific granulomatous reaction with pseudoepitheliomatous hyperplasia is seen.[21,54] The gold standard for making a diagnosis is tissue culture, with S schenckii grown in mycelial phase at 25°C and converted to yeast form at 37°C.[55] In most cases, the organism grows within 8 days after initiating cultures.[50] A recent enzyme-linked immunosorbent assay test directed toward detecting antibodies to SsCBF, a cell wall antigen of S schenckii, was developed in Brazil and demonstrated fairly high sensitivity and specificity[56] but has seen limited use to date, whereas older serologic tests have not been commercialized. Similarly, molecular (PCR based) techniques are research based at present but seem to be promising for rapid diagnosis in the future.[57]

Consensus guidelines for the treatment of sporotrichosis were published 4 years ago by the Infectious Diseases Society of America.[50] For cutaneous and lymphocutaneous sporotrichosis, the recommended first-line agent was itraconazole to be given for up to 3 to 6 months, with terbinafine and saturated solution of potassium iodide considered for nonresponders. Fluconazole and local hyperthermia were reserved for patients who could not be safely prescribed the previous antifungals. Amphotericin B was not recommended because of toxicity and inconvenience of administration and also because these were non-life-threatening infections.[50] A recently published open-label study showed that terbinafine at a lower dose (250 mg daily) had equivalent outcomes compared with oral itraconazole for cutaneous sporotrichosis.[58] In contrast to other subcutaneous mycoses, treatment outcomes are generally excellent for cutaneous and lymphocutaneous sporotrichosis, and surgery is usually unnecessary. The fungi are susceptible to the newer azoles in vitro, but there have been no clinical studies to date.[50]

FUNGAL INFECTIONS IN RETURNING TRAVELERS

Travelers, particularly those to the tropics, are at risk for a wide range of infectious diseases. Except for superficial and cutaneous mycoses, however, other forms of fungal infections are rare. Dermatophytosis accounts for 4% of all dermatologic conditions in travelers,[59–61] but there are surveillance limitations because individuals who do not view their symptoms as significant may not seek medical advice.

Systemic and endemic mycoses have been reported in areas of nonendemicity because travelers are involved in a range of activities that increase their risks for acquiring such infections. Most infections manifest soon after travel, although delayed presentations are seen among migrants and long stayers from endemic regions. Histoplasmosis is the most commonly reported endemic mycosis affecting travelers, followed by coccidioidomycosis and scattered cases of paracoccidioidomycosis, blastomycosis, and cryptococcosis.

Histoplasmosis in travelers can be difficult to diagnose, presenting most frequently as a self-limiting illness of fever, dry cough, and headache in immunocompetent individuals. Severe pulmonary symptoms can occur in high-inoculum exposure, and immunocompromised individuals may present with disseminated disease. Clusters and outbreaks have been reported among groups that have gone spelunking in Costa Rica, Ecuador, and Peru.[62–69] Immigrants or expatriates from endemic countries tend to present with disease reactivation, often associated with immunosuppressive conditions such as human immunodeficiency virus (HIV) infection.[70,71] The number of reported cases of histoplasmosis in travelers is likely an underestimate because of the self-limiting nature of acute pulmonary histoplasmosis. Case clusters highlight the lack of awareness of risks of this disease among more adventurous travelers. Potential spelunkers and cave explorers should be informed about the risks of acquiring histoplasmosis, with the use of face/surgical masks during cave exploration being the most important preventive strategy.[6] Immigrants with HIV infection and undifferentiated fever from endemic countries should be investigated for histoplasmosis.

Coccidioidomycosis is caused by inhalation of the fungi in areas where it is endemic.[6] Around 40% of those infected develop symptomatic illness, the most common of which is a nondescript flulike illness. Immunocompromised individuals such as those with HIV infection or who are on immunosuppressive drugs are at risk of disseminated disease, whereas African Americans, pregnant women, and diabetic patients may develop severe pulmonary disease.[72] Outbreaks of coccidioidomycosis have been reported in travelers who have returned from endemic areas.[73,74] Sporadic cases have been reported in travelers from Japan, Australia, and India,[75,76] whereas some Indian nationals who had previously resided in endemic parts of Arizona have also been diagnosed with the disease.[77,78] Common risk factors were activities related to construction or working in a dusty environment in endemic areas. During the Model Airplane Flying World Championship in Lost Hills, California, in 2001, several participants from various parts of the world, including Australia, United Kingdom, and Finland, developed coccidioidomycosis.[79]

Penicillium marneffei is endemic in Southeast Asia, with most cases being reported from northern Thailand.[80] Global travel and migration have resulted in cases of penicilliosis exported from these countries among individuals with HIV infection.[81–84] Antinori and coworkers[82] reviewed 36 cases of penicilliosis reported outside endemic regions from 1998 to 2004. These were mainly in travelers to and from endemic regions such as Thailand and Myanmar. There were few cases with no links to an endemic region, an African patient who had spent 4 months in a microbiology laboratory in Paris, and an HIV-infected Ghanaian who was diagnosed in Germany.[84]

Paracoccidioidomycosis is endemic in South America, in rural areas surrounding the Amazon River. As with the other endemic mycoses, infections have been reported in Netherlands, Austria, Spain, and Germany, primarily in individuals who are either migrants from South America or who have resided in an endemic area for a prolonged period.[71,85-87]

Cryptococcal infections are rarely seen in travelers. However, sporadic cases of *Cryptococcus gattii* have been reported from travel to Vancouver Island in Canada, where the fungus is now considered endemic following an outbreak since 1999.[88-90] Blastomycosis is also rare in travelers; imported cases with pulmonary or cutaneous disease have been described, however.[91,92]

SUMMARY

The spectrum of fungal infections is greater in the tropics, as is the burden of disease. For many conditions, especially the subcutaneous mycoses, the best treatment strategies remain unclear because of the lack of proper therapeutic trials. The export of tropical fungal infections via travelers and migrants is increasingly prevalent as international travel becomes easier. Travelers and physicians need to be aware of the risk factors for infection, and the prolonged latency of illness in conditions such as paracoccidioidomycosis highlights the need for detailed travel history. Enhanced surveillance for fungal infections can lead to early diagnosis and an understanding of the epidemiology of the fungal infections among travelers.

REFERENCES

1. Hay RJ. Fungal infections. In: Cook GC, Zumla A, editors. Manson's tropical diseases. 22nd edition. Philadelphia: WB Saunders; 2008. p. 1169–89. Chapter 71.
2. International Organization for Migration. World migration report 2010. Available at: http://publications.iom.int/bookstore/free/WMR2010_summary.pdf. Accessed August 13, 2011.
3. World Tourism Organization. Historical perspective of world tourism. Available at: http://www.unwto.org/facts/eng/historical.htm. Accessed August 13, 2011.
4. Freedman DO, Weld LH, Kozarsky PE, et al. Spectrum of disease and relation to place of exposure among ill returned travelers. N Engl J Med 2006;354:119–30.
5. Walsh TJ, Dixon DM. Spectrum of Mycoses. In: Baron S, editor. Medical microbiology. 4th edition. Galveston (TX): The University of Texas Medical Branch; 1996. Chapter 75. Available at: http://www.ncbi.nlm.nih.gov/books/NBK7902/. Accessed February 29, 2012.
6. Hsu LY, Ng ES, Koh LP. Common and emerging fungal pulmonary infections. Infect Dis Clin North Am 2010;24:557–77.
7. Chakrabarti A, Slavin MA. Endemic fungal infections in the Asia-Pacific region. Med Mycol 2011;49:337–44.
8. Colombo AL, Tobon A, Restrepo A, et al. Epidemiology of endemic systemic fungal infections in Latin America. Med Mycol 2011;49:785–98.
9. Havlickova B, Czaika VA, Friedrich M. Epidemiological trends in skin mycoses worldwide. Mycoses 2008;51(Suppl 4):2–15.
10. Gupta AK, Batra R, Bluhm R, et al. Pityriasis versicolor. Dermatol Clin 2003;21: 413–29.
11. Padilla-Desgarenes MC. Pityriasis versicolor. Dermatologia Rev Mex 2005;49: 157–67.
12. Bonifaz A, Gomez-Daza F, Paredes V, et al. Tinea versicolor, tinea nigra, white piedra, and black piedra. Dermatol Clin 2010;28:140–5.

13. Perez C, Colella MT, Olaizola C, et al. Tinea nigra: report of twelve cases in Venezuela. Mycopathologia 2005;160:235–8.
14. Xavier MH, Ribeiro LH, Duarte H, et al. Dermatoscopy in the diagnosis of tinea nigra. Dermatol Online J 2008;14:15.
15. Ameen M. Epidemiology of superficial fungal infections. Dermatol Clin 2010;28: 197–201.
16. Millikan LE. Current concepts in systemic and topical therapy for superficial mycoses. Dermatol Clin 2010;28:212–6.
17. Ilkit M. Favus of the scalp: an overview and update. Mycopathologia 2010;170: 143–54.
18. Bonifaz A, Vázquez-González D. Tinea imbricate in the Americas. Curr Opin Infect Dis 2011;24:106–11.
19. Silva JP, de Souza W, Rozenthal S. Chromoblastomycosis: a retrospective study of 325 cases on Amazonic region (Brazil). Mycopathologia 1998;143:171–5.
20. Nakausavariya P, Chaiprasert A, Sivayathorn A, et al. Deep fungal and higher bacterial skin infections in Thailand: clinical manifestations and treatment regimens. Int J Dermatol 1999;38:279–84.
21. Lupi O, Tyring SK, McGinnis MR. Tropical dermatology: fungal tropical diseases. J Am Acad Dermatol 2005;53:931–51.
22. Sharma A, Hazarika NK, Gupta D. Chromoblastomycosis in sub-tropical regions of India. Mycopathologia 2010;169:381–6.
23. Queiroz-Telles F, McGinnis MR, Salkin I. Subcutaneous mycoses. Infect Dis Clin North Am 2003;17:59–85.
24. Torres E, Lievanos Z. Chromoblastomycosis associated with a lethal squamous cell carcinoma. An Bras Dermatol 2010;85:267–70.
25. Ameen M. Managing chromoblastomycosis. Trop Doct 2010;40:65–7.
26. Bonifaz A, Paredes-Solis V, Saul A. Treating chromoblastomycosis with systemic antifungals. Expert Opin Pharmacother 2004;5:247–54.
27. Castro LG, Pimental ER, Lacaz CS. Treatment of chromomycosis by cryosurgery with liquid nitrogen: 15 years' experience. Int J Dermatol 2003;42: 408–12.
28. Kikuchi Y, Kondo M, Yaguchi H, et al. A case of chromomycosis caused by Fonsecaea pedrosoi presenting as a small plaque on the left upper arm: a review of reported cases of dematiaceous fungal infection in Japan. Nihon Ishinkin Gakkai Zasshi 2007;48:85–9 [in Japanese].
29. Negroni R, Tobon A, Bustamante B, et al. Posaconazole treatment of refractory eumycetoma and chromoblastomycosis. Rev Inst Med Trop Sao Paulo 2005;47: 339–46.
30. Sran HS, Narula IM, Agarwal RK, et al. History of mycetoma. Indian J Hist Med 1972;17:1–7.
31. Granica M, Nucci M, Queiroz-Telles F. Difficult mycoses of the skin: advances in the epidemiology and management of eumycetoma, phaeohyphomycosis and chromoblastomycosis. Curr Opin Infect Dis 2009;22:559–63.
32. Maslin J, Morand JJ, Civatte M. The eumycetomas (fungal mycetomas with black or white grains). Med Trop (Mars) 2001;61:111–4.
33. Ahmed AO, van Leeuwen W, Fahal A, et al. Mycetoma caused by *Madurella mycetomatis*: a neglected infectious burden. Lancet Infect Dis 2004;4:566–74.
34. Sarris I, Berendt AR, Athanasous N, et al. MRI of mycetoma of the foot: two cases demonstrating the dot-in-circle sign. Skeletal Radiol 2003;32:179–83.
35. Afroz N, Khan N, Siddiqui FA, et al. Eumycetoma versus actinomycetoma: diagnosis on cytology. J Cytol 2010;27:133–5.

36. Ahmed AO, Desplaces N, Leonard P, et al. Molecular detection and identification of agents of eumycetoma: detailed report of two cases. J Clin Microbiol 2003;41: 5813–6.
37. Djeng MT, Sy MH, Diop BM, et al. Mycetoma: 130 cases. Ann Dermatol Venereol 2003;130:16–9.
38. Fahal AH, Hassan MA. Mycetoma. Br J Surg 1992;79:1138–41.
39. Lobo J. Um caso de blastomicose produzido por uma especie nova encontrada em Recife. Rev Med Pernambucana 1931;1:763–75 [in Portugese].
40. Vilela R, Mendoza L, Rosa PS, et al. Molecular model for studying the uncultivated fungal pathogen *Lacazia loboi*. J Clin Microbiol 2005;43:3657–61.
41. Haubold EM, Cooper CR Jr, Wen JW, et al. Comparative morphology of *Lacazia loboi* (syn. *Loboa loboi*) in dolphins and humans. Med Mycol 2000;38:9–14.
42. Burns RA, Roy JS, Woods C, et al. Report of the first human case of lobomycosis in the United States. J Clin Microbiol 2000;38:1283–5.
43. Ramos-E-Silva M, Aguiar-Santos-Vilela F, Cardoso-de-Brito A, et al. Literature review and future perspectives. Actas Dermosifiliogr 2009;100(Suppl 1):92–100.
44. Camargo ZP, Baruzzi RG, Maeda SM, et al. Antigenic relationship betwcen *Loboa loboi* and *Paracoccidiodes brasiliensis* as shown by serological methods. Med Mycol 1998;36:413–7.
45. Fischer M, Chrusciak Talhari A, Reinel D, et al. Successful treatment with clofazimine and itraconazole in a 46 year old patient after 32 years duration of disease. Hautarzt 2002;53:677–81.
46. Carneiro FP, Maia LB, Moraes MA, et al. Lobomycosis: diagnosis and management of relapsed and multifocal lesions. Diagn Microbiol Infect Dis 2009;65:62–4.
47. Bustamente B, Campos PE. Endemic sporotrichosis. Curr Opin Infect Dis 2001; 14:145–9.
48. López-Romero E, Reyes-Montes Mdel R, Pérez-Torres A, et al. *Sporothrix schenckii* complex and sporotrichosis, an emerging health problem. Future Microbiol 2011;6:85–102.
49. Hay RJ, Morris-Jones R. Outbreaks of sporotrichosis. Curr Opin Infect Dis 2008; 21:119–21.
50. Kauffman CA, Bustamante B, Chapman SW, et al. Clinical practice guidelines for the management of sporotrichosis: 2007 update by the Infectious Diseases Society of America. Clin Infect Dis 2007;45:1255–65.
51. Kohler A, Weber L, Gall H, et al. Sporotrichosis—fixed cutaneous and lymphocutaneous form. Hautarzt 2000;51:09–12.
52. De Araujo T, Marques AC, Kerdel F. Sporotrichosis. Int J Dermatol 2001;40: 737–42.
53. Schwendiman MN, Johnson RP, Henning JS. Subcutaneous nodules with sporotrichoid spread. Dermatol Online J 2009;15:11.
54. Maslin J, Morand JJ, Civatte M. Sporotrichosis. Med Trop (Mars) 2002;62:9–11.
55. Mendoza M, Diaz AM, Hung MB, et al. Production of culture filtrates of *Sporothrix schenckii* in diverse culture media. Med Mycol 2002;40:447–54.
56. Bernardes-Engemann AR, Costa RC, Miguens BR, et al. Development of an enzyme-linked immunosorbent assay for the serodiagnosis of several clinical forms of sporotrichosis. Med Mycol 2005;43:487–93.
57. Hu S, Chung WH, Hung SI, et al. Detection of *Sporothrix schenckii* in clinical samples by a nested PCR assay. J Clin Microbiol 2003;41:1414–8.
58. Francesconi G, Francesconi do Valle AC, Passos SL, et al. Comparative study of 250 mg/day terbinafine and 100 mg/day itraconazole for the treatment of cutaneous sporotrichosis. Mycopathologia 2011;171:349–54.

59. Lederman ER, Weld LH, Elyazar IR, et al. Dermatologic conditions of the ill returned traveler: an analysis from the GeoSentinel Surveillance Network. Int J Infect Dis 2008;12:593–602.
60. Herbinger KH, Siess C, Nothdurft HD, et al. Skin disorders among travellers returning from tropical and non-tropical countries consulting a travel medicine clinic. Trop Med Int Health 2011;16:1457–64.
61. Ansart S, Perez L, Jaureguiberry S, et al. Spectrum of dermatoses in 165 travelers returning from the tropics with skin diseases. Am J Trop Med Hyg 2007;76:184–6.
62. Lyon GM, Bravo AV, Espino A, et al. Histoplasmosis associated with exploring a bat-inhabited cave in Costa Rica, 1998-1999. Am J Trop Med Hyg 2004;70:438–42.
63. Centers for Disease Control and Prevention. Outbreak of histoplasmosis among travelers returning from El Salvador–Pennsylvania and Virginia, 2008. MMWR Morb Mortal Wkly Rep 2008;57:1349–53.
64. Nasta P, Donisi A, Cattane A, et al. Acute histoplasmosis in spelunkers returning from Mato Grosso, Peru. J Travel Med 1997;4:176–8.
65. Valdez H, Salata RA. Bat-associated histoplasmosis in returning travelers: case presentation and description of a cluster. J Travel Med 1999;6:258–60.
66. Salomon J, Flament Saillour M, De Truchis P, et al. An outbreak of acute pulmonary histoplasmosis in members of a trekking trip in Martinique, French West Indies. J Travel Med 2003;10:87–93.
67. Gascon J, Torres JM, Luburich P, et al. Imported histoplasmosis in Spain. J Travel Med 2000;7:89–91.
68. Ohno H, Ogata Y, Suguro H, et al. An outbreak of histoplasmosis among healthy young Japanese women after traveling to Southeast Asia. Intern Med 2010;49: 491–5.
69. Weinberg M, Weeks J, Lance-Parker S, et al. Severe histoplasmosis in travelers to Nicaragua. Emerg Infect Dis 2003;9:1322–5.
70. Norman FF, Martin-Davila P, Fortun J, et al. Imported histoplasmosis: two distinct profiles in travelers and immigrants. J Travel Med 2009;16:258–62.
71. Buitrago MJ, Bernal-Martinez L, Castelli MV, et al. Histoplasmosis and paracoccidioidomycosis in a non-endemic area: a review of cases and diagnosis. J Travel Med 2011;18:26–33.
72. Rosenstein NE, Emery KW, Werner SB, et al. Risk factors for severe pulmonary and disseminated coccidioidomycosis: Kern County, California, 1995-1996. Clin Infect Dis 2001;32:708–15.
73. Cairns L, Blythe D, Kao A, et al. Outbreak of coccidioidomycosis in Washington state residents returning from Mexico. Clin Infect Dis 2000;30:61–4.
74. Centers for Disease Control and Prevention. Coccidioidomycosis in travelers returning from Mexico–Pennsylvania, 2000. MMWR Morb Mortal Wkly Rep 2000;49: 1004–6.
75. Ogiso A, Ito M, Koyama M, et al. Pulmonary coccidioidomycosis in Japan: case report and review. Clin Infect Dis 1997;25:1260–1.
76. Kumar KS, Narasimhan A, Gopalakrishnan R, et al. Coccidioidomycosis in Chennai. J Assoc Physicians India 2011;59:122–4.
77. Bharucha NE, Ramamoorthy K, Sorabjee J, et al. All that caseates is not tuberculosis. Lancet 1996;348:1313.
78. Verghese S, Arjundas D, Krishnakumar KC, et al. Coccidioidomycosis in India: report of a second imported case. Med Mycol 2002;40:307–9.
79. Centers for Disease Control and Prevention. Coccidioidomycosis among persons attending the world championship of model airplane flying—Kern County, California, October 2001. MMWR Morb Mortal Wkly Rep 2001;50:1106–7.

80. Sirisanthana T, Supparatpinyo K. Epidemiology and management of penicilliosis in human immunodeficiency virus-infected patients. Int J Infect Dis 1998;3:48–53.
81. Perlman DC, Carey J. Prevention of disseminated *Penicillium marneffei* in human immunodeficiency virus-infected travelers. J Travel Med 2006;13:386.
82. Antinori S, Gianelli E, Bonaccorso C, et al. Disseminated *Penicillium marneffei* infection in an HIV-positive Italian patient and a review of cases reported outside endemic regions. J Travel Med 2006;13:181–8.
83. Carey J, Hofflich H, Amre R, et al. *Penicillium marneffei* infection in an immuno-compromised traveler: a case report and literature review. J Travel Med 2005; 12:291–4.
84. Lo Y, Tintelnot K, Lippert U, et al. Disseminated *Penicillium marneffei* infection in an African AIDS patient. Trans R Soc Trop Med Hyg 2000;94:187.
85. Ginarte M, Pereiro M Jr, Toribio J. Imported paracoccidioidomycosis in Spain. Mycoses 2003;46:407–11.
86. Horre R, Schumacher G, Alpers K, et al. A case of imported paracoccidioidomy-cosis in a German legionnaire. Med Mycol 2002;40:213–6.
87. Van Damme PA, Bierenbroodspot F, Telgtt DS, et al. A case of imported paracoc-cidioidomycosis: an awkward infection in The Netherlands. Med Mycol 2006;44: 13–8.
88. Hagen F, van Assen S, Luijckx GJ, et al. Activated dormant *Cryptococcus gattii* infection in a Dutch tourist who visited Vancouver Island (Canada): a molecular epidemiological approach. Med Mycol 2010;48:528–31.
89. Georgi A, Schneemann M, Tintelnot K, et al. *Cryptococcus gattii* meningoen-cephalitis in an immunocompetent person 13 months after exposure. Infection 2009;37:370–3.
90. Datta K, Bartlett KH, Baer R, et al. Spread of *Cryptococcus gattii* into Pacific Northwest region of the United States. Emerg Infect Dis 2009;15:1185–91.
91. Velazquez R, Munoz-Hernandez B, Arenas R, et al. An imported case of *Blasto-myces dermatitidis* infection in Mexico. Mycopathologia 2003;156:263–7.
92. Rodriguez-Mena A, Mayorga J, Solis-Ledesma G, et al. Blastomycosis: report of an imported case in Mexico, with only cutaneous lesions. Rev Iberoam Micol 2010;27:210–2 [in Spanish].

Laboratory Diagnosis of Tropical Infections

Bryan H. Schmitt, DO[a], Jon E. Rosenblatt, MD[a],
Bobbi S. Pritt, MD, MSc, (D)TMH[b],*

KEYWORDS

- Tropical medicine • Malaria • Parasitology • Travel medicine

KEY POINTS

- Microscopy remains the cornerstone of diagnosis for tropical infections.
- Partnership between the clinical team and the laboratory is important so that the most efficacious, expedient, and cost-effective diagnostic methods may be identified.
- It is important to understand the limitations and proper use of available diagnostic tests.

INTRODUCTION

The content of this article is limited to the laboratory diagnosis of infections that occur predominantly in the tropics. The discussion includes the diagnosis of blood and tissue parasites, intestinal parasites, and tropical infections caused by fungi, bacteria, and mycobacteria. Special sections detailing laboratory performance of techniques for the identification of intestinal parasites and for specimen collection for virology testing are also included.

Although tuberculosis is prevalent in tropical countries, it is a worldwide infection, and the discussion of mycobacteria focuses on the diagnosis of leprosy and Buruli ulcer. Similarly, viral diagnostics is limited to dengue, yellow fever, human T-lymphocyte virus 1 (HTLV-1), and so forth rather than those viruses that can be common in the tropics (human immunodeficiency virus [HIV], hepatitis viruses, and others) but also cause infection worldwide. The same theme follows for all other types of microbial infections. In addition, the authors do not discuss those rare organisms that can cause severe disease in the tropics but require specialized investigative resources for their diagnosis (ie, Ebola virus, Marburg virus, and so forth).

[a] Division of Clinical Microbiology, Department of Laboratory Medicine and Pathology, Mayo Clinic, 200 First Street Southwest, Rochester, MN 55905, USA; [b] Clinical Parasitology and Virology, Division of Clinical Microbiology, Department of Laboratory Medicine and Pathology, Mayo Clinic, 200 First Street Southwest, Rochester, MN 55905, USA
* Corresponding author.
E-mail address: pritt.bobbi@mayo.edu

Infect Dis Clin N Am 26 (2012) 513–554
doi:10.1016/j.idc.2012.03.011
0891-5520/12/$ – see front matter © 2012 Elsevier Inc. All rights reserved.

Because many clinical laboratories have limited experience with the organisms causing tropical infections, it is important for clinicians to discuss the suspected diagnoses with the laboratory as a general rule. Providing this information will allow the laboratory to identify the necessary resources and collect and preserve the appropriate samples. Many tests are routinely available in clinical laboratories, whereas others are only available from laboratories of the Centers for Disease Control and Prevention (CDC), the World Health Organization (WHO), or other reference laboratories. Some of the discussed tests are only available by special arrangement with research and developmental centers. Whichever testing source is used, it is important to have enough information about the validity of the method used to have confidence in the results. In an effort to provide more rapid results, some laboratories may perform simple commercially available immunochromatographic assays (ICTs), or dipstick tests, if diseases, such as malaria, are suspected. Although these may be useful as readily available screening tests, they may lack sensitivity or specificity and should be followed up with more accurate confirmatory tests, such as a morphologic preparation or polymerase chain reaction (PCR) assay, as soon as possible.

GENERAL COMMENTS REGARDING DIAGNOSTIC TESTS AVAILABLE FOR ILLNESSES ENCOUNTERED IN THE TROPICS

Table 1 contains a general list of the diagnostic tests available for illnesses possibly encountered in tropical areas of the world. Please see the specific organism sections for more detailed information. Test results are only as reliable as the experience, resources, and expertise of the laboratory performing the tests. In general, laboratories of the CDC and WHO are more likely than commercial laboratories to have the experience and volume of specimens to properly validate the more rarely performed tests. On the other hand, turnaround time for results is often faster with commercial reference laboratories. Direct communication by telephone or e-mail will sometimes hasten specimen processing and result reporting from public health laboratories, especially when there is an urgent clinical situation. Given the availability of rapid shipping methods (FedEx, UPS, and so forth) and e-mail or other electronic communication, results can also be available from laboratories in Europe and Asia in surprisingly short periods of time. It is useful to obtain shipping information from such laboratories to avoid unnecessary delays because of customs, airline regulations, or other delivery problems. The DPDx Web site (http://www.dpd.cdc.gov/dpdx/HTML/DiagnosticProcedures.htm) may be consulted for a current list of diagnostic tests for parasitic infections available from the CDC.

LABORATORY DIAGNOSIS OF INFECTIONS CAUSED BY BLOOD AND TISSUE PARASITES

Microscopy remains the cornerstone of diagnostic laboratory testing for blood and tissue parasites (see **Table 1**).[1] The microscopic examination of thick and thin peripheral blood films stained with Giemsa or other appropriate stains is used for the detection and identification of protozoans, such as the *Plasmodium, Babesia,* and *Trypanosoma* species, and the filarial nematodes, *Brugia, Mansonella, and Wuchereria,*[2] whereas the microscopic examination or culture of ulcer samples, bone marrow, tissue aspirates, and biopsies are useful in the diagnosis of African trypanosomiasis, onchocerciasis, trichinosis, and leishmaniasis.[3] The accuracy of these methods depends on the availability of well-trained and experienced technologists, and diagnosis may be hampered by the sparseness of organisms on the slide and the subjective nature of differentiating similar-appearing organisms. Furthermore, samples must be properly obtained, transported to the laboratory as quickly as possible, and

Table 1
Laboratory diagnosis of tropical infections: infectious diseases or infecting organisms that may be encountered in the tropics and available diagnostic tests

Disease/Causative Agent	Diagnostic Tests	Remarks
African histoplasmosis/*Histoplasma duboisii*	Culture (mold at 25°C, 8–15 μm yeast at 37°C) and histopathology; DNA probe for identification of *Histoplasma capsulatum* from culture cross-reacts with *Histoplasma duboisii*	Commonly mistaken for *Blastomyces dermatitidis* on tissue section but has narrow-based rather than broad-based buds
African tick-bite fever/*Rickettsia africae*	Serology from CDC or WHO Reference laboratory. Cross-reacts with other members of the spotted fever group	WHO Center for Rickettsial Reference and Research in Marseille, France, Contact Professor Didier Raoult (Didier.Raoult@medecine.univ-mrs.fr)
Amebiasis/*Entamoeba histolytica*	Stool ova and parasite microscopy, antigen detection from stool using EIA, serology for extraintestinal disease, PCR	Microscopy cannot differentiate between *Entamoeba histolytica*, *Entamoeba dispar*, and *Entamoeba moshkovkii*, whereas some antigen and PCR methods can. EIA kits are commercially available in the United States. Serology is the test of choice for disseminated disease, including amoebic liver abscess, because stool O&P may be negative.
Ascariasis/*Ascaris lumbricoides*	Stool ova and parasite microscopy; Larvae may be identified in sputum during pulmonary migration.	Characteristic macroscopic adult worms may be passed in stool or through the nose or mouth.
Babesiosis/*Babesia* species, including *Babesia microti, Babesia divergens*	Microscopy of thick and thin blood films stained with Giemsa or other appropriate stains	Real-time PCR available from CDC and referral laboratories as is serology, which does not distinguish acute from past infections.
Bartonellosis/*Bartonella bacilliformis*	Acute phase, peripheral blood film with Giemsa stain; Chronic phase, silver stain of skin lesions;	Culture using Columbia-blood agar
Brucellosis/*Brucella* species	Culture of blood, bone marrow, tissues, abscess fluid, CSF, urine, and respiratory specimens may be used. Automated culture systems give higher yield. Screening is with IgM and IgG	Cultures should be performed in biologic safety cabinet. Blood and bone marrow are the preferred specimens.

(continued on next page)

Table 1
(continued)

Disease/Causative Agent	Diagnostic Tests	Remarks
	antibodies. Confirmation is by *Brucella*-specific agglutination tests.	
Buruli ulcer/*Mycobacterium ulcerans*	AFB stain of smears from the base of lesion or biopsy; PCR testing, if available, is rapid and sensitive.	Culture requires 6–12 wk and mycobacterial media
Chikungunya/chikungunya virus	Serology from CDC (Division of Vector Borne Diseases, Ft Collins, CO; cdc.gov/ncidod/dvbid) and reference laboratories	Acute and convalescent sera may be required to show significant titer increase. In fatal cases, CDC offers PCR, histopathology with immunohistochemistry, or virus culture (BSL-3).
Chromoblastomycosis/Multiple dematiaceous fungi	Brown muriform bodies on skin biopsy histologic section, fungal culture for definitive identification and antimicrobial susceptibility testing	Caused by multiple dematiaceous fungi; causative agents cannot be distinguished by histopathology
Clonorchiasis/*Clonorchis sinensis*, *Opisthorchis* spp	Stool or duodenal aspirate ova and parasite microscopy, serology	The eggs of *Clonorchis sinensis* and *Opisthorchis* spp are morphologically indistinguishable. Adult flukes may be recovered at surgery.
Crimean-Congo hemorrhagic fever (CCHF)/CCHF virus	Viremia occurs early on in illness, during which culture, antigen detection, or RT-PCR may be performed. Serology will be positive later in disease in patients who survive.	BSL-4 facilities are required for culture, antigen detection, and RT-PCR. Contact the CDC Special Pathogens Branch http://www.cdc.gov/ncidod/dvrd/spb/index.htm
Cryptosporidiosis/*Cryptosporidium parvum, Cryptosporidium hominis*, and other species	Stool microscopy using specific stains (modified Kinyoun acid-fast) or fecal antigen detection	*Cryptosporidium* spp may be detected by routine stool microscopy but with lower sensitivity than with specific stains
Cyclosporiasis, cystoisosporiasis (isosporiasis), and sarcocystosis/*Cyclospora cayetanensis, Cystoisospora belli/Sarcocystis* spp	Ova and parasite microscopy; modified Kinyoun acid-fast or safranin stains for *Cyclospora* and *Cystoisospora*; blue autofluorescence of *Cyclospora* and *Sarcocystis* with UV microscopy	*Cryptosporidium* and *Cyclospora cayetanensis* have a similar appearance on acid-fast stains and must be differentiated by measurement (*Cryptosporidium* oocysts are smaller). Rarely sporulation assays are used to differentiate *Cyclospora* oocysts from blue-green algae.

Disease/Organism	Test	Comments
Cysticercosis/*Taenia solium*	Serology is by EIA or WB assay from CDC and reference laboratories. Sensitivity is decreased with single or healed/calcified cysts.	Western blot immunoassay is more accurate than EIA. Serology cross-reacts with *Echinococcus*.
Dengue/Dengue virus	Serology from CDC (Division of Vector Borne Diseases, Ft Collins, CO; cdc.gov/ncidod/dvbid) and reference laboratories, commercially available ELISA, and lateral-flow rapid antigen tests. PCR from specialized centers	Acute and convalescent sera may be required to show significant titer increase. In fatal cases, CDC offers PCR, histopathology with immunohistochemistry, or virus culture (BSL-2).
Echinococcosis/*Echinococcus granulosus, Echinococcus multilocularis*	Serology is by EIA or WB from CDC and reference laboratories. Sensitivity is decreased if only lung cysts are present.	WB immunoassay is more accurate than EIA. Serology cross-reacts with cysticercosis.
Eosinophilic meningitis/*Angiostrongylus cantonensis*	Serology is available at CDC or at the Department of Helminthology, Faculty of Tropical Medicine, Mahidol University, 420/6 Rajvithi Road, Bangkok 10400, Thailand (http://www.tm.mahidol.ac.th/en/special).	Eosinophilic meningitis may also be caused by *Gnathostoma* in endemic areas, but serology will differentiate the 2 different causes.
Fascioliasis and fasciolopsiasis, *Fasciola, Fasciolopsis*	Stool (or duodenal aspirate for *Fasciola*) ova and parasite microscopy, serology	The eggs of *Fasciola hepatica* and *Fasciolopsis buski* are morphology indistinguishable. *Fasciola* eggs may be transiently found in human stool caused by ingestion of infected animal liver. Repeated detection establishes infection.
Filariasis, lymphatic caused by species of *Wuchereria, Brugia,* and *Mansonella*	Microscopy of thick and thin blood films stained with Giemsa or other appropriate stains; Microscopy of concentrated (Knott) or Nuclepore-filtered blood or buffy coat (increased sensitivity). Serology or antigen detection for *Wuchereria bancrofti* (*May be* available from CDC or reference laboratory) Speciated by morphologic characteristics, such as presence/absence of sheath and position of nuclei.	Blood films may be best examined during night depending on periodicity of microfilaria (*Wuchereria bancrofti* and *Brugia malayi*). Serology does not differentiate genera and species of filaria. Contact CDC or Dr Thomas Nutman at the NIH (tnutman@niaid.nih.gov), Laboratory of Parasitic Diseases, National Institutes of Health (301) 496 - 5398. Motile adult worms may be visualized by ultrasound examination of involved lymphatics.

(continued on next page)

Table 1
(continued)

Disease/Causative Agent	Diagnostic Tests	Remarks
Filariasis, Onchocerciasis/*Onchocerca volvulus*	Microscopy of skin snip; histopathologic examination of skin biopsy	Skin snips should be from areas adjacent to nodules and should be razor thin with no visible blood present. Antibody or antigen detecting immunoassays may be available from the CDC.
Giardiasis/*Giardia intestinalis* (*Giardia lamblia*, *Giardia duodenalis*)	Stool and duodenal aspirate ova and parasite microscopy, Enterotest (HDC Diagnostics, San Jose, CA, USA), fecal antigen detection by FA or EIA	Falling-leaf motility of trophozoites on direct examination. Multiple specimens for stool examination may be required because of intermittent excretion.
Gnathostomiasis caused by *Gnathostoma spp* (may be a cause of eosinophilic meningitis)	Serology available at CDC or at the Department of Helminthology, Faculty of Tropical Medicine, Mahidol University, 420/6 Rajvithi Road, Bangkok 10400, Thailand; telephone: 662 246-0321, 662 246-9000 to 13, 662 246-5600 ext 1820; Fax: 662-643-5600; (http://www.tm.mahidol.ac.th/en/special)	Eosinophilic meningitis may also be caused by *Angiostrongylus* in endemic areas, but serology will differentiate the 2 different causes.
Hookworm/*Ancylostoma duodenale* and *Necator americanus*	Stool ova and parasite microscopy	Eggs in unpreserved stool may hatch if examination is delayed for more than 24 h and must be differentiated from *Strongyloides* larvae. Eggs of *Ancylostoma duodenale* and *Necator americanus* cannot be differentiated by morphology.
HTLV-1, HTLV-2 infection	Serology (ELISA) from reference laboratories; positives are confirmed with WB or RIPA. PCR amplification of proviral DNA is the preferred method for distinguishing subtypes.	HTLV-1 serology has extensive cross-reactivity with HTLV-2. Patients with HTLV-1 infection are at increased risk for crusted scabies and disseminated strongyloidiasis. All blood donors in the United States are tested for antibodies to HTLV-1 and 2.
Japanese encephalitis/Japanese encephalitis virus	Serology from CDC (Division of Vector Borne Diseases, Ft Collins, CO; cdc.gov/ncidod/dvbid)	In fatal cases, CDC offers PCR, histopathology with immunohistochemistry, or virus culture (BSL-3).

Organism	Diagnostic method	Comments
Leishmaniasis, cutaneous/*Leishmania* species	Microscopic examination of Giemsa-stained touch-impression smears of leading edge of ulcers; Culture may be available using special media (NNN and others) from reference laboratories or CDC.	Histopathologic microscopy of ulcer leading edge biopsies may be diagnostic but is not more sensitive than impression smears.
Leishmaniasis, visceral/*Leishmania* species	Histopathologic microscopy of Giemsa-stained bone marrow; Culture may be available using special media (NNN and others). Serology using IFA or K39 antigen is available from CDC (Fsteurer@cdc.gov) or reference laboratories.	Positive K39 serology has been reported in some patients with cutaneous leishmaniasis without evidence of visceral disease
Leprosy/*Mycobacterium leprae*	Skin biopsy with Fite stain for AFB	PCR and PGL-I antibody levels may be helpful but are only available through research laboratories.
Leptospirosis/*Leptospira* species	Culture of blood or CSF during first week of illness, urine thereafter (notify laboratory because special procedures may be required); Serology is positive after first week of symptoms.	Variety of serologic tests has been used. Most available is from reference laboratories is probably IHA; Significant elevation in titer (4-fold) between acute and convalescent sera diagnostic, but high titer single specimen may also be diagnostic ($\geq$1:100 for IHA)
Lobomycosis/*Lacazia loboi* (formerly *Loboa loboi*	Cannot be grown in fungal culture; Histologic section shows chains of uniform round-to-oval yeasts connected by narrow buds/intracellular bridges; Maltese cross birefringence on polarized light	Often mistaken as paracoccidioidomycosis, blastomycosis, or African histoplasmosis by histopathology
Malaria/*Plasmodium* species	Microscopy of thick and thin blood films stained with Giemsa or other appropriate stains; antigen (HRP2 or LDH) detecting immunochromatographic strip tests	Malaria is potentially life threatening and should be considered an STAT diagnosis. Antigen strip tests lack sensitivity when parasitemia is low and do not differentiate all species of *Plasmodium*. Real-time PCR is available from CDC and some reference laboratories and will differentiate species.

(continued on next page)

Table 1
(continued)

Disease/Causative Agent	Diagnostic Tests	Remarks
Melioidosis/*Burkholderia pseudomallei*	Blood cultures and cultures and Gram stain of skin lesions (looking for Gram negative bipolar rods suggestive of *Burkholderia pseudomallei*)	Serology by IFA from reference laboratories; IgG titers ≥1:128 for a single serum indicates exposure; IgM titer of ≥1:40 suggests recent or current infection. A 4-fold increase in IgG titer between acute and convalescent sera at least 2 wk apart confirms recent or current infection.
Microsporidiosis/multiple species, including *Enterocytozoon bieneusi*, *Encephalitozoon* spp	Microscopy of stool concentrate smears using chromotrope 2R stains, including trichrome blue stain or fluorescent Calcofluor white stain, histopathologic examination of small intestinal biopsies	Significant expertise is required for identification because of the very small size (0.8–4 μm) and morphologic similarity to yeasts. Transmission electron microscopy is considered the gold standard of microsporidian species but is expensive and not widely used.
Mycetoma/various fungi and filamentous bacteria	Microscopic examination and culture of grains from draining sinuses. Both fungi and bacteria will stain with Gram stain (positive), PAS, and GMS. Culture for identification of causative agent	Bacterial causes are approximately 4 times more common than fungal causes of mycetoma. Culture is required for antimicrobial susceptibility testing.
Paracoccidioidomycosis/*Paracoccidioides brasiliensis*	Culture of tissue or respiratory specimens; mold at 25 °C, yeast at 37°C; On histology or wet prep, multiple circumferential buds from 2–30 μm yeast make a mariner's wheel	Morphologic differential diagnosis includes *Blastomyces dermatitidis*. DNA probes for *Blastomyces dermatitidis* from culture isolates may cross-react with *Paracoccidioides brasiliensis* and cause false positive results.
Paragonimiasis/*Paragonimus westermani* and other species	Microscopy of unstained stool or sputum concentrates	Eggs in sputum may be swallowed and identified in stool. They must be differentiated from similar-appearing operculated eggs, such as eggs of *Fasciola hepatica* and *Diphyllobothrium latum*. Adult flukes may be seen in histopathologic sections of lung biopsies. Serology is available from the CDC.

Disease/Organism	Diagnostic Methods
Penicilliosis/*Penicillium marneffei*	Culture; Gray-pink mold with red reverse at 25°C, yeast at 37°C; On histology or wet prep, oval to elongated 3–6 μm yeasts with a transverse septum. Distinguished from other small yeasts, such as *Histoplasma capsulatum* by division via transverse septation rather than budding
Rickettsiosis, spotted fever group *Rickettsia rickettsii, R conorii, R akari, R africae*	Serology, generally group specific, available from CDC and reference laboratories (IFA IgG titers ≥1:256 suggest active disease). Weil-Felix reaction using cross-reacting *Proteus* antigen is generic for rickettsial infection and less useful. *R africae* demonstrates cross-reactivity with other assays for spotted fever group.
Rickettsiosis, Typhus fever group/*R typhi, R prowazekii*	Serology, generally group specific, available from CDC and reference laboratories (IFA IgG titers ≥1:256 suggest active disease). Weil-Felix reaction using cross-reacting *Proteus* antigen is generic for rickettsial infection and less useful
Rift Valley fever/Rift Valley fever virus	Serology (EIA) from CDC, Special Pathogens Branch (http://www.cdc.gov/ncidod/dvrd/spb/index.htm). Viral antigen detection and viral RNA by RT-PCR in serum or blood may be available from CDC by special request. Virus may not be detectable in blood during later stages of illness (encephalitis, retinitis).
Schistosomiasis/*Schistosoma mansoni, S hematobium,* and *S japonicum* are the main species	Stool or urine ova and parasite microscopy or microscopy of Nuclepore filter from spot urine collection; histopathology of rectal or bladder biopsy; serology. Serology from CDC and reference laboratories; CDC performs FAST-ELISA for *Schistosoma mansoni* and specific immunoblots, which can identify infecting species
Strongyloidiasis/*Strongyloides stercoralis*	Stool ova and parasite microscopy; Examination of fresh specimen, free of preservatives, is useful to identify motile larvae. In hyperinfection syndrome, examination of sputum or CSF may also show motile larvae. Serology may be helpful when multiple stool and sputum examinations fail to demonstrate the parasite. Eggs are not excreted in stool. Examination of multiple stools (up to 7) and use of special procedures, such as agar plate culture or Baermann technique, increases diagnostic sensitivity. Serology is available from CDC and reference laboratories but may cross-react with serum from patients with filariasis and other nematode infections. Microscopy is required for definitive diagnosis of active infection.

(continued on next page)

Table 1
(continued)

Disease/Causative Agent	Diagnostic Tests	Remarks
Tapeworm Infection (caused by *Taenia* species or *Diphyllobothrium latum*)	Stool ova and parasite microscopy. Gross examination of fresh stool may reveal motile proglottids.	*Taenia solium* and *Taenia saginata* eggs are morphologically indistinguishable. The 2 species can be differentiated by morphologic examination of proglottids or the scolex. Vitamin B12 deficiency may be detected with *Diphyllobothrium latum* infection.
Traveler's diarrhea (caused by *Campylobacter, Escherichia coli, Salmonella, Shigella, Vibrio*)	Stool culture for enteric pathogens (enterotoxigenic *Escherichia coli* not detected by routine culture); Notify laboratory if vibrios or enterohemorrhagic *Escherichia coli* suspected	Stool examination for presence of WBCs may be useful in differentiating bacterial from other causes of diarrhea. PCR available from some reference laboratories.
Trench Fever/*Bartonella quintana*	Indirect Immunofluorescence Assay (IFA) to detect IgG and IgM antibodies	Culture using Columbia-blood agar. PCR available from referral laboratories.
Trichinosis/*Trichinella spiralis* and other species	Serology from CDC or reference laboratories	Encysted larvae can be seen in histopathologic sections. Stool microscopy is not used for detection.
Trichuriasis/*Trichuris trichiura*	Stool ova and parasite microscopy	
Trypanosomiasis, African (sleeping sickness) caused by *Trypanosoma brucei gambiense* (West African) or *T. b. rhodesiense* (East African)	Microscopy of thick and thin blood films or buffy coat preps stained with Giemsa or other appropriate stains. CSF and aspirates of chancres and lymph nodes may also be examined.	A card agglutination test is available for serology of T. b. gambiense infection. Contact CDC or the Parasite Diagnostic Unit, Prince Leopold Institute of Tropical Medicine, Antwerp, Belgium: telephone: +32 3247.63 71; Fax: +32 3 24763 73; info@itg.be, http://www.itg.be/itg/
Trypanosomiasis, American (Chagas disease) caused by *Trypanosoma cruzi*	Microscopy of thick and thin blood films or buffy coat preps stained with Giemsa or other appropriate stains (acute infection). Serology is available for donor and diagnostic testing. Culture of blood may be available using special media (NNN and others)	During chronic infection, parasitemia is low and blood film examinations are insensitive. IgG antibody may persist for decades, and its presence is considered evidence of chronic infection. An ELISA has been developed specifically for the screening of blood donors.

Typhoid fever (infection with *Salmonella typhi*)	Blood cultures are positive in 80% of cases during first wk of illness with subsequent decreases in positivity. There is significant decreased positivity in treated patients. Culture of bone marrow may enhance recovery.	*Salmonella typhi* may be cultured from stool during third to fourth wk of illness. Notify laboratory because recovery is enhanced by use of enrichment media. Widal test and newer serologic assays are neither sensitive nor specific.
West Nile virus	Serology from CDC on blood and CSF (Division of Vector Borne Diseases, Ft Collins, CO; cdc.gov/ncidod/dvbid) and many state public health laboratories and reference laboratories	PCR is available but useful only in very early stages of the disease. WNV ELISA may cross-react with other Flaviviruses (eg Saint Louis encephalitis, dengue, yellow fever); positive ELISA tests should be confirmed by neutralization testing.
Yellow fever	Serology from CDC (Division of Vector Borne Diseases, Ft Collins, CO; cdc.gov/ncidod/dvbid)	In fatal cases, CDC offers PCR, histopathology with immunohistochemistry, or virus culture (BSL-3). Viremia occurs early in illness. Positive serology should be confirmed by neutralization testing.

Notes: Unless otherwise specified, CDC refers to the Division of Parasitic Diseases at the Centers for Disease Control, Atlanta Georgia, (770) 488-4431. Central telephone for CDC: (404) 639-3311; Available at: http://www.cdc.gov/or http://www.dpd.cdc.gov/dpdx/. Reference laboratories refers to any laboratory that performs esoteric testing not usually done in routine hospital laboratories, examples in the United States include ARUP (800) 522-2787), FOCUS Diagnostics ([703] 480-2500), and Mayo Medical Laboratories (800-533-1710). All have their own Web sites.

Abbreviations: BSL, biosafety level; CL, cutaneous leishmaniasis; CSF, cerebrospinal fluid; EIA, enzyme-linked immunoassay; ELISA, enzyme-linked immunosorbent assay; FA, fluorescent antibody; GMS, Gomori methenamine silver; H&E, hematoxylin and eosin; HAT, human African trypanosomiasis; HRP2, histidine rich protein 2; IFA, indirect fluorescent antibody; IHA, indirect hemagglutination assay; LDH, lactic dehydrogenase; MAT, microscopic agglutination test; NIH, National Institutes of Health; NNN, Novy-MacNeal-Nicolle medium; O&P, ova and parasite; PAS, periodic acid Schiff stain; PGL-I, phenolic glycolipid-I; QBC, Quantitative Buffy Coat; RBC, red blood cell; RDT, rapid diagnostic test; RIPA, radioimmunoprecipitation assay; RT-PCR, reverse transcriptase PCR; TAT, tube agglutination test; VL, visceral leishmaniasis; WB, Western blot; WBC, white blood cell.

processed in a timely fashion to preserve organism viability or morphology. The clinician can greatly aid in the laboratory diagnosis of blood and tissue parasites by providing clinical and epidemiologic information that will assist in the selection of appropriate testing and guide the interpretation of results.

Serologic assays for the detection of antibodies are available as adjunctive methods for the diagnosis of several infections. However, none of these assays are sensitive or specific enough to be used to establish the diagnosis without the consideration of the clinical presentation and the potential faults of each test.[1] In particular, assays for infection with a particular helminth will often cross-react with antibodies to a different helminth. Also, there are different types of serologic tests, each with their own inherent advantages and disadvantages. Indirect fluorescent antibody assays (IFA) can provide quantitative titer results, but reading the slides is subjective and inherently prone to variability. In comparison, enzyme-linked immunosorbent assays (ELISA) provide only qualitative positive or negative results determined by an arbitrarily set breakpoint. Thus, clinicians will not be able to determine if a positive result was a very strong positive or a very weak one without calling the laboratory for more information.

PCR assays have been developed for the diagnosis of many blood and tissue parasites, including malaria[4] and leishmania.[5] Although these assays typically demonstrate good sensitivity and specificity, the costs of performing the assay may be prohibitive and availability may be restricted because many of the assays are currently only being performed on a research basis. The diseases for which PCR assays have been developed and their availability are discussed in their respective sections.

LABORATORY DIAGNOSIS OF MALARIA

The standard method for the diagnosis of malaria is microscopy of Giemsa-stained thick and thin blood films.[1] Wright, Wright-Giemsa, or a rapid stain, such as Field, may also be used as long as white blood cells (WBCs; which stain the same as parasites) are adequately stained. Although this method requires a minimum amount of resources (staining materials and high-quality microscopes), well-trained and experienced technologists must be available. Blood film examinations for *Plasmodium* should be considered statim procedures, and ideally the slides should be examined within 2 to 3 hours of being obtained from patients.[3] In addition, if blood is collected in EDTA tubes, parasite morphology may be altered by delays in preparation of the slides.[1,3]

The thick blood film is essentially a lysed concentrate of red blood cells (RBCs) and is, therefore, the most sensitive preparation for the microscopic identification of *Plasmodium* and *Babesia* parasites (**Fig. 1**).[1]

Thick films do not generally allow for the definitive identification of the infecting species[2]; however, the thin film can be used for speciation and determining the degree of parasitemia (**Fig. 2**). Several excellent atlases are available for describing the characteristic features of each *Plasmodium* species.[3,6]

Parasitemia is usually expressed as a percentage of RBCs parasitized and may be used to direct initial therapy, especially in malaria caused by *Plasmodium falciparum*, and to follow the response to therapy. It is important to remember that the persistence of gametocytes is common in adequately treated malaria when nongametocidal drugs are used and does not indicate a failure of therapy.[7] Therefore, the laboratory should indicate when parasitemia is predominantly caused by the presence of gametocytes versus other forms. Recently, human infections with the simian parasite, *Plasmodium knowlesi,* have been described.[8] This organism has morphologic features similar to *Plasmodium malariae* but may cause severe clinical infections. Because it is difficult

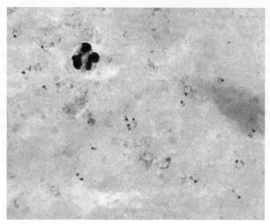

Fig. 1. Thick film containing *Plasmodium falciparum* parasites. The numerous small purple-blue dots, some with attached ringlike structures, are parasites. The RBCs have been lysed so that no intact cells are visible, but there is a single WBC in the upper left hand corner (Giemsa, original magnification ×1000).

to specifically identify on blood films, molecular testing may be useful.[8] It is important to remember that *Babesia* and *Plasmodium* may at times be indistinguishable on blood films and that both can be transmitted by transfusion so each can occur in atypical clinical settings.

Depending on the laboratory setting, tests other than traditional thick and thin blood films may be available. The Quantitative Buffy Coat (QBC Diagnostics, Port Matilda, PA, USA) method is a morphologic diagnostic method that detects fluorescently stained parasites within RBCs.[9] Positive QBC results should be followed by the preparation of a thin blood film to specifically identify the infecting species and determine the percent parasitemia.

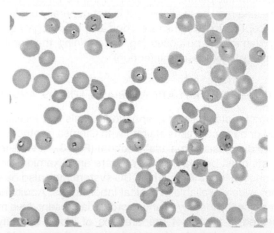

Fig. 2. Thin blood film containing *Plasmodium falciparum* parasites. Note that the RBCs are intact and the parasites contained within can be examined for morphologic features consistent with *Plasmodium* species (Giemsa, original magnification ×1000).

Rapid antigen diagnostics tests (RDTs) are also commercially available. The Binax-Now (Inverness Medical, Scarborough, ME, USA) rapid diagnostic test for the diagnosis of malaria is currently the only Food and Drug Administration (FDA)-approved test and is a rapid ICT card (or dipstick) assay that uses monoclonal antibodies to detect the histidine-rich protein 2 (HRP-2) antigen of *Plasmodium falciparum* and an aldolase common to all species of *Plasmodium*. The use of RDTs has been shown to be preferable to routine microscopy in some studies.[10] Positive RDTs should be confirmed by blood films, which are also necessary to determine which species other than *Plasmodium falciparum* (if the assay is aldolase positive but HRP-2 negative) is present and to determine the degree of parasitemia. It may also be used to help differentiate malaria from babesiosis. This RDT is somewhat less sensitive than a thick blood film and may be falsely negative in cases with very low degrees of parasitemia.[11] However, the sensitivity is comparable with blood films in patients with symptomatic malaria in endemic areas[12] but this may not be true for nonimmune patients who may be symptomatic at very low levels of parasitemia. In addition, RDTs may be falsely positive for several days after the eradication of intact parasites because antigens may still be detected. Therefore, the assay should not be used to follow patients after adequate therapy has been given. The RDT should not be viewed as a replacement for blood films but rather as a substitute in situations whereby reliable blood films will not be readily available or when the clinical situation is critical and an immediate diagnosis is required (eg, stat laboratory in the emergency department).[13] Quality thick and thin blood films should follow RDT testing as soon as possible. A negative RDT in a clinical setting suggesting malaria must be followed-up by adequate blood films without delay.

Rapid real time PCR assays for the diagnosis of malaria have also been developed[4,14] and are available from commercial referral laboratories and the CDC. Many methods are comparable in sensitivity to the thick blood film and may be useful in the accurate diagnosis of acute infection if films are negative or difficult to interpret and in the differentiation of malaria parasites from *Babesia* or nonparasitic artifacts. PCR may also confirm the diagnosis in cases empirically treated without prior laboratory diagnosis through the detection of remnant nucleic acid. Asplenic patients are less able to clear the infection, and PCR tests may remain persistently positive with all forms of *Plasmodium falciparum* being seen in the peripheral blood.[15]

Finally, IFA for malaria may be available but is not generally useful for the diagnosis of acute disease except perhaps in the rare tropical splenomegaly syndrome. It is also widely used for epidemiologic purposes (eg, determining the number of individuals that have been previously exposed to infection).

LABORATORY DIAGNOSIS OF LYMPHATIC FILARIASIS, LOIASIS, AND ONCHOCERCIASIS

The standard method for diagnosis of lymphatic filariasis and loiasis is microscopy of thick and thin blood or buffy coat films stained with Giemsa or other appropriate stains (see the "Laboratory diagnosis of malaria" section) (**Fig. 3**).[2,3] Well-trained and experienced technologists must be available to prepare and examine these slides for the presence of these unusual organisms. The QBC system may also be used to enhance sensitivity but is not widely available in clinical laboratories. Additional thin films may be required to determine the identity of any microfilaria present. Live motile microfilaria may also be observed in fresh wet preparations of blood or buffy coat samples. Concentration methods, such as the Knott technique or the use of Nuclepore polycarbonate filters (Capitol Scientific, Inc., Austin, TX, USA), can increase the sensitivity of light microscopy.[3] *Wuchereria bancrofti* and *Brugia malayi* may have nocturnal

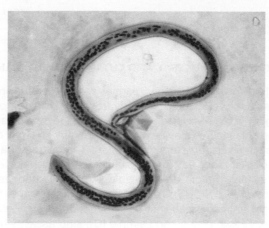

Fig. 3. Microfilaria of *Wuchereria bancrofti*. Microfilariae are differentiated by morphologic features, such as the presence of a sheath and placement of internal nuclei. In this case, a poorly stained sheath is present, and the nuclei do not extend to the tip of the tail, which is classic for this species. (Giemsa, thick blood film, original magnification ×1000).

periodicity (depending on geographic origin of infection) and blood may be best examined in samples taken from 10 PM to 2 AM.[16,17]

In comparison with the blood-borne microfilariae, the standard method for laboratory diagnosis of onchocerciasis is microscopy of multiple Giemsa-stained skin snips, which can demonstrate microfilaria.[18] Skin snips are minute bloodless biopsies taken down to the dermal papillae using a razor blade or corneoscleral biopsy instrument. Multiple (up to 6), thin, 1- to 2-mg snips of skin are needed for a reliable diagnosis. They can be taken from the tissue surrounding nodules suspected of containing adult worms or at random sites overlying the scapula or iliac crest. Fresh unstained wet preps of skin snips can be examined immediately and should also be examined after incubation in saline at 37° C for 2 to 24 hours.[19] Less commonly, microfilaria can be seen in histopathologic sections of skin biopsies stained with hematoxylin and eosin (H&E), although this is not a preferred method of identification.

In some instances, identification of adult filarial worms can be performed through either gross examination or microscopic examination of histopathologic sections. Adult worms of *Loa loa* can sometimes be observed in the subconjunctival space of the eye, permitting a presumptive clinical diagnosis. These worms can be extracted from the eye or subcutaneous nodules (Calabar swellings), permitting definitive identification. Similarly, adults of *Onchocerca volvulus* can be observed in the gross or histopathologic study of surgically removed or biopsied skin nodules (onchocercomas).[20]

Filarial serology is available from referral laboratories (FOCUS Diagnostics, http://www.focusdx.com/) and can detect filarial immunoglobulin (Ig) G4 antibodies. Antigens of *Dirofilaria immitis* or *Brugia malayi* are typically used, which cross-react with all filarial species. Because of this, the assay is nonspecific and provides only qualitative positive or negative results.[1] Antibodies may not be detectable in chronic lymphatic filariasis (elephantiasis). Antigen-detecting immunoassays performed at the CDC are an adjunct to detecting microfilaremia caused by *Wuchereria bancrofti*. An ICT card test (BinaxNow ICT) and an Og43C ELISA (Filariasis CELISA, Cellabs,

Sydney, Australia) are reported to be both sensitive and specific,[16,21] although neither of these commercial assays is approved by the FDA.

LABORATORY DIAGNOSIS OF VISCERAL AND CUTANEOUS LEISHMANIASIS

The standard method for the laboratory diagnosis of visceral leishmaniasis (VL) is microscopy of Giemsa- or H&E-stained aspirates and biopsies of bone marrow, spleen, or liver (**Fig. 4**).[3,22] Well-trained and experienced technologists must be available because tissue amastigotes may be difficult to identify and may be confused with other organisms, such as *Histoplasma capsulatum*. The culture of aspirates of bone marrow or spleen or liver biopsies can be useful if the Novy-MacNeal-Nicolle (NNN) medium or other suitable media are available. An IFA immunoassay is available from referral laboratories (FOCUS Diagnostics and others) and the CDC, which detects IgG and IgM antibodies against *Leishmania donovani, Leishmania tropica,* and *Leishmania braziliensis*. A rapid and simple ICT strip assay, which detects antibodies against the rK39 antigen of *Leishmania donovani,* is commercially available and is more than 90% sensitive and specific for VL in India but may be less accurate in other regions.[22] Sensitivity is diminished in patients infected with HIV or other immunocompromised patients. These serologic assays should not be used in the diagnosis of cutaneous leishmaniasis (CL), although CL has been associated with a reactive rK39 assay result in some US servicepeople without clinical evidence of VL.[23]

The standard method for laboratory diagnosis of CL and mucocutaneous leishmaniasis is the microscopy of Giemsa- or H&E-stained scrapings, impression smears, aspirates, or biopsies of skin ulcers or mucosal lesions.[3,22,24]

Subsurface needle aspirates, scrapings, or biopsy of the advancing edge of the skin ulcer should be performed while avoiding the purulent center of the ulcer. Biopsy is most practical for mucosal lesions. The addition of culture to microscopy increases the sensitivity of diagnosis to 85%. Serologic assays developed for the diagnosis of VL are not adequately sensitive or specific for routine use in the diagnosis of CL. PCR methods have been described for the diagnosis of VL and CL in Italy, Africa, and South America but are not generally available for patient diagnostic testing.[25–27]

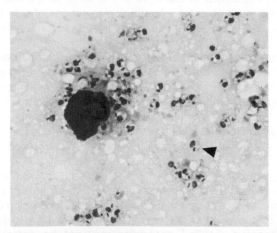

Fig. 4. *Leishmania* species amastigotes. Multiple intracellular and extracellular oval-shaped amastigotes are seen on this touch-preparation of liver tissue from a patient with visceral leishmaniasis. Note that each amastigote (*arrow*) has a nucleus and smaller rod-shaped kinetoplast. (Giemsa, original magnification ×1000).

LABORATORY DIAGNOSIS OF CYSTICERCOSIS, ECHINOCOCCOSIS, AND TRICHINOSIS

The laboratory diagnosis of these infections, which are caused by tissue invasion of the larval form of the parasites, is primarily serologic and supported by clinical, epidemiologic, and radiographic findings. For cysticercosis and echinococcosis, enzyme immunoassays (EIA) and Western blot (WB) immunoassays are commercially available.[28–30] These assays have decreased sensitivity when lesions are calcified and presumably inactive when only one cysticercus is present or when echinococcal cysts are located only in organs other than the liver. There is also a high degree of cross-reactivity between assays for these 2 organisms but this is rarely a problem because the clinical diseases and epidemiology are quite different. Microscopic examination of histopathologic sections of tissue biopsies or cyst aspirates may reveal characteristic larval cestode organisms, tissue remnants, or hooklets (**Fig. 5**).

The diagnosis of trichinosis depends heavily on clinical suspicion arising from patient symptoms and a history of ingestion of raw or inadequately cooked pork or bear meat. The suspect meat will often have been home processed and is a good source for microscopy of muscle tissue. Eosinophilia is invariably present. A positive patient muscle biopsy will establish the diagnosis but is seldom available. A positive serology is an adjunct to diagnosis in highly suspect cases, but the specificity of commercial assays is not optimal and the clinician should be wary of false positive results in patients with an atypical clinical picture.[31] The lack of quantitative results with ELISAs can be problematic in that very low or borderline positives will only be recognized as positive results by clinicians. In cases with a questionable ELISA result, the laboratory may be able to provide additional information indicating whether the result was borderline, low positive, or strong positive.

LABORATORY DIAGNOSIS OF AFRICAN TRYPANOSOMIASIS AND AMERICAN TRYPANOSOMIASIS

The standard method for diagnosis of human African trypanosomiasis (HAT, sleeping sickness, caused by *Trypanosoma brucei, ss rhodesiense, ss gambiense*) during the acute phase of infection is the microscopy of thick and thin blood or buffy coat films stained with Giemsa or other appropriate stains (see section, Laboratory Diagnosis of Malaria) (**Fig. 6**).[2,3] Well-trained and experienced technologists must be available to

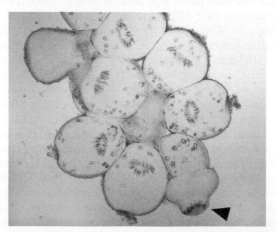

Fig. 5. *Echinococcus* sp protoscoleces in aspirated cyst fluid. A single protoscolex has everted, revealing a row of apical hooklets (unstained, original magnification ×1000).

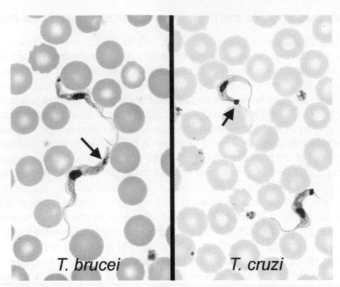

T. brucei   *T. cruzi*

Fig. 6. Motile forms (trypomastigotes) of *Trypanosoma brucei* (*left*) and *Trypanosoma cruzi* (*right*). The trypomastigotes are differentiated primarily by the size of their kinetoplast (*arrows*). Peripheral blood thin film (Giemsa, original magnification ×1000).

thoroughly examine the slide because parasites are often few in number and may be unexpectedly detected on the blood submitted for suspicion of malaria. Live motile trypanosomes may also be observed in fresh wet preparations of blood or buffy coat samples as well as aspirates of enlarged lymph nodes. It must be emphasized that live trypanosomes are highly infectious and specimens must be handled with care using standard precautions, including the use of gloves and other personal protective measures. Microscopy of blood is less useful during the later meningoencephalitic stages of infection when parasitemias are low. Although trypanosomes are rare and difficult to detect in cerebrospinal fluid (CSF), sensitivity may be enhanced by double centrifugation of the CSF before examining the sediment. The presence of mononuclear WBCs and Mott cells (large plasma cells containing immunoglobulin) in CSF is highly suggestive of HAT in the appropriate clinical and epidemiologic setting.[32,33] Serologic or PCR assays may be available from the CDC in the United States or provincial laboratories in Canada. Another valuable resource of information on the diagnosis of HAT is the Department of Parasitology, Prince Leopold Institute of Tropical Medicine in Antwerp Belgium (Institute of Tropical Medicine, Nationalestraat 155, B-2000 Antwerpen, Belgium; telephone: +32-3-247 62 00; Fax: +32-3-237 67 31; e-mail: dir@itg.be; Web site: www.itg.be). A card agglutination test with good sensitivity and specificity is available for the diagnosis of Gambian HAT.

The standard method for the diagnosis of American trypanosomiasis (Chagas disease caused by *Trypanosoma cruzi*) during the acute phase of infection is microscopy of thick and thin blood or buffy coat films stained with Giemsa or other appropriate stains (see "Laboratory diagnosis of malaria") (see **Fig. 6**).[2,3] Live motile trypanosomes may also be observed in fresh wet preparations of blood or buffy coat samples, which must be handled with care using standard precautions, including the use of gloves and other personal protective measures, because the organisms are highly infectious. Microscopy is less useful during the latent and chronic stages of infection when rates of parasitemia are very low and the nonmotile (amastigote) intracellular form of *Trypanosoma cruzi* predominates. The diagnosis in these stages may be established serologically or by the microscopic examination and culture of tissue aspirates or biopsies.[32] Culture of appropriate blood or tissue specimens using NNN or Evan's modified Tobie's medium during the acute and chronic stages may aid the sensitivity of the laboratory diagnosis. Serology by commercially available ELISA kits is of greatest use during the latent and chronic stages of the disease.[34] Separate assays are used for patient diagnosis and blood donor screening. Positive results are considered evidence of active infection and would exclude blood/tissue donors because the infection has been transmitted by transfusion and transplantation.[35] Rapid real-time PCR assays have recently been developed but are available only in research laboratories.

LABORATORY DIAGNOSIS OF EOSINOPHILIC MENINGITIS CAUSED BY *ANGIOSTRONGYLUS* AND *GNATHOSTOMA* SPECIES

Angiostrongylus and *Gnathostoma* are nematodes (roundworms) that cause human infections by migration of the larval forms through the blood stream and tissues. These infections are found predominantly in the Far East and are associated with eating raw fish, frogs, crabs, and so forth or contaminated vegetables. Recently, infections have occurred in the Caribbean and South and Central America. The most common clinical disease is eosinophilic meningitis[36,37]; however, *Gnathostoma spinigerum* may also cause intermittent migratory subcutaneous nodules or swellings. *Angiostrongylus cantonensis* (rat lungworm) is the most common microbiologic cause of eosinophilic meningitis. Diagnosis is suspected with the findings of peripheral and CSF eosinophilia associated with neurologic signs of meningoencephalitis. Larvae are rarely seen in the CSF, and specific diagnosis is based on serology, which is not widely available but may be obtained from the CDC or the Department of Helminthology, Faculty of Tropical Medicine, Mahidol University, 420/6 Rajvithi Road, Bangkok 10400, Thailand (http://www.tm.mahidol.ac.th/en/special).

LABORATORY DIAGNOSIS OF TROPICAL INTESTINAL PARASITES

The most common method for identifying intestinal parasites is by the macroscopic and microscopic examination of stool specimens, commonly referred to as the ova and parasite or O&P examination. This method allows for the identification of both protozoan (eg, *Giardia intestinalis)* and helminth infections (eg, *Ascaris lumbricoides*) and may be performed in a variety of laboratory settings, including the field laboratory. Although most intestinal parasites can be readily detected by the O&P examination, some require alternative or additional techniques for optimal detection (eg, *Strongyloides stercoralis, Cryptosporidium* spp).

   In general, serology is most useful in detecting parasites with a disseminated or invasive stage, such as amebiasis (ie, liver abscess), schistosomiasis, strongyloidiasis, and trichinosis. In contrast, serology is not useful for the detection of infections without a significant invasive component (eg, ascariasis, trichuriasis, giardiasis) because these parasites do not generate a detectable immune response. For infections in which serology is used, cross-reactivity between helminth infections is common.[38] Common intestinal parasites and the preferred tests for diagnosis are listed in **Table 1**.

COLLECTION OF FECES FOR O&P EXAMINATION

Stool specimens should be collected in a clean, dry, leak-proof container without contaminating water or urine because these could negatively impact parasite morphology or introduce contaminating organisms. Unfixed specimens are used to detect motility patterns of some organisms (eg, protozoan trophozoites and helminth larvae), but the specimen must be transported immediately to the laboratory to avoid parasite degradation. If the specimen cannot be analyzed in the laboratory within several hours of collection (something that is challenging even when the laboratory is adjacent to the clinic), it should be placed immediately into a fixative, such as formalin, to preserve parasite morphology. All specimens should be treated as potentially infectious because they may contain infective parasite forms (eg, *Strongyloides stercoralis* larvae, *Enterobius vermicularis* eggs), bacteria (eg, *Shigella* or *Salmonella* species), and viruses (eg, HIV, hepatitis viruses).[39] The use of a fixative, such as formalin, will minimize but not fully eliminate the infectious risk from stool specimens.

Because many parasites or their ova are shed sporadically, the examination of 3 or more specimens is recommended.[3] Some parasites, such as *Giardia intestinalis* (*lamblia, duodenalis*), *Entamoeba histolytica*, and *Strongyloides stercoralis* may require more than 3 stool specimens for optimal detection by microscopy.[39] Multiple stool collections are not always clinically feasible, and alternate techniques are available for some parasites (see **Table 1**).

IMPORTANT COMPONENTS OF THE O&P EXAMINATION

At the laboratory, specimens are first examined macroscopically for the presence of round worms and cestode (tapeworm) proglottids. At the time of macroscopic examination, the consistency of the specimen (liquid, semiformed, formed) and the presence of blood, mucus, and pus can also be noted because this information may provide useful clinical information.

When fresh specimens are received, a direct wet preparation of the specimen can be made and examined for motile organisms.[3] The presence of motility may help increase sensitivity of parasite detection, whereas the type of motility (eg, falling-leaf motility of *Giardia intestinalis*) observed can provide information regarding identification of the parasite.[40]

Direct (nonconcentrated) specimens are usually adequate for the detection of intestinal parasites, such as hookworm, *Ascaris lumbricoides*, and *Trichuris trichiura*, at clinically significant levels.[3] Important exceptions to this rule are schistosoma and strongyloides stercoralis infections, which may require fecal concentration and ancillary detection methods for optimal detection.[3] Fecal concentration is also important in settings where the detection of all parasites is important, even when present at subclinical levels (eg, in travelers returning from endemic areas) because concentration methods greatly increase the sensitivity of stool parasite detection. Stool is typically concentrated by sedimentation or flotation techniques, with the formol ether sedimentation technique being most widely used in diagnostic laboratories worldwide.[41] For fieldwork, more simplistic methods, such as the Kato-Katz technique,[42] provide partial concentration of specimens and allow for semiquantitation of helminth eggs. Concentration techniques remove a significant portion of fecal debris while concentrating helminth eggs, larvae, and protozoan forms for more ready microscopic identification. Preparations are usually viewed without stain or with a simple iodine solution to enhance protozoan characteristics. There are many excellent atlases available for differentiation of common and uncommon helminth eggs.[3,40,43] An example of an unstained concentrated stool specimen preparation (sedimentation concentration method) containing multiple helminth eggs is shown in **Fig. 7**.

The permanently stained stool preparation is the final component of a complete stool O&P examination (**Fig. 8**). Although not performed in all laboratories worldwide,

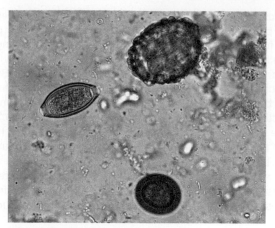

Fig. 7. Ova of *Ascaris lumbricoides* (*upper right*), *Trichuris trichiura* (*upper left*), and *Taenia* sp (*bottom*) (Concentrate, original magnification ×400). Bacteria, yeast, and fecal debris are also seen.

it is a mandatory component of all O&Ps performed in the United States and provides the greatest sensitivity for the detection of protozoa,[3,44] including *Dientamoeba fragilis*. Trichrome and iron-hematoxylin are the most commonly used stains. *Cryptosporidium* species and microsporidia are not reliably detected by routine O&P and require special concentration and staining processes.

INTERPRETATION OF STOOL O&P EXAMINATION RESULTS

The interpretation of the stool O&P must always be taken in the context of the individual patient. The presence of pathogenic parasites in the stool specimen indicates infection with these agents and treatment is typically recommended. Other parasites, however, are not considered human pathogens and their presence alone does not

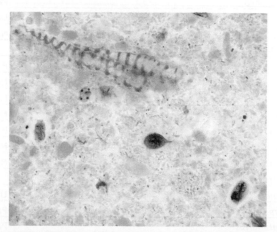

Fig. 8. Stool preparation showing a classic *Giardia intestinalis* trophozoite (*center*) and 2 cysts (*left* and *bottom right*). At the top, a spiral form of partially digested food material is seen (trichrome, original magnification ×1000).

necessitate the use of antiparasitic drugs (**Table 2**). The value in knowing that a nonpathogenic parasite is present is that it serves as a marker for patient exposure to contaminated food or water sources, and, thus, additional testing for pathogenic parasites may be indicated.

Other possible findings from the O&P examination include RBCs, WBCs, and Charcot-Leyden crystals. Gross pus or microscopic WBCs indicate intestinal inflammation and may be seen in cases of bacterial and amoebic dysentery[1] in addition to some noninfectious processes (eg, inflammatory bowel disease).[45] Other signs of dysentery include RBCs and mucus. If gross blood is present, it is helpful to know if it is admixed with the specimen or limited to the stool surface because the latter indicates rectal/anal bleeding rather than dysentery. Charcot-Leyden crystals may be seen in stool (and sputum) specimens in parasitic infections and represent breakdown products of eosinophils (**Fig. 9**). Finally, pale or fatty-appearing (eg, frothy) specimens are commonly described with giardiasis, malabsorption, and obstructive jaundice.[39]

PARASITES REQUIRING SPECIALIZED STAINS AND TECHNIQUES FOR OPTIMAL DETECTION

Although many parasites can be identified via routine O&P examination, the identification by additional or alternative methods may be indicated for optimal detection or confirmation of some parasites. Important examples of these parasites are discussed later.

Table 2
Pathogenic status of intestinal protozoa

Parasite	Pathogenic Status
Amoebae	
Endolimax nana	Nonpathogen
Entamoeba coli	Nonpathogen
Entamoeba dispar	Nonpathogen
Entamoeba hartmanni	Nonpathogen
Entamoeba histolytica	Pathogen
Entamoeba moshkovkii	Uncertain
Iodamoeba butschlii	Nonpathogen
Ciliates and flagellates	
Balantidium coli	Pathogen
Chilomastix mesnili	Nonpathogen
Dientamoeba fragilis	Pathogen
Enteromonas hominis	Nonpathogen
Giardia intestinalis	Pathogen
Pentatrichomonas (Trichomonas) hominis	Nonpathogen
Retortamonas intestinalis	Nonpathogen
Coccidia and others	
Blastocystis hominis	Uncertain
Cryptosporidium species	Pathogen
Cyclospora cayetanensis	Pathogen
Cystoisospora (Isospora) belli	Pathogen
Sarcocystis species	Pathogen

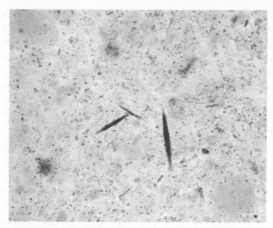

Fig. 9. Charcot Leyden crystals (trichrome stain, original magnification ×1000).

Cryptosporidium spp, Cyclospora Cayetanensis, Cystoisospora (Isospora) Belli, and Sarcocystis spp

With the exception of *Cryptosporidium*, these parasites may be readily identified on routine O&P because of their characteristic morphology. The use of a modified Kinyoun (acid fast) or Safranin stain may increase the sensitivity of detection of *Cryptosporidium* and provide a useful confirmatory tool for cryptosporidium, cyclospora cayetanensis, and cystoisospora oocysts (**Fig. 10**).

The oocysts of *Cyclospora* and the sarcocysts of *Sarcocystis* also exhibit blue autofluorescence using UV fluorescence microscopy. Rarely, sporulation assays are used to confirm the diagnosis of *Cyclospora cayetanensis* and differentiate the oocysts from similar-appearing blue-green algae.

Microsporidia

Because of their small size (0.8–4.0 μm in length) and close resemblance to yeast cells on stool preparations, the spores of this organism (now considered a highly

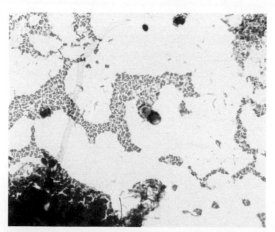

Fig. 10. Two oocysts of *Cyclospora cayetanensis* (*center*) are stained red-pink (modified Kinyoun stain, original magnification × 1000). It is common to see stained and unstained oocysts in the same preparation.

specialized fungus) are best identified through the use of chromotrope 2R stains, such as strong trichrome blue. With these preparations, the oval spores stain bright red and may have a central band running perpendicular to the long axis (**Fig. 11**). Even with chromotrope stains, these spores may still be extremely difficult to correctly identify. Therefore, molecular methods are becoming the diagnostic test of choice. Transmission electron microscopy is rarely used clinically but is the traditional gold standard for species identification.[46]

Entamoeba Histolytica

The cysts and trophozoites are readily identified in the O&P examination but cannot be differentiated from the morphologically identical forms of the nonpathogenic amoeba, *Entamoeba dispar*, or from *Entamoeba moshkovkii*, which has uncertain pathogenicity. Only when ingested RBCs are seen within morphologically characteristic trophozoites can a presumptive diagnosis of *Entamoeba histolytica* be made (**Fig. 12**).[47] Because of differences in pathogenicity, *Entamoeba histolytica* should be differentiated from other amoebae whenever possible. This differentiation is best accomplished through the use of antigen detection kits or PCR. Not all commercially available antigen detection kits can differentiate between *Entamoeba histolytica* and *Entamoeba dispar*, so it is important to be familiar with the characteristics of the test being used. Trophozoites may also be identified on biopsy; the characteristic pattern of invasion into the colon mucosa causing the so-called flask-shaped ulcer is diagnostic for this organism.[48] For the detection of disseminated disease (eg, amoebic liver abscess), serology is the test of choice. Many patients with disseminated disease do not have detectable parasites in stool preparations, and recognizable organisms are rarely seen in aspirated abscess material.[49]

Strongyloides Stercoralis

The laboratory diagnosis of this invasive nematode can be challenging because organisms are not regularly shed in the stool and multiple stool specimens (>3) may be required to identify the parasite.[50] Therefore, fecal concentration techniques and serology are widely used adjunctive tests. Serology is helpful for determining if patients have been previously exposed but cannot be used to diagnose current

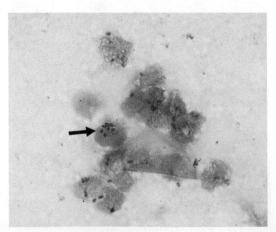

Fig. 11. Microsporidian species (trichrome blue stain, original magnification ×1000). Note the tiny size and occasional perpendicular band (*arrow*).

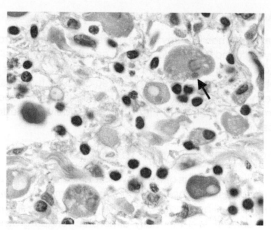

Fig. 12. *Entamoeba histolytica* (hematoxylin and eosin, original magnification ×1000). Note ingested RBCs (*arrow*).

infection. Cross-reactivity with other nematodes, including microfilariae, is common. A positive antibody test should prompt additional procedures for microscopic identification of the parasite. Antibody levels can be used to monitor the response to treatment in immunocompetent individuals because they typically decrease over a 6-month period following successful treatment.

Fecal concentration methods for *Strongyloides stercoralis* include the Baermann funnel technique,[3] Harada-Mori filter culture,[51] and agar culture.[52] Of these, agar culture is more sensitive for the detection of *Strongyloides stercoralis* than the Baermann technique and is the most easily performed in the laboratory.[53] In agar culture, stool is placed on nutrient agar in a Petri dish and covered securely with a taped lid.[52] The agar plate is then examined daily for the presence of *Strongyloides* larvae, which are identified by the trails of bacteria that are dragged with them as they migrate through the agar (**Fig. 13**).

Finally, the microscopic examination of sputum may reveal characteristic filariform larvae in the hyperinfection syndrome of strongyloidiasis.[54,55] This result should be reported immediately because of the potentially fatal course of disseminated disease.

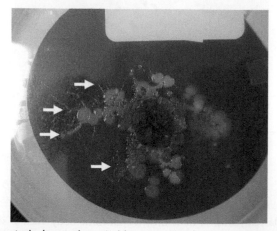

Fig. 13. Trails of bacteria (*arrows*) carried by migrating larvae are seen radiating from the central stool specimen on the agar plate.

LABORATORY DIAGNOSIS OF TROPICAL FUNGAL INFECTIONS

Fungal infections are common in many areas of the subtropics and tropics and include infections that may be found worldwide, such as candidiasis, aspergillosis, cryptococcosis, and tinea (dermatophyte infection). This section focuses on fungal infections that are geographically restricted to tropical regions. All fungal agents described here are cultivable in culture except *Lacazia loboi*, the agent of lobomycosis. Therefore, tissue specimens should be submitted for fungal culture in addition to histopathology when possible.

LABORATORY DIAGNOSIS OF AFRICAN HISTOPLASMOSIS

This chronic progressive mycosis is caused by *Histoplasma duboisii*, also known as the large-cell form of *Histoplasma capsulatum,* or *Histoplasma capsulatum* var. *duboisii*. Diagnosis is accomplished by fungal culture or histologic examination of infected tissue. *Histoplasma duboisii* is a thermally dimorphic fungus growing as a white or tan mold at 25°C and as yeast at 37°C. Confirmation of culture isolate identification can be performed with commercially available DNA probes for *Histoplasma capsulatum* because these probes cross-react with *Histoplasma duboisii*. On tissue section, many yeasts within phagocytic cells are seen, typically associated with granulomatous inflammation.[56] Yeasts in culture or histologic preparations measure 8 to 15 μm in diameter compared with the 2 to 5 μm diameter of *Histoplasma capsulatum*, although both produce buds on a narrow base. Because of their larger size, *Histoplasma duboisii* is commonly mistaken for *Blastomyces dermatitidis*, although the latter multiplies by broad-based rather than narrow-based budding.

LABORATORY DIAGNOSIS OF CHROMOBLASTOMYCOSIS

The hallmark laboratory feature of this unique warty chronic skin lesion is the identification of naturally pigmented (dematiaceous) thick brown fungal cells called muriform bodies (also known as sclerotic bodies, medlar bodies or copper pennies) on histologic sections of skin biopsies or wet preparations of tissue scrapings. Muriform bodies measure 5 to 12 μm in diameter and divide into 1 or 2 planes by the intersection of the septa **(Fig. 14)**.[1,56] Fungal culture of skin biopsies may grow one of several

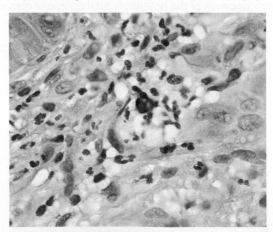

Fig. 14. Chromoblastomycosis. A dark brown muriform body with 2 septations is seen (*center*), associated with scattered neutrophils (hematoxylin and eosin, original magnification ×1000).

dematiaceous fungi, including *Fonsecaea pedrosoi*, *Cladosporium* spp, *and Phialophora verrucosa*. The identification of most species is performed by the examination of morphologic features in culture or ribosomal gene sequencing.

LABORATORY DIAGNOSIS OF LOBOMYCOSIS

Lobomycosis is caused by an unusual fungus called *Lacazia loboi* (formerly *Loboa loboi*), which cannot be grown in fungal culture.[56] Therefore, the diagnosis is based on histologic sections with observation of the classic chains of thick-walled, uniform, round to lemon-shaped yeasts measuring 5 to 12 μm in diameter, connected by intracellular bridges (**Fig. 15**).[56] The yeasts are highlighted by fungal stains, such as Gomori methenamine silver (GMS) and periodic acid Schiff (PAS). Based on the histologic appearance, the differential diagnosis includes blastomycosis, African histoplasmosis (caused by *H duboisii*), and paracoccidioidomycosis. Some fungal cells demonstrate birefringence using polarized light, producing a so-called Maltese-cross appearance (**Fig. 16**).

LABORATORY DIAGNOSIS OF MYCETOMA

This chronic infection produces subcutaneous swelling and draining sinuses with discharge containing grains of organism (either a fungus or Gram positive filamentous bacterium). Fungal causes of mycetoma include *Curvularia* spp, *Exophiala jeanselmei, Madurella mycetomatis*, and *Pseudallescheria boydii*, whereas bacterial causes include *Nocardia* spp, *Nocardiopsis* spp, *Streptomyces* spp, and *Actinomadura* spp (the cause of Madura foot). A provisional diagnosis can be obtained from the microscopic examination of the crushed grains in 10% sodium hydroxide or with Gram stain to determine if they contain fungal hyphae or long branching bacterial filaments.[57] Culture is required for definitive diagnosis and antimicrobial susceptibility testing. Tissue for culture should be obtained from a deep biopsy, with specimen also submitted for histopathology if possible.[57] The identification of most species is performed by the examination of morphologic features in culture or ribosomal gene sequencing. Both bacterial and fungal organisms are highlighted with GMS and PAS stains (**Fig. 17**). *Nocardia* spp will also stain red with a modified acid-fast stain (Kinyoun or Fite).

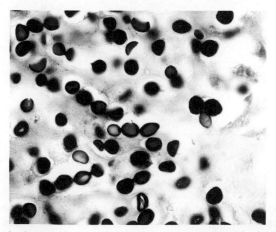

Fig. 15. Lobomycosis. Section from a skin biopsy showing chainlike budding of round to lemon-shaped cells (GMS, original magnification ×1000).

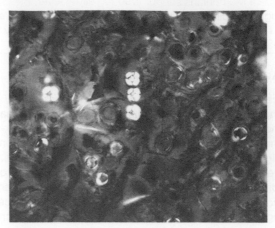

Fig. 16. Using polarized light, several yeasts from the same section as earlier demonstrating birefringence in a Maltese cross pattern (hematoxylin and eosin stain, original magnification ×1000).

LABORATORY DIAGNOSIS OF PARACOCCIDIOIDOMYCOSIS

Paracoccidioidomycosis, otherwise known as South American blastomycosis, is caused by the thermally dimorphic fungus *Paracoccidioides brasiliensis*. This fungus grows slowly as a white to brown mold at 25°C and gradually converts to a thick-walled yeast stage with multiple circumferential narrow-based buds at 37°C.[56] Yeasts vary in diameter from 2 to 30 μm. On biopsy or wet preps, the classic circumferential budding produces the so-called mariner's wheel appearance (**Fig. 18**). The morphologic differential diagnosis includes blastomycosis and cryptococcosis. Because there is no commercially available

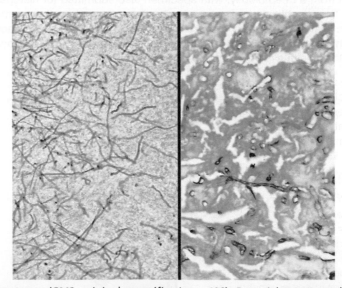

Fig. 17. Mycetoma, (GMS, original magnification ×400). Bacterial mycetoma is shown on the left, while fungal mycetoma is shown on the right. Both are comprised of branching filaments, but note the much smaller diameter of the bacteria compared with the fungal hyphae.

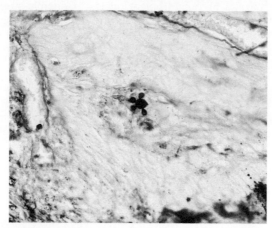

Fig. 18. Paracoccidioidomycosis. Shown is the classic mariner's wheel form (*center*) with multiple circumferential narrow-based buds coming from the larger mother yeast cell (GMS, original magnification ×400).

DNA probe for the identification of *P brasiliensis* culture isolates, yeast conversion or histology are the definitive means of diagnosis. It is important to note, however, that false positive results may occur with blastomyces dermatitidis probes on culture isolates and caution must be used in interpreting results.

LABORATORY DIAGNOSIS OF PENICILLIOSIS

Although multiple members of the genus *Penicillium* can be isolated in the clinical mycology laboratory, these usually represent environmental contaminants. *Penicillium marneffei* is the only member of the genus that grows as a thermally dimorphic fungus and is the etiologic agent of an endemic mycosis in Southeast Asia.[56] *P marneffei* will grow readily on standard fungal media at 25°C and produces a characteristic gray to pink mold with a deep red color on reverse (seen by examining the underside of the culture plate).[56] At 37 °C, the fungus will convert to a yeast stage with soft tan convoluted colonies. An exoantigen test can be performed on the isolate for rapid identification. Unlike other human pathogens, *P marneffei* divides by binary fission rather than budding. Therefore, the yeasts have a classic appearance on direct culture or histologic preparations as small, 3 to 6 μm diameter, oval to elongated forms with a transverse septum (**Fig. 19**).[56]

LABORATORY DIAGNOSIS OF TROPICAL VIRAL INFECTIONS

In addition to the many common viruses that an individual may encounter worldwide, such as influenza A and B viruses, hepatitis A to E, and HIV, an individual in the tropics or subtropics may also be exposed to many viruses that are geographically restricted, such as yellow fever virus, dengue virus, Crimean-Congo hemorrhagic fever virus, HTLV-1, and Japanese encephalitis virus. These tropical viruses are responsible for a diverse spectrum of clinical manifestations, including hemorrhagic fever, flaccid paralysis, encephalitis, hepatitis, and malignancy.[58] Despite the number of organ systems potentially involved by these viruses, most cannot be grown in routine cell culture or pose significant hazards to laboratory personnel; therefore, laboratory identification is typically accomplished by IgM and IgG class antibody detection rather

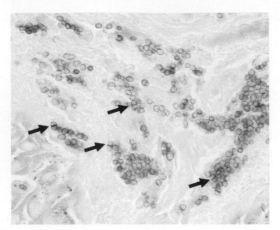

Fig. 19. Penicilliosis caused by *Penicillium marneffei*. Tissue section shows small yeasts with occasional transverse septa (*arrows*) (GMS, original magnification × 1000).

than organ-specific testing with culture. Less commonly, PCR, antigen detection, or histology with specific immunohistochemistry may be performed. Common tropical viruses and their means of diagnosis are outlined in **Table 1**.

SPECIMEN COLLECTION

Because of the risks that many tropical viruses pose to exposed individuals and the lack of effective therapy for many infections, safe handling necessitates that special precautions be observed.[59] If a tropical virus is suspected, it is essential to notify the laboratory before sending the specimen so that the degree of risk may be assessed. In many cases, the specimen will not be analyzed at the local or even reference laboratory level and will be sent directly to an appropriate public health laboratory, such as the CDC or the WHO reference laboratory. In particular, many agents of viral hemorrhagic fever are manipulated only in biosafety level 3 or 4 laboratories, which provide the necessary level of biologic containment. Specimens for viral culture should be taken as early as possible following symptom onset and should be placed in viral transport media to help maintain infectivity and prevent bacterial and fungal overgrowth. If a delay of more than 1 hour is anticipated between the time of specimen collection and culture, then the specimen should be refrigerated at 4°C.[60] In contrast to culture, PCR does not require viable virus so long as the template DNA or RNA is intact.

Laboratory personnel can offer advice on how to collect and transport specimens for PCR to avoid introducing potential PCR inhibitors or RNAses into the specimens. A discussion of 2 specific tropical virus groups and special considerations related to their laboratory diagnosis follows.

LABORATORY DIAGNOSIS OF ARBOVIRUSES

Many tropical viruses fall in the taxonomically diverse group of arboviruses (arthropod-borne viruses). The diagnosis of most viruses in this group is accomplished by serologic testing performed by a reference or public health laboratory. IgM and IgG antibodies are typically detectable after the initial febrile stage.[57] The viremic stage is generally short, therefore, limiting the usefulness of viral culture or nucleic acid detection from the blood of symptomatic individuals.[57] Dengue and yellow fever viruses are important exceptions in that they tend to have higher and more prolonged levels of viremia[61]; thus, nucleic acid or antigens can be detected during the febrile stage of the illness. Antigen detection methods, such as ELISAs and lateral-flow rapid tests, are commercially available for the detection of dengue virus in acute-stage blood specimens. Some tests are capable of differentiating dengue virus from other viruses, such as Japanese encephalitis virus, with high specificity.[61] Culture and nucleic acid detection of these 2 viruses is generally restricted to specialized centers such as the CDC.

In select cases, arbovirus diagnosis can be made from tissue using immunohisto-chemical staining, nucleic acid detection, or electron microscopy. The CDC and other specialized reference centers, such as the University of Texas Medical Branch in Galveston, may accept fresh or formalin-fixed tissue for detection of certain arboviruses, such as dengue virus, Crimean-Congo hemorrhagic fever virus, and Japanese encephalitis virus.[61]

LABORATORY DIAGNOSIS OF HTLV-1 AND 2

HTLV-1 and 2 retroviruses differ from many other tropical viruses in their chronic nature of infection and the association of HTLV-1 with adult T-cell leukemia and increased risk of disseminated strongyloidiasis and crusted (Norwegian) scabies. Like most other tropical viruses, serology is the primary means of detection. Serologic tests are also used to screen blood donors for the presence of antibodies to HTLV-1 and HTLV-2.[61] Screening assays include EIA and chemiluminescence immunoassays, which are sensitive means for detecting antibodies to HTLV-1 and 2 in serum or plasma. These assays cannot differentiate between the 2 types, and positive results should be (ideally) repeated and then confirmed by WB or radioimmunoprecipitation assay.[60] Nucleic acid detection is the method of choice of distinguishing between the 2 types. Serology can be repeated at 3 months if HTLV-1 and 2 infections are highly suspected and initial test results are negative or indeterminate. Of note, individuals with HTLV-1 and 2 viruses do not have false positive results with screening or confirmatory assays for HIV.[60]

LABORATORY DIAGNOSIS OF TROPICAL BACTERIAL AND RICKETTSIAL INFECTIONS

This discussion of bacterial and rickettsial diseases focuses on specific disease entities that may be encountered primarily in the tropics. Although culture continues to be a mainstay of diagnosis in bacterial infections, in many situations culture may have poor sensitivity, require impractical conditions or special media, be time consuming, or a combination. It is in these situations that alternate testing methods, such as serology or PCR, may play a greater role in helpful clinical diagnostics for patients. Diagnostic tests helpful in the diagnosis of tropical bacterial and rickettsial illnesses are outlined in **Table 1**.

LABORATORY DIAGNOSIS OF MELIOIDOSIS

Because of the lack of sensitive and specific rapid testing for *Burkholderia pseudomallei*, the causative agent of melioidosis, culture and gram stain continue to be the gold standard for diagnosis. Gram stain of lesional material will demonstrate Gram negative bipolar rods, whereas culture may reveal the causative agent. *Burkholderia pseudomallei* is classified as a biosafety level 3 agent, and safe handling requires the use of the appropriate biosafety level equipment and facilities. Therefore, it is essential to communicate to the laboratory when *Burkholderia pseudomallei* is suspected. *Burkholderia pseudomallei* has not been documented as normal flora[62]; therefore, isolation of *Burkholderia pseudomallei* from any sample, including from potentially colonized sites (urine, respiratory secretions, superficial skin swabs, and so forth), should be viewed as highly suspicious for infection with *Burkholderia pseudomallei* in the proper clinical context. The bacteria grow slowly and can, therefore, be easily overgrown in mixed cultures. Recovery, especially from nonsterile sites, can be greatly enhanced with the use of selective agars, including Ashdown medium, burkholderia pseudomallei selective agar, and commercially prepared *Burkholderia cepacia* selective agar.[63]

Specimens from patients receiving appropriate antimicrobial therapy may fail to grow *Burkholderia pseudomallei*, so a diagnosis of melioidosis should still be considered if clinical suspicion remains, despite a negative culture.[64]

PCR assays are being investigated for the diagnosis of melioidosis but are not currently in clinical use; moreover, their sensitivity have not been shown to be significantly better than culture.[65,66] Serodiagnosis in melioidosis-endemic areas is of limited value because seropositivity in the healthy population is likely to be high. Serologic testing in travelers, however, is of diagnostic utility, particularly in those who have no history of residence in a region where melioidosis is endemic or who have made only a small number of short visits during which exposure may have occurred. In this setting, paired sera (acute and convalescent samples at least 2 weeks apart) demonstrating rising antibody titers to *Burkholderia pseudomallei* support the diagnosis of melioidosis.

The most commonly used serodiagnostic test is the indirect hemagglutination assay (IHA), which may be obtained from several reference laboratories worldwide. Although interpretations may vary,[67] IgG titers greater than or equal to 1:128 for a single serum generally indicates exposure, whereas IgM titers of greater than or equal to 1:40 suggests recent or current infection. A 4-fold increase in IgG titer between acute and convalescent sera at least 2 weeks apart supports a diagnosis of a recent or active infection.[68]

LABORATORY DIAGNOSIS OF BRUCELLOSIS

The gold standard in the laboratory diagnosis of brucellosis is a positive culture of the organism. Although potentially hazardous to laboratory personnel, culture also remains essential for evaluating antimicrobial susceptibility and for determination of species. As with many tropical infections, the laboratory should be notified whenever infection with *Brucella* is suspected so that proper precautions can be taken. The timeframe required for organism recovery depends largely on the culture method used and the type and volume of specimen. Traditional culture methods using biphasic mediums often required up to 30 days to obtain maximum recovery of organisms, but the use of continuously monitored blood culture systems, such as the Bactec (BD Diagnostics, Sparks, Maryland), have been shown to have higher sensitivity than conventional culture methods and to hasten the detection of bacterial growth. Most cases can be recovered within 7 days,[69] although most laboratories using continuously monitored blood culture systems will hold specimens for brucella culture for up to 14 days to ensure optimal recovery of the organism. Some studies have reported that the utilization of bone marrow culture may be superior to blood culture under the appropriate circumstances, resulting in 15% to 20% higher yields than peripheral blood,[69] faster culture times, and increased sensitivity in patients who have been previously treated with antibiotics.[70]

Serologic assays are the most commonly used tests for the laboratory diagnosis of brucellosis. Enzyme immunoassay detection of antibrucella IgM and IgG antibodies has been demonstrated to be a sensitive screening method, although all specimens producing a positive EIA result should be confirmed by a brucella-specific agglutination method. One method, the tube agglutination test (TAT), uses a combined IgG and IgM brucella antibody against brucella abortus antigen. This procedure detects antibodies to the A and M antigens of the *Brucella* species and cross-reacts with all species except *Brucella canis*. Because of the cross-reactivity, this test is useful for confirming serologic response to *Brucella* species but cannot differentiate among them. Cross-reactivity is also known to occur with Francisella antigen. IgM antibodies appear during the first week of infection, followed by a switch to IgG synthesis during the second week.

The most accurate serologic determination of acute infection is made by simultaneous testing of acute and convalescent serum specimens collected 3 to 4 weeks apart. A 4-fold increase in titer is considered significant. When testing single specimens only, a titer of 1:160 indicates a *Brucella* infection at some time but does not allow for the determination of a current or recent infection and a titer of less than 1:160 does not necessarily rule out brucellosis. Low levels of IgG may be present for up to 1 year after the infection, whereas persistently high titers of IgG in the serum may be seen in cases of chronic brucellosis.

Molecular diagnostic methods have shown promise in the evaluation of suspected cases of brucellosis and could potentially significantly reduce turnaround time and the hazards associated with cultivation of the organism. Further studies and standardization will be necessary before they are widely used in clinical practice.[71]

LABORATORY DIAGNOSIS OF TYPHOID FEVER

The diagnosis of typhoid (enteric) fever caused by *Salmonella typhi* in developed countries relies heavily on blood culture. The sensitivity of blood culture is highest during the first week of illness with significant declines in sensitivity afterward.[72] Bone marrow cultures may be performed and have been reported to have superior sensitivity, particularly in partially treated patients,[73] but the practical obstacles to obtaining a bone marrow specimen may outweigh the benefits.

Salmonella typhi can be cultured from stool and urine during the third and fourth weeks of illness and is the preferred method within this time interval. The microbiology laboratory should be notified if typhoid fever is suspected because special media will be required to enhance recovery of the organism.

The Widal test has been the mainstay of serologic diagnosis for more than a century; however, a lack of sensitivity and specificity and difficulty in the establishment of baseline titers in endemic regions significantly reduces the clinical utility.[74] Newer serologic tests demonstrate better performance than the Widal test; however, they still do not offer acceptable sensitivity and specificity.[75,76]

PCR tests of blood for *Salmonella Typhi*,[77] and for both *Salmonella typhi* and *Salmonella paratyphi* have been developed[78]; however, these tests are currently only available on a research basis at specialized centers.

LABORATORY DIAGNOSIS OF OTHER BACTERIAL ENTERIC PATHOGENS

Stool cultures, as performed in most clinical laboratories, will detect the most common organisms responsible for infectious gastroenteritis in travelers, which includes *Salmonella, Shigella,* and *Campylobacter*.[72] One important caveat, however, is that the most common bacterial cause of travelers diarrhea, enterotoxigenic *Escherichia coli* (ETEC), cannot be identified by culture and, therefore, diagnoses are typically made based on clinical history and symptoms. Laboratory assays for the detection of ETEC involve the detection of the associated heat-labile and heat-stable enterotoxins, usually by EIA, but are not widely available. PCR assays have been developed for the detection of non-typhi *Salmonella sp*, *Shigella sp*, *Campylobacter sp*, and *Vibrio sp* and are available from some reference laboratories.

LABORATORY DIAGNOSIS OF TRENCH FEVER

Culture of *Bartonella quintana*, the etiologic agent of trench fever, can be performed from tissue or blood and is considered the gold standard for definitive diagnosis. However, the bacteria are difficult to grow, requiring special media and a lengthy incubation period of at least 21 days and possibly up to 45 days.[6]

The traditional diagnosis of trench fever caused by *Bartonella quintana* by serologic testing (eg, the Weil-Felix test) has largely been supplanted by the more sensitive and specific indirect immunofluorescence assay. In general, IFA IgG titers of 1:256 and greater are considered presumptive evidence of recent infection and endpoint titers of 1:128 are considered evidence of infection at an undetermined time. IgG endpoint titers less than 1:128 suggest that the patient does not have a current infection. IgM endpoint titers of 1:20 and greater are considered presumptive evidence of recent infection, whereas lower than 1:20 suggests that the patient does not have a current infection. Sensitive and specific qualitative PCR testing of tissue or blood using probes specific to *Bartonella quintana* is available through commercial reference laboratories (FOCUS Diagnostics, http://www.focusdx.com/).

LABORATORY DIAGNOSIS OF OROYA FEVER AND VERRUGA PERUANA

Diagnosis of *Bartonella bacilliformis* infection, during the acute phase (Oroya fever) can be made most rapidly through microscopic examination of a Giemsa-stained peripheral blood film for characteristic blue extraerythrocytic and intraerythrocytic bacilli, provided an experienced laboratory technician is available.[79] Culture of *Bartonella bacilliformis* during the acute phase of the disease is successful approximately 70% of the time; however, blood cultures may take up to 29 days to grow and require special media.[80,81]

Diagnosis during the chronic phase (verruga peruana) of the infection can be made through microscopic examination of lesional skin biopsies using a specialized silver stain, such as the Warthin-Starry or Dieterle stains.

LABORATORY DIAGNOSIS OF LEPROSY

Mycobacterium leprae, the etiologic agent of leprosy, cannot be grown in routine in vitro culture; thus, the diagnosis of leprosy is typically made on clinical grounds. Microscopic examination of lesional biopsies provides definitive diagnosis through characteristic morphologic features and the presence of acid-fast bacilli using a modified acid-fast tissue stain, such as a Fite stain. The classic Ziehl-Neelsen stain may not stain these partially acid-fast mycobacteria. Although both lepromatous and tuberculoid forms of the disease have characteristic histopathologic features, it is not uncommon that biopsies demonstrate overlapping or nonspecific features, thus requiring correlation with clinical findings for interpretation.

Although clinical and morphologic methods remain the mainstay of diagnosis of leprosy, serologic and molecular-based methods show promise as primary or adjunctive laboratory-based diagnostics and may be available commercially in the future. Specifically, serologic tests for the detection of antibodies to *Mycobacterium leprae*–specific phenolic glycolipid-I (PGL-I) have been shown to detect antibodies in 90% of patients with untreated lepromatous leprosy and 40% to 50% of patients with paucibacillary disease. Following initiation of therapy, PGL-I antibody levels typically decrease, allowing their use in monitoring chemotherapy effectiveness.[82] Unfortunately, serology is only available in the research setting at this time. PCR methods targeting 16s ribosomal RNA have also been developed to detect *Mycobacterium leprae*; however, like PGL-I, these assays are currently only available through research laboratories. PCR methods will likely prove most helpful when acid-fast bacilli are detected, but the clinical or histopathologic features are not characteristic of the disease. Prolonged formalin fixation decreases the sensitivity of PCR assays in general and biopsies to be submitted for PCR should either be fixed in alcohol or processed rapidly.[83]

LABORATORY DIAGNOSIS OF BURULI ULCER

Necrotizing cutaneous infections caused by *Mycobacterium ulcerans* (Buruli ulcer) are traditionally diagnosed on a clinical basis. However, Buruli ulcer can present with nonspecific features and may be mistaken for other disease entities; therefore, additional laboratory methods are useful for providing of a definitive diagnosis.[84] A simple method is to perform microscopic examination for acid-fast bacilli on direct smears from the necrotic base of the lesion, using Ziehl-Neelsen or auramine O stains. Positive cases will typically demonstrate clumps of acid-fast bacilli. Microscopic examination has been shown to have a sensitivity of only 40%; direct smears from surgically obtained tissue have recently been shown to increase sensitivity up to 60%.[85]

Biopsies for histologic evaluation have shown a sensitivity ranging between approximately 65% and greater than 90%.[86,87] The disease features are often nonspecific and may be dependent on the clinical stage of the disease.[63]

For definitive diagnosis, *Mycobacterium ulcerans* can be cultured from ulcer exudate or fresh tissue. Cultures require special media, such as Lowenstein-Jensen, and incubation at 29°C to 33 °C[87]; therefore, communication with the laboratory regarding suspected organisms will be helpful in ensuring that appropriate conditions are used for isolation. Because of the slow growth rate of this organism, cultures may require an incubation period of 6 to 12 weeks. The isolation rate of *Mycobacterium ulcerans* from patients ranges from 20% to 60% because of the difficulties in culturing the organism.[87,88]

Although only currently available through select research laboratories, PCR is a rapid, sensitive, and specific method for the identification of mycobacteria, including *Mycobacterium ulcerans*. PCR generally can provide results within 2 days and has been shown to be highly sensitive (90%–98%).[89] Dry reagent–based PCR assays have also been developed and show sensitivities comparable with conventional PCR methods.[90]

LABORATORY DIAGNOSIS OF LEPTOSPIROSIS

The standard method of establishing the diagnosis of leptospirosis is isolation of the microorganism from body fluids or human tissue. Following infection, the leptospires can be isolated from the blood for the first 7 to 10 days, after which the organism migrates to the kidneys and can be found most reliably in fresh urine where it may be excreted for up to 4 weeks.[6,72] Although the organism may be found in other body fluids, such as CSF, the timeframe to reliably isolate them is shorter. Cultures may also be performed from blood, serum, fresh urine, and fresh kidney biopsy specimens. Culture of *Leptospira sp* requires special media and may require incubation for up to 6 weeks with examination by darkfield microscopy at weekly intervals.[6] The sensitivity of blood culture is additionally reported to be low: approximately 45% in one study.[91]

Serologic screening for leptospirosis is most commonly performed by the use of IHA, which is widely available from reference laboratories. IgM antibody will typically be detectable following the first week of symptomatic illness. Significant elevation in titer (4-fold) between acute and convalescent sera is diagnostic but high titer single specimen may also be diagnostic (≥1:100 for IHA).

The gold standard for the diagnosis of leptospirosis is the microscopic agglutination test (MAT), which is performed by the CDC laboratory in the United States. The MAT typically requires paired acute and convalescent serum specimens for confirmation of the diagnosis. Acute sera are typically collected 1 to 2 weeks after the onset of symptoms and convalescent sera are collected 2 weeks following. A standard panel of 23 leptospire antigens is used and a diagnosis of leptospirosis is confirmed after a 4-fold increase in titer between acute and convalescent sera is seen with one or more of the antigens. Although the MAT is highly specific, the time required between testing of acute and convalescent sera and the requirement of a 4-fold increase in titer renders the test most useful for retrospective confirmation of the disease.[92]

Darkfield microscopy alone may be performed on blood, CSF, or urine if a skilled microscopist is available. Although potentially rapid, results must be interpreted with caution because artifact, particularly problematic in blood samples, may be easily misinterpreted as spirochetes.[6] Identification of spirochetes on darkfield microscopy, in the proper clinical setting, may be strongly suggestive of leptospirosis.

LABORATORY DIAGNOSIS OF RICKETTSIAL DISEASES

This discussion of diagnostic modalities for rickettsial diseases centers on the diagnosis of rickettsial disease entities typically encountered outside of Western countries. The mainstay of diagnostic methods for the diagnosis of rickettsial diseases, including Mediterranean spotted fever and African tick-bite fever, are serologic testing by indirect IFA, which is available from several reference laboratories worldwide. It should be noted that these assays are group specific, with antibodies to the spotted fever group, including *Rickettsia rickettsii*, *Rickettsia conorii*, *Rickettsia akari*, *Rickettsia sibirica*, and *Rickettsia australis*, and antibodies to the typhus fever group, including *Rickettsia typhi* and *Rickettsia prowazekii*. Interpretation of antibody titers between the groups is identical with IFA IgG titers greater than or equal to 1:256 suggesting active disease and IgM titers greater than or equal to 1:64 suggestive of recent infection. A 4-fold or greater increase in IgG titer between 2 serum samples drawn 1 to 2 weeks apart and tested in parallel is considered presumptive evidence of recent or current infection. Antibody can be absent for 1 to 2 weeks after onset of symptoms and, therefore, an initial negative titer should not be used to exclude the diagnosis of rickettsial disease. A second serum specimen should be obtained 10 to 14 days later to establish the diagnosis in such patients.

Rickettsia africae is one of the most recently described human pathogens of the spotted fever group and is the cause of African tick-bite fever. IFA specific for *Rickettsia africae* is not currently available; however, because of the extensive cross-reaction, commercial assays for the spotted fever group can be used with the caveat that diagnostic antibody titers are most often seen in the later stages of the illness, frequently greater than 3 weeks after symptoms begin, and may be undetectable in mild or treated cases.[93]

If the group identification is inadequate, serologic confirmation of rickettsial diseases, including African tick-bite fever and Mediterranean spotted fever, can be performed by the WHO Collaborative Center for Rickettsial Reference and Research in Marseille,

France or by submission to the CDC through state health departments within the United States.

Although still widely used, the Weil-Felix reaction using cross-reacting *Proteus* antigen is generic for rickettsial infections and demonstrates less sensitivity and specificity than current serologic methods.[94] The Weil-Felix test is, therefore, not recommended if newer serologic testing methods are available.

SUMMARY

An array of microscopic, serologic, and molecular assays has been developed for the diagnosis of tropical diseases. Although microscopy remains key to the diagnosis, particularly in the field, the increasing use and availability of RDTs and molecular assays are changing the way that we approach these infections, allowing for more rapid and accurate diagnoses and increased specificity in the identification of infectious organisms. These advantages are important not only for patient care in the clinical setting but also for epidemiology and global public health. As molecular techniques continue to develop and emerging technologies, such as mass spectrometry, become more commonplace in the laboratory, this trend will continue at a rapid pace, but the importance of understanding the available diagnostic tests remains. Finally, partnership between the clinical team and the laboratory can be of the utmost importance if these diseases are suspected clinically so that the most efficacious, expedient, and cost-effective diagnostic methods may be identified.

REFERENCES

1. Versalovic J, American Society for Microbiology. Manual of clinical microbiology. 10th edition. Washington, DC: ASM Press; 2011.
2. Garcia LS, Bullock-Iacullo SL, Fritche TR, et al. Laboratory diagnosis of blood-borne parasitic diseases; approved guideline. NCCLS document M15-A, vol. 20. Wayne (PA): NCCLS (now CLSI); 2000.
3. Garcia LS. Diagnostic medical parasitology. 5th edition. Washington, DC: ASM Press; 2007. p. 142–180.
4. Swan H, Sloan L, Muyombwe A, et al. Evaluation of a real-time polymerase chain reaction assay for the diagnosis of malaria in patients from thailand. Am J Trop Med Hyg 2005;73(5):850–4.
5. Wortmann G, Hochberg L, Houng HH, et al. Rapid identification of leishmania complexes by a real-time pcr assay. Am J Trop Med Hyg 2005;73(6):999–1004.
6. Winn WC, Koneman EW. Koneman's color atlas and textbook of diagnostic microbiology. 6th edition. Philadelphia: Lippincott Williams & Wilkins; 2006.
7. Tangpukdee N, Krudsood S, Srivilairit S, et al. Gametocyte clearance in uncomplicated and severe plasmodium falciparum malaria after artesunate-mefloquine treatment in thailand. Korean J Parasitol 2008;46(2):65–70.
8. Putaporntip C, Hongsrimuang T, Seethamchai S, et al. Differential prevalence of plasmodium infections and cryptic plasmodium knowlesi malaria in humans in thailand. J Infect Dis 2009;199(8):1143–50.
9. Moody A. Rapid diagnostic tests for malaria parasites. Clinical microbiology reviews 2002;15(1):66–78.
10. Kahama-Maro J, D'Acremont V, Mtasiwa D, et al. Quality of routine microscopy for malaria at different levels of the health system in dar es salaam. Malaria J 2011; 10:322.

11. Stauffer WM, Newberry AM, Cartwright CP, et al. Evaluation of malaria screening in newly arrived refugees to the united states by microscopy and rapid antigen capture enzyme assay. Pediatr Infect Dis J 2006;25(10):948–50.
12. Ochola LB, Vounatsou P, Smith T, et al. The reliability of diagnostic techniques in the diagnosis and management of malaria in the absence of a gold standard. Lancet Infect Dis 2006;6(9):582–8.
13. Stauffer WM, Cartwright CP, Olson DA, et al. Diagnostic performance of rapid diagnostic tests versus blood smears for malaria in us clinical practice. Clin Infect Dis 2009;49(6):908–13.
14. Persing DH, Mathiesen D, Marshall WF, et al. Detection of babesia microti by polymerase chain reaction. J Clin Microbiol 1992;30(8):2097–103.
15. Guerrant RL, Walker DH, Weller PF. Tropical infectious diseases: Principles, pathogens & practice. 3rd edition. Philadelphia: Elsevier; 2011.
16. Taylor MJ, Hoerauf A, Bockarie M. Lymphatic filariasis and onchocerciasis. Lancet 2010;376(9747):1175–85.
17. McPherson RA, Pincus MR, Henry JB. Henry's clinical diagnosis and management by laboratory methods. 21st edition. Philadelphia: Saunders Elsevier; 2007.
18. Udall DN. Recent updates on onchocerciasis: Diagnosis and treatment. Clin Infect Dis 2007;44(1):53–60.
19. Kale OO, Bammeke AO, Ayeni O. An evaluation of skin snip techniques used in the quantitative assessment of microfilarial densities of onchocerca volvulus. Bull World Health Organ 1974;51(5):547–9.
20. Okulicz JF, Stibich AS, Elston DM, Schwartz RA. Cutaneous onchocercoma. Int J Dermatol 2004;43(3):170–2.
21. Weil GJ, Lammie PJ, Weiss N. The ict filariasis test: a rapid-format antigen test for diagnosis of bancroftian filariasis. Parasitol Today 1997;13(10):401–4.
22. Murray HW, Berman JD, Davies CR, et al. Advances in leishmaniasis. Lancet 2005;366(9496):1561–77.
23. Hartzell JD, Aronson NE, Weina PJ, et al. Positive rk39 serologic assay results in us servicemen with cutaneous leishmaniasis. Am J Trop Med Hyg 2008;79(6):843–6.
24. Ramirez JR, Agudelo S, Muskus C, et al. Diagnosis of cutaneous leishmaniasis in colombia: The sampling site within lesions influences the sensitivity of parasitologic diagnosis. J Clin Microbiol 2000;38(10):3768–73.
25. de Oliveira CI, Bafica A, Oliveira F, et al. Clinical utility of polymerase chain reaction-based detection of leishmania in the diagnosis of american cutaneous leishmaniasis. Clin Infect Dis 2003;37(11):e149–53.
26. Antinori S, Calattini S, Longhi E, et al. Clinical use of polymerase chain reaction performed on peripheral blood and bone marrow samples for the diagnosis and monitoring of visceral leishmaniasis in hiv-infected and hiv-uninfected patients: A single-center, 8-year experience in italy and review of the literature. Clin Infect Dis 2007;44(12):1602–10.
27. Deborggraeve S, Laurent T, Espinosa D, et al. A simplified and standardized polymerase chain reaction format for the diagnosis of leishmaniasis. J Infect Dis 2008;198(10):1565–72.
28. White AC Jr. Neurocysticercosis: Updates on epidemiology, pathogenesis, diagnosis, and management. Annu Rev Med 2000;51:187–206.
29. Garcia HH, Gonzalez AE, Evans CA, et al. Taenia solium cysticercosis. Lancet 2003;362(9383):547–56.
30. Zhang W, Li J, McManus DP. Concepts in immunology and diagnosis of hydatid disease. Clinical Microbiology Reviews 2003;16(1):18–36.

31. Gottstein B, Pozio E, Nockler K. Epidemiology, diagnosis, treatment, and control of trichinellosis. Clinical Microbiology Reviews 2009;22(1):127–45.
32. Barrett MP, Burchmore RJ, Stich A, et al. The trypanosomiases. Lancet 2003; 362(9394):1469–80.
33. Brun R, Blum J, Chappuis F, et al. Human african trypanosomiasis. Lancet 2010; 375(9709):148–59.
34. Rassi A Jr, Rassi A, Marin-Neto JA. Chagas disease. Lancet 2010;375(9723): 1388–402.
35. Blood donor screening for chagas disease–United States, 2006-2007. MMWR Morb Mortal Wkly Rep 2007;56(7):141–3.
36. Ramirez-Avila L, Slome S, Schuster FL, et al. Eosinophilic meningitis due to angiostrongylus and gnathostoma species. Clinical Infectious Diseases 2009; 48(3):322–7.
37. Katchanov J, Sawanyawisuth K, Chotmongkoi V, et al. Neurognathostomiasis, a neglected parasitosis of the central nervous system. Emerg Infect Dis 2011; 17(7):1174–80.
38. Ishida MM, Rubinsky-Elefant G, Ferreira AW, et al. Helminth antigens (taenia solium, taenia crassiceps, toxocara canis, schistosoma mansoni and echinococcus granulosus) and cross-reactivities in human infections and immunized animals. Acta Trop 2003;89(1):73–84.
39. Cheesbrough M, Tropical Health Technology (Firm). District laboratory practice in tropical countries. 2nd edition. Cambridge (United Kingdom): Cambridge University Press; 2005.
40. Ash LR, Orihel TC. Ash & Orihel's atlas of human parasitology. 5th edition. Chicago: ASCP Press; 2007.
41. Suwansaksri J, Nithiuthai S, Wiwanitkit V, et al. The formol-ether concentration technique for intestinal parasites: Comparing 0.1 n sodium hydroxide with normal saline preparations. Southeast Asian J Trop Med Public Health 2002;33(Suppl 3): 97–8.
42. Tarafder MR, Carabin H, Joseph L, et al. Estimating the sensitivity and specificity of kato-katz stool examination technique for detection of hookworms, ascaris lumbricoides and trichuris trichiura infections in humans in the absence of a gold standard. Int J Parasitol 2010;40(4):399–404.
43. Ash LR, Orihel TC, Salvioli L. Bench aids for the diagnosis of intestinal parasites. Geneva (Switzerland): World Health Organization publications; 1994.
44. Scholten TH, Yang J. Evaluation of unpreserved and preserved stools for the detection and identification of intestinal parasites. Am J Clin Pathol 1974;62(4):563–7.
45. Surawicz CM. What's the best way to differentiate infectious colitis (acute self-limited colitis) from ibd? Inflamm Bowel Dis 2008;14(Suppl 2):S157–8.
46. Garcia LS. Laboratory identification of the microsporidia. J Clin Microbiol 2002; 40(6):1892–901.
47. WHO/PAHO/UNESCO report. A consultation with experts on amoebiasis. Mexico city, Mexico 28-29 January, 1997. Epidemiol Bull 1997;18(1):13–4.
48. Ralston KS, Petri WA. Tissue destruction and invasion by entamoeba histolytica. Trends Parasitol 2011;27(6):253–62.
49. Salles JM, Moraes LA, Salles MC. Hepatic amebiasis. Braz J Infect Dis 2003;7(2): 96–110.
50. Nielsen PB, Mojon M. Improved diagnosis of strongyloides stercoralis by 7 consecutive stool specimens. Zbl Bakt-Int J Med M 1987;263(4):616–8.
51. Harada Y, Mori O. A new method for culturing hookworm. Yonago Acta Med 1995; 1(17).

52. Koga K, Kasuya S, Khamboonruang C, et al. A modified agar plate method for detection of strongyloides-stercoralis. American Journal of Tropical Medicine and Hygiene 1991;45(4):518–21.

53. Salazar SA, Gutierrez C, Berk SL. Value of the agar plate method for the diagnosis of intestinal strongyloidiasis. Diagn Microbiol Infect Dis 1995;23(4): 141–5.

54. Sidoni A, Polidori GA, Alberti PF, et al. Fatal strongyloides stercoralis hyperinfection diagnosed by papanicolaou-stained sputum smears. Pathologica 1994; 86(1):87–90.

55. Grapsa D, Petrakakou E, Botsoli-Stergiou E, et al. Strongyloides stercoralis in a bronchial washing specimen processed as conventional and thin-prep smears: Report of a case and a review of the literature. Diagn Cytopathol 2009;37(12): 903–5.

56. Chandler FW, Watts JC. Pathologic diagnosis of fungal infections. Chicago: ASCP Press; 1987.

57. Gill GV, Beeching N. Lecture notes on tropical medicine. 5th edition. Malden (MA): Blackwell Pub; 2004.

58. Tsai TF, Halstead SB. Tropical viral infections. Curr Opin Infect Dis 1998;11(5): 547–53.

59. Biosafety in microbiological and biomedical laboratories. U.S. Dept. of Health and Human Services, Public Health Service, Centers for Disease Control and Prevention, National Institutes of Health. Available at: http://purl.access.gpo.gov/GPO/LPS124402. Accessed February 7, 2012.

60. Storch GA. Essentials of diagnostic virology. New York: Churchill Livingstone; 2000.

61. Versalovic J, Carroll KC, Funke G, et al. Manual of clinical microbiology. Washington, DC: ASM Press; 2011.

62. Kanaphun P, Thirawattanasuk N, Suputtamongkol, et al. Serology and carriage of pseudomonas pseudomallei: A prospective study in 1000 hospitalized children in northeast thailand. J Infect Dis 1993;167(1):230–3.

63. Peacock SJ, Chieng G, Cheng AC, et al. Comparison of ashdown's medium, burkholderia cepacia medium, and burkholderia pseudomallei selective agar for clinical isolation of burkholderia pseudomallei. J Clin Microbiol 2005;43(10): 5359–61.

64. Limmathurotsakul D, Jamsen K, Arayawichanont A, et al. Defining the true sensitivity of culture for the diagnosis of melioidosis using bayesian latent class models. PLoS One 2010;5(8):e12485.

65. Chantratita N, Wuthiekanun V, Limmathurotsakul D, et al. Prospective clinical evaluation of the accuracy of 16s rrna real-time pcr assay for the diagnosis of melioidosis. Am J Trop Med Hyg 2007;77(5):814–7.

66. Meumann EM, Novak RT, Gal D, et al. Clinical evaluation of a type iii secretion system real-time pcr assay for diagnosing melioidosis. J Clin Microbiol 2006; 44(8):3028–30.

67. Limmathurotsakul D, Peacock SJ. Melioidosis: a clinical overview. Br Med Bull 2011;99:125–39.

68. Ip M, Osterberg LG, Chau PY, et al. Pulmonary melioidosis. Chest 1995;108(5): 1420–4.

69. Araj GF. Update on laboratory diagnosis of human brucellosis. Int J Antimicrob Agents 2010;36(Suppl 1):S12–7.

70. Franco MP, Mulder M, Gilman RH, et al. Human brucellosis. Lancet Infect Dis 2007;7(12):775–86.

71. Queipo-Ortuno MI, Tena F, Colmenero JD, et al. Comparison of seven commercial DNA extraction kits for the recovery of brucella DNA from spiked human serum samples using real-time pcr. Eur J Clin Microbiol Infect Dis 2008;27(2):109–14.
72. Murray PR, Baron EJ, American Society for Microbiology. Manual of clinical microbiology. 8th edition. Washington, DC: ASM Press; 2003.
73. Gasem MH, Dolmans WM, Isbandrio BB, et al. Culture of salmonella typhi and salmonella paratyphi from blood and bone marrow in suspected typhoid fever. Trop Geogr Med 1995;47(4):164–7.
74. Olopoenia LA, King AL. Widal agglutination test - 100 years later: Still plagued by controversy. Postgrad Med J 2000;76(892):80–4.
75. Olsen SJ, Pruckler J, Bibb W, et al. Evaluation of rapid diagnostic tests for typhoid fever. J Clin Microbiol 2004;42(5):1885–9.
76. Wain J, Hosoglu S. The laboratory diagnosis of enteric fever. J Infect Dev Ctries 2008;2(6):421–5.
77. Hatta M, Smits HL. Detection of salmonella typhi by nested polymerase chain reaction in blood, urine, and stool samples. Am J Trop Med Hyg 2007;76(1):139–43.
78. Ali A, Haque A, Sarwar Y, et al. Multiplex pcr for differential diagnosis of emerging typhoidal pathogens directly from blood samples. Epidemiol Infect 2009;137(1):102–7.
79. Maguina C, Guerra H, Ventosilla P. Bartonellosis. Clin Dermatol 2009;27(3):271–80.
80. Maguina C, Gotuzzo E. Bartonellosis. New and old. Infect Dis Clin North Am 2000;14(1):1–22, vii.
81. Maguina C, Garcia PJ, Gotuzzo E, et al. Bartonellosis (carrion's disease) in the modern era. Clin Infect Dis 2001;33(6):772–9.
82. Silva EA, Iyer A, Ura S, et al. Utility of measuring serum levels of anti-pgl-i antibody, neopterin and c-reactive protein in monitoring leprosy patients during multi-drug treatment and reactions. Trop Med Int Health 2007;12(12):1450–8.
83. Bang PD, Suzuki K, Phuong le T, et al. Evaluation of polymerase chain reaction-based detection of mycobacterium leprae for the diagnosis of leprosy. J Dermatol 2009;36(5):269–76.
84. van der Werf TS, Stienstra Y, Johnson RC, et al. Mycobacterium ulcerans disease. Bull World Health Organ 2005;83(10):785–91.
85. Affolabi D, Bankole H, Ablordey A, et al. Effects of grinding surgical tissue specimens and smear staining methods on buruli ulcer microscopic diagnosis. Trop Med Int Health 2008;13(2):187–90.
86. Guarner J, Bartlett J, Whitney EA, et al. Histopathologic features of mycobacterium ulcerans infection. Emerg Infect Dis 2003;9(6):651–6.
87. Buruli ulcer: Diagnosis of mycobacterium ulcerans disease. In: Johnson P, Portaels F, Meyers WM, editors. A manual for healthcare providers. Geneva (Switzerland): World Health Organization; 2001.
88. Meyers WM, Shelly WM, Connor DH, et al. Human mycobacterium ulcerans infections developing at sites of trauma to skin. Am J Trop Med Hyg 1974;23(5):919–23.
89. Phillips RO, Sarfo FS, Osei-Sarpong F, et al. Sensitivity of pcr targeting mycobacterium ulcerans by use of fine-needle aspirates for diagnosis of buruli ulcer. J Clin Microbiol 2009;47(4):924–6.
90. Siegmund V, Adjei O, Nitschke J, et al. Dry reagent-based polymerase chain reaction compared with other laboratory methods available for the diagnosis of buruli ulcer disease. Clin Infect Dis 2007;45(1):68–75.

91. Sasaki DM, Pang L, Minette HP, et al. Active surveillance and risk factors for leptospirosis in hawaii. Am J Trop Med Hyg 1993;48(1):35–43.
92. Effler PV, Domen HY, Bragg SL, et al. Evaluation of the indirect hemagglutination assay for diagnosis of acute leptospirosis in hawaii. J Clin Microbiol 2000;38(3): 1081–4.
93. Jensenius M, Fournier PE, Kelly P, et al. African tick bite fever. Lancet Infect Dis 2003;3(9):557–64.
94. Kularatne SA, Gawarammana IB. Validity of the weil-felix test in the diagnosis of acute rickettsial infections in sri lanka. Trans R Soc Trop Med Hyg 2009;103(4): 423–4.

Index

Note: Page numbers of article titles are in **boldface** type.

A

Infect Dis Clin N Am 26 (2012) 555–574
doi:10.1016/S0891-5520(12)00029-3
0891-5520/12/$ – see front matter © 2012 Elsevier Inc. All rights reserved.

N

Moving?

Make sure your subscription moves with you!

To notify us of your new address, find your **Clinics Account Number** (located on your mailing label above your name), and contact customer service at:

Email: journalscustomerservice-usa@elsevier.com

800-654-2452 (subscribers in the U.S. & Canada)
314-447-8871 (subscribers outside of the U.S. & Canada)

Fax number: 314-447-8029

Elsevier Health Sciences Division
Subscription Customer Service
3251 Riverport Lane
Maryland Heights, MO 63043

*To ensure uninterrupted delivery of your subscription, please notify us at least 4 weeks in advance of move.

Printed and bound by CPI Group (UK) Ltd, Croydon, CR0 4YY

03/10/2024

01040446-0012